# Therapeutic Advances in Hospital Medicine

## A FOCUS ON THE OLDER ADULT

# Therapeutic Advances in Hospital Medicine

## A FOCUS ON THE OLDER ADULT

SERIES EDITOR

### Peter Manu, MD

Professor of Medicine

Donald and Barbara Zucker School of Medicine at
Hofstra/Northwell

Hempstead, New York

Editor-in-Chief

American Journal of Therapeutics

EDITOR

### Liron D. Sinvani, MD

Assistant Professor of Medicine

Donald and Barbara Zucker School of Medicine at
Hofstra/Northwell

Hempstead, New York

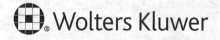 Wolters Kluwer

Philadelphia • Baltimore • New York • London
Buenos Aires • Hong Kong • Sydney • Tokyo

*Acquisitions Editor:* Rebecca Gaertner
*Development Editor:* Ashley Fischer
*Editorial Coordinator:* Lindsay Ries
*Marketing Manager:* Rachel Mante-Leung
*Production Project Manager:* Barton Dudlick
*Design Coordinator:* Holly McLaughlin
*Manufacturing Coordinator:* Beth Welsh
*Prepress Vendor:* S4Carlisle Publishing Services

9 8 7 6 5 4 3 2 1

Printed in Mexico

**Library of Congress Cataloging-in-Publication Data**

ISBN-13: 978-1-4963-9993-9
ISBN-10: 1-4963-9993-5

Cataloging-in-Publication data available on request from the Publisher.

shop.lww.com

# Contents

# SECTION 3
## Therapeutic Advances in the Management of Common Geriatric Conditions

# SECTION 4
## Therapeutic Advances in Sub-Specialty Geriatric Care

# SECTION 5
## Therapeutic Advances in Advanced Care Planning

# Contributors

**Sam Anandan, MD**
Assistant Professor
Division of Hospital Medicine
Department of Medicine
Donald and Barbara Zucker School of
    Medicine at Hofstra/Northwell
Hempstead, New York

**Olawumi Babalola, MD**
Assistant Professor
Division of Hospital Medicine
Department of Medicine
Donald and Barbara Zucker School of
    Medicine at Hofstra/Northwell
Hempstead, New York

**Judith L. Beizer, PharmD, CGP,
FASCP, AGSF**
Professor
Department of Medicine
College of Pharmacy and Health Sciences
St. John's University
Queens, New York
Division of Geriatrics and Palliative Care
Northwell Health
Manhasset, New York

**Brooke Calabrese, MD**
Medicine Resident
Division of Hospital Medicine
Department of Medicine
Donald and Barbara Zucker School of
    Medicine at Hofstra/Northwell
Hempstead, New York

**Maria Torroella Carney, MD**
Associate Professor
Division of Geriatric and Palliative
    Medicine
Department of Medicine
Donald and Barbara Zucker School of
    Medicine at Hofstra/Northwell
Hempstead, New York

**Melissa Chamblain, MD**
Medicine Resident
Division of Hospital Medicine
Department of Medicine
Donald and Barbara Zucker School of
    Medicine at Hofstra/Northwell
Hempstead, New York

**Alicia Chionchio, MD**
Medicine Resident
Division of Hospital Medicine
Department of Medicine
Donald and Barbara Zucker School of
    Medicine at Hofstra/Northwell
Hempstead, New York

**Zunaira Choudhary, MD**
Medicine Resident
Division of Hospital Medicine
Department of Medicine
Donald and Barbara Zucker School of
    Medicine at Hofstra/Northwell
Hempstead, New York

**Jessica Cohen, MD**
Assistant Professor
Division of Hospital Medicine
Department of Medicine
Donald and Barbara Zucker School of
    Medicine at Hofstra/Northwell
Hempstead, New York

**Nicolas Fausto, PharmD**
Pharmacist
Department of Clinical Health
    Professionals
Huntington Hospital
Huntington, New York

**Sheila Firoozan, MD**
Medicine Resident
Division of Hospital Medicine
Department of Medicine
Donald and Barbara Zucker School of
    Medicine at Hofstra/Northwell
Hempstead, New York

**Patricia Garnica, ANP-BC, CDE, CDTC**
Nurse Practitioner
Division of Endocrinology
Department of Medicine
Donald and Barbara Zucker School of
    Medicine at Hofstra/Northwell
Hempstead, New York

**Mark Goldin, MD**
Assistant Professor
Division of Hospital Medicine
Department of Medicine
Donald and Barbara Zucker School of
    Medicine at Hofstra/Northwell
Hempstead, New York

**Matthew Gorski, MD**
Assistant Professor
Department of Ophthalmology
Donald and Barbara Zucker School of
    Medicine at Hofstra/Northwell
Hempstead, New York

**Gregory J. Hughes, PharmD, BCPS, CGP**
Division of Hospital Medicine
Department of Medicine
Donald and Barbara Zucker School of
    Medicine at Hofstra/Northwell
Hempstead, New York
Associate Professor
Department of Clinical Health
    Professions
College of Pharmacy and Health Sciences
St. John's University
Queens, New York

**Corey Karlin-Zysman, MD**
Assistant Professor
Division of Hospital Medicine
Department of Medicine
Donald and Barbara Zucker School of
    Medicine at Hofstra/Northwell
Hempstead, New York

**Kinga Kiszko, DO**
Geriatric Fellow
Division of Hospital Medicine
Department of Medicine
Donald and Barbara Zucker School of
    Medicine at Hofstra/Northwell
Hempstead, New York

**Courtney Kluger, MD**
Assistant Professor
Division of Hospital Medicine
Department of Medicine
Donald and Barbara Zucker School of
    Medicine at Hofstra/Northwell
Hempstead, New York

**Sean LaVine, MD**
Assistant Professor
Division of Hospital Medicine
Department of Medicine
Donald and Barbara Zucker School of
    Medicine at Hofstra/Northwell
Hempstead, New York

**Tara Liberman, DO**
Assistant Professor
Division of Geriatric and Palliative Medicine
Department of Medicine
Donald and Barbara Zucker School of Medicine at Hofstra/Northwell
Hempstead, New York

**Huei-Wen Lim, MD**
Medicine Resident
Division of Hospital Medicine
Department of Medicine
Donald and Barbara Zucker School of Medicine at Hofstra/Northwell
Hempstead, New York

**Jason Ling, MD**
Endocrinology Fellow
Division of Endocrinology
Department of Medicine
Donald and Barbara Zucker School of Medicine at Hofstra/Northwell
Hempstead, New York

**Evangelos Loukas, DO**
Assistant Professor
Division of Hospital Medicine
Department of Medicine
Donald and Barbara Zucker School of Medicine at Hofstra/Northwell
Hempstead, New York

**Adrienne H. Ma, PharmD**
Pharmacist
Department of Clinical Health Professionals
Medstar Montgomery Medical Center
Olney, Maryland

**Chinedu Madu, MD**
Medicine Resident
Division of Hospital Medicine
Department of Medicine
Donald and Barbara Zucker School of Medicine at Hofstra/Northwell
Hempstead, New York

**Nicole Maisch, PharmD**
Associate Professor
Department of Clinical Health Professionals
College of Pharmacy and Health Sciences
St. Johns University
Queens, New York

**Sutapa Maiti, MD**
Geriatric Fellow
Division of Hospital Medicine
Department of Medicine
Donald and Barbara Zucker School of Medicine at Hofstra/Northwell
Hempstead, New York

**Nichol Martinez, MD**
Medicine Resident
Division of Hospital Medicine
Department of Medicine
Donald and Barbara Zucker School of Medicine at Hofstra/Northwell
Hempstead, New York

**Jacqueline Moore, MD**
Medicine Resident
Division of Hospital Medicine
Department of Medicine
Donald and Barbara Zucker School of Medicine at Hofstra/Northwell
Hempstead, New York

**Samantha Moore, PharmD**
Assistant Professor
Department of Clinical Health Professions
College of Pharmacy and Health Sciences
St. John's University
Queens, New York

**Colm Mulvany, BS**
Research Assistant
Division of Hospital Medicine
Department of Medicine
Donald and Barbara Zucker School of
    Medicine at Hofstra/Northwell
Hempstead, New York

**Neal Murphy, MD**
Medicine Resident
Division of Hospital Medicine
Department of Medicine
Donald and Barbara Zucker School of
    Medicine at Hofstra/Northwell
Hempstead, New York

**Alyson Myers, MD**
Assistant Professor
Division of Endocrinology
Department of Medicine
Donald and Barbara Zucker School of
    Medicine at Hofstra/Northwell
Hempstead, New York

**Laura Palazzolo, MD**
Ophthalmology Resident
Department of Ophthalmology
SUNY Downstate Medical Center
Brooklyn, New York

**Karishma Patel, MD**
Geriatrician
Division of Hospital Medicine
Department of Medicine
Donald and Barbara Zucker School of
    Medicine at Hofstra/Northwell
Hempstead, New York

**Raj Patel, MD**
Medicine Resident
Division of Hospital Medicine
Department of Medicine
Donald and Barbara Zucker School of
    Medicine at Hofstra/Northwell
Hempstead, New York

**Michele Pisano, PharmD**
Assistant Professor
Department of Medicine
College of Pharmacy and Health Sciences
St. John's University
Queens, New York
Division of Geriatrics and Palliative Care
Northwell Health
Manhasset, New York

**Ryann Quinn, MD**
Medicine Resident
Division of Hospital Medicine
Department of Medicine
Donald and Barbara Zucker School of
    Medicine at Hofstra/Northwell
Hempstead, New York

**Siddharth Raghavan, MD**
Assistant Professor
Division of Hospital Medicine
Department of Medicine
Donald and Barbara Zucker School of
    Medicine at Hofstra/Northwell
Hempstead, New York

**Maha Saad, PharmD**
Associate Professor
Department of Clinical Health
    Professionals
College of Pharmacy and Health Sciences
St. Johns University
Queens, New York

**Hira Shafeeq, PharmD, BCPS**
Division of Hospital Medicine
Department of Medicine
Donald and Barbara Zucker School of
    Medicine at Hofstra/Northwell
Hempstead, New York
Assistant Professor
Department of Clinical Health
    Professions
College of Pharmacy and Health Sciences
St. John's University
Queens, New York

**Shikha Sheth, MD**
Medicine Resident
Division of Hospital Medicine
Department of Medicine
Donald and Barbara Zucker School of
Medicine at Hofstra/Northwell
Hempstead, New York

**Jonathan Silver, MD**
Assistant Professor
Division of Hospital Medicine
Department of Medicine
Donald and Barbara Zucker School of
Medicine at Hofstra/Northwell
Hempstead, New York

**Liron D. Sinvani, MD**
Assistant Professor
Division of Hospital Medicine
Department of Medicine
Donald and Barbara Zucker School of
Medicine at Hofstra/Northwell
Hempstead, New York

**Philip Solomon, MD**
Assistant Professor
Division of Hospital Medicine
Department of Medicine
Donald and Barbara Zucker School of
Medicine at Hofstra/Northwell
Hempstead, New York

**Sara Tariq, MD**
Medicine Resident
Division of Hospital Medicine
Department of Medicine
Donald and Barbara Zucker School of
Medicine at Hofstra/Northwell
Hempstead, New York

**Shankar Thampi, MD**
Medicine Resident
Division of Hospital Medicine
Department of Medicine
Donald and Barbara Zucker School of
Medicine at Hofstra/Northwell
Hempstead, New York

**Ali Torbati, MD**
Geriatrician
Division of Hospital Medicine
Department of Medicine
Donald and Barbara Zucker School of
Medicine at Hofstra/Northwell
Hempstead, New York

**Pooja Vyas, DO**
Medicine Resident
Division of Hospital Medicine
Department of Medicine
Donald and Barbara Zucker School of
Medicine at Hofstra/Northwell
Hempstead, New York

**Benny Wong, MD**
Medical Student
Division of Hospital Medicine
Department of Medicine
Donald and Barbara Zucker School of
Medicine at Hofstra/Northwell
Hempstead, New York

**Shu Yang, MD**
Assistant Professor
Division of Hospital Medicine
Department of Medicine
Donald and Barbara Zucker School of
Medicine at Hofstra/Northwell
Hempstead, New York

# Preface

*So Nature deals with us, and takes away*
*Our playthings one by one, and by the hand*
*Leads us to rest so gently, that we go*
*Scarce knowing if we wish to go or stay*

**Henry Wadsworth Longfellow, Nature, Book of Sonnets, Part II, 1878**

Annual death rates for the noninstitutionalized elderly in the United States range from 2.3% for those aged 65-74 to 12.7% for persons 85 years old or older. Poverty, living alone, requiring help with activities of daily living, and having two or more chronic medical conditions correlate with a significantly higher death rate.[1] Heart disease, malignancies, chronic lower respiratory pathology, cerebrovascular disorders, and Alzheimer dementia have been identified as the cause of more than 80% of the deaths in this age group.[2] Close to one-third (31.8%) of these deaths occur within 30 days of discharge from an inpatient hospital stay. The hospital mortality of the geriatric population in the United States is 17.5%.[1]

Any attempt to improve the outcome of hospitalizations in the elderly must take into account the age-related deterioration in function, as well as the diminished physiologic reserve in many or all organ systems. The biologic decline and increased vulnerability to the effects of acute and chronic illnesses are considered to represent the frailty syndrome. This distinct pathologic entity is diagnosed in the presence of three or more of the following clinical findings: unintentional weight loss, low level of physical activity, fatigue, slowness, and weakness.[3] Frailty is more prevalent in African Americans and in women, and increases with age.[4] The common biologic predictors of frailty are anemia, hypoalbuminemia, and azotemia.[5] Among the proposed mechanisms are immune activation and chronic inflammation, dysregulations of the hypothalamic-pituitary-adrenal axis or of the growth hormone-insulin–like growth factor somatotropic axis, and involuntary malnutrition.[3] As an independent predictor of mortality in elderly patients admitted for intensive care, frailty is stronger than the presence of cardiac arrest or brain injury before admission, and than widely used severity illness scores.[6]

In taking care of the hospitalized geriatric patient, clinicians cannot treat frailty with specific pharmacologic interventions. Instead, they must rely on insight, wisdom, discrimination, and tenacity in taking the challenge of meticulous correction of pathologic entities. This book tells us how far to go, and when to stop, in helping our old patients fight for their life.

The book starts with in-depth reviews of issues related to medication management in the elderly and highlights important advances in caring for patients with anticoagulant-induced bleeding and diabetes. It continues with chapters focused on common geriatric hospital presentations, such as heart failure, complicated urinary tract infections, symptomatic hyponatremia, orthostatic hypotension, delirium, chronic pain, and insomnia. An important part of the book evaluated the effect of improved interdisciplinary collaboration for perioperative care, nutritional support, and advanced care planning.

The work inaugurates the *Therapeutic Advances* series, a collaboration between *American Journal of Therapeutics* and *Lippincott Williams & Wilkins*, a publication and an imprint of Wolters Kluwer, Philadelphia. The text has been available online in the January 2018 issue of the journal. I am delighted to see it now published in book format and congratulate my colleagues on their outstanding accomplishment.

PETER MANU

## References

1. Gorina Y, Pratt LA, Kramarow EA, Elgaddal N. Hospitalization, readmission, and death experience of noninstitutionalized Medicare fee-for-service beneficiaries aged 65 and older. National Health Statistics Reports, Number 84, September 28, 2015.

2. National Center for Health Statistics. *Health, United States, 2016: With Chart Book on Long-Term Trends in Health.* Hyattsville, MD: NCHS; 2017.

3. Chen X, Mao G, Leng SX. Frailty syndrome: an overview. *Clin Interv Aging.* 2014;9:433-441.

4. Shamlyian T, Talley KM, Ramakrishnan R, Kane RL. Association of frailty with survival: a systematic literature review. *Ageing Res Rev.* 2013;12:719-736.

5. Manu P, Asif M, Khan S, et al. Risk factors for medical deterioration of psychiatric inpatients: opportunities for early recognition and prevention. *Compr Psychiatry.* 2012;53(7):968-974.

6. Le Maguet P, Roquilly A, Lasocki S, et al. Prevalence and impact of frailty on mortality in elderly ICU patients: a prospective, multicenter, observational study. *Intensive Care Med.* 2014;40(5):674-682.

# Introduction

As a geriatrician hospitalist, I often encounter the consequences of inadequate geriatric care provision in the hospital setting, and I am passionate about improving the short-term and the long-term outcomes of this vulnerable population. With the increasing number of older adults occupying hospital beds and the scarcity of geriatricians in hospital medicine, there is a pressing need to "geriatricize" hospital care.[1] This special edition of the *American Journal of Therapeutics* will address innovative therapeutic strategies for common geriatric conditions and special considerations for this vulnerable population.

Today, Medicare patients account for approximately 50% of hospital days, with annual health care costs exceeding $1 trillion.[2,3] Yet acute care facilities are unprepared and ill-equipped to care for older adults.[4] Hospitalization in this vulnerable population often results in poor outcomes including functional and cognitive decline, readmissions, institutionalization, and premature death.[5-9] Although geriatric models of care such as Acute Care for Elderly units have demonstrated success, widespread implementation has been limited because of staffing barriers, costs, and pressure to fill open beds.[10] Furthermore, despite the obvious complexity of treating the elderly in acute care settings, most hospital providers have never received geriatric training.[4] Indeed, the number of geriatric health care providers dedicated to the care of hospitalized vulnerable older adults is currently insufficient.[11,12]

The care of hospitalized older adults proves challenging at every step. Initially, these older patients present to the emergency department with acute conditions requiring immediate medical treatment, in addition to their multiple underlying complex chronic conditions and baseline functional and cognitive impairment. Once admitted, they are at risk for the numerous hazards of hospitalization, including hospital-associated disability, delirium, falls, medication discrepancies, use of potentially inappropriate medications, and transition fragmentation.[5,13-17] The very therapeutic interventions that will prove to be lifesaving may further decrease the compromised physiologic functions of their kidneys and liver, increase their risk for adverse drug events, and ultimately jeopardize their goals of care and quality of life.

As the proportion of older adults continues to rise, hospital medicine will be shaped by the ability to standardize better processes of care to improve outcomes.[18] *Therapeutic Advances in Hospital Medicine: A Focus on the Older Adult* will address established and innovative therapeutic approaches to conditions and diagnoses common to the older population to ensure that all providers can serve the needs of this vulnerable population.

LIRON D. SINVANI

## References

1. Friedman SM, Gillespie SM, Medina-Walpole AM, et al. "Geriatricizing" hospitalists: identifying educational opportunities. *Gerontol Geriatr Educ.* 2013;34:409-420.

2. Weiss AJ, Elixhauser A. Overview of hospital stays in the United States, 2012: statistical brief #180. 2006. http://europepmc.org/abstract/med/25506966. Accessed January 9, 2017.

3. National Center for Health Statistics (US). Health, United States, 2015: with special feature on racial and ethnic health disparities [Internet]. Hyattsville, MD: National Center for Health Statistics (US); 2016. http://www.ncbi.nlm.nih.gov/books/NBK367640. Accessed January 9, 2017.

4. Retooling for an aging America: building the health care workforce [Internet]. *Inst Med.* 2017. http://www.nationalacademies.org/hmd/Reports/2008/Retooling-for-an-Aging-America-Building-the-Health-Care-Workforce.aspx. Accessed January 9, 2017.

5. Creditor MC. Hazards of hospitalization of the elderly. *Ann Intern Med.* 1993;118:219.

6. Forster AJ, Murff HJ, Peterson JF, et al. The incidence and severity of adverse events affecting patients after discharge from the hospital. *Ann Intern Med.* 2003;138:161-167.

7. Jencks SF, Cuerdon T, Burwen DR, et al. Quality of medical care delivered to Medicare beneficiaries: a profile at state and national levels. *JAMA.* 2000;284:1670-1676.

8. Jencks SF, Williams MV, Coleman EA. Rehospitalizations among patients in the Medicare fee-for-service program. *N Engl J Med.* 2009;360:1418-1428.

9. Wachter R. *Understanding Patient Safety*. New York, NY: McGraw Hill Professional; 2012.

10. Palmer RM, Landefeld CS, Kresevic D, et al. A medical unit for the acute care of the elderly. *J Am Geriatr Soc.* 1994;42:545-552.

11. Boult C, Counsell SR, Leipzig RM, et al. The urgency of preparing primary care physicians to care for older people with chronic illnesses. *Health Aff (Millwood).* 2010;29:811-818.

12. Warshaw GA, Bragg EJ, Thomas DC, et al. Are internal medicine residency programs adequately preparing physicians to care for the baby Boomers? A national survey from the association of directors of geriatric academic programs status of geriatrics Workforce study. *J Am Geriatr Soc.* 2006;54:1603-1609.

13. Covinsky KE, Pierluissi E, Johnston CB. Hospitalization-associated disability: "she was probably able to ambulate, but I'm not sure." *JAMA.* 2011;306:1782-1793.

14. Leslie DL, Marcantonio ER, Zhang Y, et al. One-year health care costs associated with delirium in the elderly population. *Arch Intern Med.* 2008;168:27-32.

15. Maher RL, Hanlon J, Hajjar ER. Clinical consequences of polypharmacy in elderly. *Expert Opin Drug Saf.* 2014;13:57-65.

16. Coleman EA, Smith JD, Raha D, et al. Posthospital medication discrepancies: prevalence and contributing factors. *Arch Intern Med.* 2005;165:1842-1847.

17. Coleman EA, Berenson RA. Lost in transition: challenges and opportunities for improving the quality of transitional care. *Ann Intern Med.* 2004;141:533-536.

18. Walke LM, Tinetti ME. ACE, MACE, and GRACE: time to put the pieces together: comment on "effects of an acute care for elders unit on costs and 30-day readmissions." *JAMA Intern Med.* 2013;173:987-989.

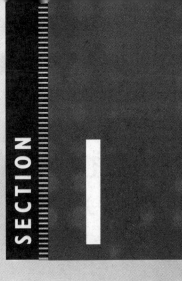

# Therapeutic Advances in Medication Management

# Optimizing Medication Management in the Hospitalized Older Adult

Michele Pisano, PharmD and Judith L. Beizer, PharmD

CHAPTER 1

## BACKGROUND

The world's older population continues to grow at an exceptional rate. Today, 8.5% of people worldwide (617 million) are aged 65 years and older.[1] According to a new report, this percentage is projected to jump to nearly 17% of the world's population by 2050 (1.6 billion).[1] As this population ages, a higher prevalence of multiple chronic disease states must be managed concurrently. According to the Centers for Disease Control and Prevention (CDC), patients aged 65 years and older are the largest consumers of prescription and nonprescription medications in the United States, and the use of medications among this group has more than doubled since 1990 and continues to rise.[2] **Polypharmacy**, which is the use of multiple medications, is of great concern for older adults because of the burden it can place on patients and society. Unfortunately, there is no agreed-on definition of **polypharmacy**, although some will use five or more medications as the cut-off. An alternate definition for **polypharmacy** can be the use of more medications than are medically necessary. The US Center for Medicare and Medicaid Services (CMS) estimates that **polypharmacy** costs the nation's health plans more than $50 billion annually.[3] A population-based survey of community-dwelling persons aged 57 to 85 years found that 37.1% of men and 36% of women between the ages of 75 and 85 years took at least five medications. Of this older group, 89.7% reported the use of prescription medication, 47.3% used an over-the-counter medication, and 54.2% a dietary supplement.[4]

Older adults often necessitate more medications because they commonly suffer from multiple chronic conditions such as congestive heart failure, diabetes mellitus, chronic obstructive pulmonary disease, and chronic renal disease. Therefore, older adults are at a higher risk of **polypharmacy** and adverse drug reactions.[5] It is imperative to consider the patient's drug treatment as the possible cause of any new signs and symptoms. The "prescribing cascade" begins when an adverse drug reaction is misinterpreted as a new medical condition, and another drug is prescribed. An example of this would be that a patient on a nonsteroidal anti-inflammatory drug develops a rise in blood pressure (a common side effect), and then an antihypertensive is prescribed. A case-control study, involving 9000 patients older than 65 years, reviewed patients newly started on antihypertensive medications. It concluded that the use of nonsteroidal anti-inflammatory drugs may increase the risk associated with starting an antihypertensive in older adults (odds ratio 1.66, 95% confidence interval, 1.54-1.80).[6]

In addition, with advancing age, pharmacokinetics and pharmacodynamics change. There is a progressive functional decline in organ systems, leading to changes in the way medications are absorbed, metabolized, and eliminated. Pharmacodynamic changes cause the aging population to become more sensitive to certain medications such as anticoagulants, benzodiazepines, and opioid analgesics.[6] Patients previously stabilized on certain doses of medications may begin to develop side effects because of these changes.[7]

There is limited evidence to guide prescribing for older people on multiple medications because of the low inclusion of this population in clinical studies.[8] Although older adults are the greatest consumers of medications, exclusion criteria limit their enrollment in these trials. Most evidence on the effects of medications in frail older adults are from observational studies and not from randomized controlled trials.[9]

# AREAS OF UNCERTAINTY

## Consequences of Polypharmacy

Multiple medications are often necessary to cure or slow the progression of disease, reduce symptoms of disease, improve quality of life, and/or decrease complications, but they can also lead to adverse consequences in older adults.

## Adverse Drug Reactions

Patients who take multiple medications are at a higher risk for adverse drug events (ADEs) and drug interactions, which can lead to increased hospitalizations.[9] One study used adverse event data to estimate the frequency and rates of hospitalizations after an emergency department (ED) visit for an ADE in older adults from 2007 to 2009. An estimated 265,802 ED visits occurred annually among adults older than 65 years. An estimated 37.5% of these visits required inpatient admission. Nearly half of hospitalizations for ADEs involved adults 80 years of age or older.[10] In a population-based study, community-dwelling older adults taking five or more medications had an 88% increased risk of experiencing an ADE compared with those taking less.[9] A retrospective cohort study evaluating hospitalizations in older veterans found that patients taking more than five medications were almost four times as likely to be hospitalized from an ADE.[11] Patients at higher risk for ADEs are those prescribed the greatest number of drugs or high-risk drugs, such as antithrombotic, oral hypoglycemic agents, cardiovascular, and central nervous system drugs.[12] A recent study examining multimorbidity and **polypharmacy** in self-reported chronic obstructive pulmonary disease (COPD) patients found that more than half (52%) reported **polypharmacy** (>5 medications). The data also demonstrated that those with COPD were more likely than those without to be prescribed multiple medications, with similar ADEs such as increased risk of falls, renal injury, constipation, and bleeding.[13] ADEs, such as falls, delirium, lethargy, and depression, account for 20% of ADEs in hospitalized older patients but often go unrecognized. Instead, because of their high frequency in this population, these syndromes are attributed to other medical causes.[14]

## Falls

Certain medications, as well as combinations of medications, can potentiate falls in the elderly. There is a strong correlation between the risk of falls and medication class. Central nervous system drugs, including antipsychotics, antiparkinsonian drugs, and narcotic analgesics, are considered to be the most strongly associated with falls.[15] In one prospective cohort study of community-dwelling elders, increased risk of falling and recurrent falls was linked to the use of four or more medications.[16] A retrospective observation study of nursing home residents looked at the incidence of falls in persons taking psychotropic medications and found that the prescription of psychotropic drugs on a scheduled basis was associated with an increased risk of falls.[17] One hospital-based study of 204 patients ≥60 years demonstrated that drug–drug interactions along with the number of medications were significantly associated with falls among the frail elderly. Last, **polypharmacy** and increased number of medications that can potentiate falls on discharge were associated with future falls.[18]

## Increase Health Care Costs

**Polypharmacy** has been associated with greater health care costs to both the patient and the health care system. A retrospective cohort study found that **polypharmacy** was linked to an increased risk of patients taking potentially inappropriate medications (PIMs), causing an approximate 30% increase in medical costs.[19]

## Medication Nonadherence

**Polypharmacy** has been associated with nonadherence because of complicated regimens, which can lead to treatment failure and hospitalizations.[19] In one observational study, when a patient is taking four or more medications, the rate of patient adherence was 35%.[20]

# THERAPEUTIC ADVANCES

## Interventions to Decrease Polypharmacy

Inappropriate prescribing in the elderly is considered an important public health issue because of its negative outcomes, such as increased morbidity and mortality, ADEs, and health care costs. Appropriate prescribing in older adults entails individualizing therapy. The medication regimen should be routinely reviewed to ensure that preventive therapies in those with a poor survival prognosis are avoided and only drugs with a favorable risk:benefit ratio are chosen. In what follows, we discuss various interventions devised to improve the appropriateness of medication selection. Several lists of explicit criteria for choosing or avoiding medications in older adults have been developed. The most well known of these in the United States are the Beers criteria for PIM use in older adults. Other lists have been developed in Europe, including the STOPP/START (Ireland) and the PRISCUS (Germany).[21]

## Beers Criteria

The Beers criteria for PIM use in older adults were originally compiled in 1991 by Dr Mark Beers, with the intent of identifying medications to avoid in nursing homes residents.[22] The criteria were later updated to apply to all older adults regardless of where they reside or receive care. Starting in 2012, the American Geriatrics Society (AGS) assumed the responsibility of maintaining and updating the Beers criteria every 3 years.[23] The list of medications is prepared by a multidisciplinary panel of health professionals with expertise in **geriatrics**, using an evidence-based approach. Current literature is reviewed and graded as to the quality of the evidence and the strength of the recommendation. A modified Delphi approach is used to reach consensus. Medications are maintained or added to the Beers criteria when there is enough evidence of potential harm to older adults or not enough evidence of benefit. The main tables of the AGS 2015 Beers criteria are summarized in Table 1.1.

It is beyond the scope of this chapter to discuss all the classes of medications included in the AGS Beers criteria. The reader is referred to the full Beers article for specific recommendations of drugs to avoid in the elderly.[23]

Along with the 2015 update, an article was published on potential alternatives to some of the Beers medications, as well as a "how to use" article.[22,23] All resources on the Beers criteria, including patient education materials, are available for download on the AGS website.[26]

## START Criteria

START (Screening Tool to Alert doctors to the Right Treatment) is a screening tool devised from evidence-based prescribing indicators that was prepared and validated to

**TABLE 1.1 • Summary of the Main Table of the 2015 AGS Beers Criteria**

| Table Number | Table Title | Note |
|---|---|---|
| 2 | 2015 AGS Beers Criteria for PIM Use in Older Adults | Consistent with 2012 AGS Beers Criteria. |
| 3 | 2015 AGS Beers Criteria for PIM Use in Older Adults Due to Drug–Disease or Drug–Syndrome Interactions That May Exacerbate the Disease or Syndrome | Consistent with 2012 AGS Beers Criteria. |
| 4 | 2015 AGS Beers Criteria for PIM to Be Used with Caution in Older Adults | Consistent with 2012 AGS Beers Criteria. |
| 5 | 2015 AGS Beers Criteria for Potentially Clinically Important Non-Anti-infective Drug–Drug Interactions That Should Be Avoided in Older Adults | New addition to the 2015 AGS Beers Criteria. |
| 6 | 2015 AGS Beers Criteria for Non-Anti-Infective Medications That Should Be Avoided or Have Their Dosage Reduced with Varying Levels of Kidney Function in Older Adults | New addition to the 2015 AGS Beers Criteria. |

identify prescribing omissions in older adults. Twenty-two evidence-based common prescribing indicators for elderly patients were identified and arranged according to physiologic system into a systematic list. An expert panel was comprised and invited to participate in the Delphi process. The validated version of START was applied to concurrent active medical problems and prescription information in a prospective cohort of 600 community-dwelling patients, aged 65 years and older, on admission to the hospital. Once an omission was identified, the patient's medical record was examined for a valid reason for the omission. Almost 58% of patients were found to have one or more prescribing omissions. The most common were HMG-CoA reductase inhibitors in atherosclerotic disease and warfarin for atrial fibrillation.[27]

## STOPP Criteria

STOPP (Screening Tool of Older Person's potentially inappropriate Prescriptions), another screening tool of older patients' medications, was developed to identify PIMs. To validate STOPP, 18 experts in geriatric pharmacotherapy were recruited to establish the content validity of STOPP by a Delphi process. STOPP incorporates commonly encountered instances of PIMs prescribing in older people, including drug–drug and drug–disease interactions, drugs that increase fall risk, and duplicate drug class prescriptions. To evaluate the performance of STOPP, 715 consecutive older patients, 65 years and older, who were admitted with acute illness to a teaching hospital were studied over a 4-month period in 2007. In this study, STOPP and Beers criteria were used to identify PIMs on admission. STOPP criteria identified a considerably higher percentage of patients requiring hospitalization as a result of a PIM-related adverse event than did Beers criteria (11.5% and 6%, respectively, $P < 0.001$).[28]

STOPP/START version 2 criteria have been expanded and updated for the purpose of minimizing inappropriate prescribing in older people. This represents an overall 31% increase in STOPP/START criteria compared with version 1. In version 2, several new STOPP categories were added, such as antiplatelet/anticoagulant drugs, drugs affecting or affected by renal function, and drugs that increase anticholinergic burden; new START categories include urogenital system drugs, analgesics, and vaccines.[29]

## How to Use Explicit Criteria in Prescribing

A key principle in applying either the AGS Beers criteria or the STOPP criteria is to remember that these medications are potentially inappropriate. There may be circumstances when the medication in question is appropriate to use, such as in palliative care. The intent of the criteria is to make the prescriber stop and think about the appropriateness of the medication for their older patient. In order for the prescriber to fully understand why the medication is potentially inappropriate, he or she should read the rationale for why the medication is a PIM and the caveats for use or avoidance. It is important to consider pharmacologic and nonpharmacologic alternatives to the Beers or STOPP medications. In older adults who have been treated with a Beers or STOPP medication, it is important to not just review that medication but to do a full review of the entire medication regimen. Clinical decision support systems can help identify PIMs during prescribing or medication reviews. In the study entitled "Collaborative approach to Optimise MEdication use for Older people in Nursing homes (COME-ON)," a software application was developed that automatically detected PIMs from a research database. The study is a multicenter cluster-controlled trial whose primary outcome relates to the appropriateness of prescribing using STOPP/START version 2 and Beers 2015 criteria in 63 nursing homes. An algorithm was developed for each criterion but not without difficulties. For example, some criteria are not as explicit as they should be. Consensus is required to more clearly define STOPP/START, version 2. Also, specific patient information, often unavailable in patient records, is required for several criteria. STOPP criteria, more often than Beers criteria, required information on medical history. Last, adding conditions to the explicit criteria can help to improve their specificity.[30]

## Deprescribing

**Deprescribing** is the process of tapering or stopping drugs, with the goal of decreasing **polypharmacy**, decreasing costs, and improving outcomes.[12,31] In one trial, 332 different drugs (on average 2.8 drugs per patient) were discontinued in 119 disabled geriatric patients. This led to reductions in 1-year mortality (21% vs 45%, $P < 0.001$), referral rates to acute care facilities (12% vs 30% $P < 0.002$), and drug costs, without significant adverse effects.[32] Another study used retrospective Medicare claims data to identify patients who were prescribed inappropriate drugs. Once identified, prescribers were notified, and this led to discontinuation of 49% of these drugs.[33]

There are four steps to discontinuing medications: (1) recognizing an indication for discontinuing a medication, such as diminished benefit or increased risk to patient because of drug interaction and ADE; (2) identifying and prioritizing the medication to be targeted for discontinuation; (3) discontinuing the medication along with proper planning and communication with the patient and other clinicians involved; and (4) monitoring the patient for both beneficial and harmful effects.[31] When discontinuing medications, it is important to note that some drugs, particularly those affecting the cardiovascular and central nervous systems, need a cautious tapering regimen to avoid adverse drug withdrawal events.[34] Adverse drug withdrawal events are defined as "a clinically significant set of symptoms or signs caused by the removal of a drug."[34] It can be a true withdrawal side effect, an exacerbation of a treated condition, or a new set of symptoms.

# MEDICATION MANAGEMENT AT TRANSITIONS OF CARE

## Medication Reconciliation

Patients often receive new medications or have changes to their existing regimen at times of transitions of care, such as on hospital admission, transfer from one unit to another, or discharge from the hospital to home or another facility.[35] Medication reconciliation is the process of creating and maintaining the most accurate list of all medications a patient is taking, including drug name, dose, frequency, and route.[35] The goal is to provide correct medications to the patient at all transition points within the hospital. The Joint Commission has included medication reconciliation in its annual patient safety goals.[36] All medications should be assessed and actively continued, discontinued, held, or modified at each transition point.[35] Each time a patient moves from one setting to another, all medications should be reviewed, and any difference should be reconciled. Poor communication of medical information at transition points is responsible for as many as 50% of all medication errors and up to 20% of ADEs in the hospital.[35] The medication reconciliation process involves three steps: verification, which is the collection of the medication history; clarification, which is checking to ensure that all medications and doses are appropriate; and reconciliation, defined as the documentation of changes in the orders. Table 1.2 reviews the steps of the medication reconciliation process. In one study, a series of interventions, including medication reconciliation, successfully decreased the rate of medication errors by 70% and reduced adverse events by over 15%.[37] Hospital-based physicians may not have access to preadmission medications, so they may be unintentionally omitted at the time of discharge. These discrepancies place patients at risk for ADEs. It is essential to also review all over-the-counter medications, vitamins, and herbal supplements on admission to hospital (Table 1.3).

**TABLE 1.2 • Steps to Take for Medication Reconciliation During Transitions of Care**

*1. Verification*

Collect a list of all medications the patient is taking

• Sources of information: Patient or caregiver; primary care provider; community pharmacy

*2. Clarification*

Assess all medications to ensure they are dosed appropriately and should be continued, resumed, or discontinued at every transition

• Consult the home medication list, current medication orders, and the transfer orders

• At discharge, review all the home medications and current medication orders and compare them

*3. Reconciliation*

Communicate to the next provider and patients any changes that were made and document any changes. Make sure patient understands the changes and knows which home medications need to be discarded, if any.

Garfinkel D, Zur-Gil S, Ben-Israel J. The war against polypharmacy: a new cost-effective geriatric-palliative approach for improving drug therapy in disabled elderly people. *Isr Med Assoc J*. 2007;9:430-434.

When performing medication reconciliation, all medications should be reviewed to ensure that drug toxicity is not the cause of patients' symptoms or reason for hospitalization. The START/STOPP and/or Beers criteria can be used to assess the appropriateness of choice of medication and also ensure appropriate dosing. Estimating life expectancy is also important in determining goals of care and the long-term value of many medications. A decrease in pill burden would be beneficial for patients with advanced dementia or end-stage organ disease.[12] When active disease, such as depression, is no longer present, medications should be tapered off and discontinued. It is also important to estimate the benefit:risk ratio for all medications; for instance, is the patient's risk of bleeding higher than his or her risk of stroke?[12] Be sure that there is no duplication of therapy with home medications because of formulary changes that occurred in hospital. Last, make sure that the patient is aware of any change and knows which home medications should be restarted or discarded.

**TABLE 1.3 • Useful Resources**

| Resource | Author | Website | Journal (If Applicable ) |
|---|---|---|---|
| BEERS Criteria | Beers et al. | https://www.ncbi.nlm.nih.gov/pubmed/26446832 | *Journal of American Geriatrics Society* 2015 |
| START /STOPP Criteria Version 2 | O'Mahony et al. | https://www.ncbi.nlm.nih.gov/pmc/articles/PMC4339726/pdf/afu145.pdf | *Age and Aging* 2015 |
| Deprescribing | | http://deprescribing.org | |
| Polypharmacy | | http://polypharmacy.ca/about-this-project/introduction/ | |
| Geriatrics Care Online | The American Geriatrics Society | https://geriatricscareonline.org | |

## Patient Education

Patients and/or family members sometimes receive conflicting recommendations, confusing medication regimens, and unclear instructions about follow-up, contributing to ineffective transitions of patient care. Patients who have a clear understanding of their after-hospital care instructions, including how to take medications and when to make follow-up appointments, are 30% less likely to be readmitted or visit the EDs than patients who lack this information.[38]

One program to educate patients about their posthospital care plans is called the Re-Engineered Hospital Discharge Program, or Project RED. The program used specially trained nurses to help patients arrange follow-up appointments, confirm medication routines, and understand their diagnoses using a personalized instruction booklet. A pharmacist then contacted patients between 2 and 4 days after hospital discharge to reinforce the medication plan and answer any question. Thirty days after their hospital discharge, the 370 patients who participated in the RED program had 30% fewer emergency visits and readmissions than the 368 patients who did not. Of the patients who participated in the RED program, 94% left the hospital with a follow-up appointment with their primary care physician, compared with 35% for patients who did not participate.[39]

Another program called the Pharm2Pharm model was implemented across six hospitals in Hawaii between 2013 and 2014. Patients were selected if they were 65 years old or older and had a medication-related admission based on the International Classification of Diseases (ICD) code. The Pharm2Pharm model is a care transition and care coordination service designed to reduce preventable medication-related hospital care, by having hospital pharmacists collaborate with community pharmacists, who follow patients for 1-year after discharge. These pharmacists would engage patients and collaborate with prescribers to identify and resolve drug-related problems to improve medication management. This model was associated with an estimated 36% reduction in medication-related hospitalization rate for older adults.[40]

## Teach-Back Method

The teach-back method is a way of checking a patient's comprehension of the information given to them. Patients are asked to state in their own words what they need to do about their health or how to take their medications. It is a way to confirm that the prescriber or pharmacist explained things in a way that the patient or family can understand. The teach-back method can help improve patient understanding and adherence and patient outcomes. It is to test not the patient's knowledge, but rather his or her comprehension, and if needed, the provider will re-explain and check again.[41]

# SUMMARY

**Polypharmacy** is the use of multiple medications and is of great concern for older adults because of the burden it can place on patients and society. Older adults often necessitate more medications because they commonly suffer from multiple chronic conditions.

Multiple medications are often necessary to cure or slow the progression of disease, reduce symptoms of disease, improve quality of life, and/or decrease complications. However, they can also lead to adverse consequences in older adults, such as ADEs, falls, increase in health care costs, and medication nonadherence.

Optimizing the medication regimen of an elderly patient starts with appropriate choice of medications, focusing on minimizing adverse effects, and simplifying the regimen to increase adherence. Medications should be evaluated for PIMs for elderly patients, utilizing Beers criteria and START/STOPP criteria. It is also important to de-prescribe medications when appropriate. **Deprescribing** is the process of tapering or stopping drugs, with the goal of decreasing **polypharmacy**, decreasing costs, and improving outcomes. Medication reconciliation should be performed at every transition point, and any change should be communicated to the patient, caregiver, and primary care provider. The teach-back method can be used to ensure proper comprehension by the patient and/or caregiver.

The challenge that all health care professionals face is to determine the most appropriate drug therapy regimen that will enhance the patient's quality of life without compromising the patient's ability to function or increasing the risk of adverse reactions.

## References

1. The National Institute of Aging. Worlds Older Population Grows Dramatically, 2016. https://www.nih.gov/news-events/news-releases/worlds-older-population-grows-dramatically. Accessed September 6, 2018.
2. Centers for Disease Control and Prevention. The state of aging and health in America, 2004. https://www.cdc.gov/aging/pdf/State_of_Aging_and_Health_in_America_2004.pdf. Accessed December 10, 2016.
3. Fillit HM, Futterman R, Orland BI et al. Polypharmacy management in medicare managed care: changes in prescribing by primary care physicians resulting from a program promoting medication reviews. *Am J Manag Care.* 1999;5:587-594.
4. Qato DM, Alexander GC, Conti R, Johnson M, Schumm P, Lindau ST. Use of prescription and over-the-counter medications and dietary supplements among older adults in the United States. *JAMA.* 2008;300:2867-2878.
5. Vrettos I, Voukelatou P, Katsoras A, Theotoka D, Kalliakmanis, A. Diseases linked to polypharmacy in elderly patients. *Curr Gerontol Geriatr Res.* 2017;2017:1-5.
6. Rochon PA, Gurwitz JH. Optimizing drug treatment for elderly people: the prescribing cascade. *BMJ.* 1997;315:1096-1099.
7. Sera LC, McPherson ML. Pharmacokinetics and pharmacodynamics changes associated with aging and implications for drug therapy. *Clin Geriatr Med.* 2012;28:273-286.

8. Hilmer SN, Gnjidic D. The effects of polypharmacy in older adults. *Clin Pharmacol Ther.* 2009;85:86-88.

9. Bourgeois FT, Shannon MW, Valim C, Mandl KD. Adverse drug events in the outpatient setting: an 11-year national analysis. *Pharmacoepidemiol Drug Saf.* 2010;19:901-910.

10. Budnitz DS, Lovegrove MC, Shehab N, Richards CL. Emergency hospitalizations for adverse drug events in older Americans. *N Engl J Med.* 2011;365:2002-2012.

11. Marcum ZA, Amuan ME, Hanlon JT, et al. Prevalence of unplanned hospitalizations caused by adverse drug reactions in older veterans. *J Am Geriatr Soc.* 2012;60:34-41.

12. Scott IA, Gray LC, Martin JH, Pillans PI, Mitchell CA. Deciding when to stop: towards evidence-based deprescribing of drugs in older populations. *Evid Based Med.* 2013;18:121-124.

13. Hanlon P, Nicholl BI, Jani BD, et al. Examining patterns of multimorbidity, polypharmacy and risk of adverse drug reactions in chronic obstructive pulmonary disease: a cross-sectional UK Biobank study. *BMJ Open.* 2018;8:e018404.

14. Klopotowska JE, Wierenga PC, Smorenberg SM, et al. Recognition of adverse drug events in older hospitalized medical patients. *Eur J Clin Pharmacol.* 2013;69:75-85.

15. Shuto H, Imakyure O, Matsumoto J, et al. Medication use as a risk factor for inpatient falls in an acute care hospital: a case-crossover study. *Br J Clin Pharmacol.* 2010;69:535-542.

16. Tromp AM, Pluijm SM, Smit JH, Deeg DJ, Bouter LM, Lips P. Fall-risk screening test: a prospective study on predictors for falls in community-dwelling elderly. *J Clin Epidemiol.* 2001;54:837-844.

17. Cox CA, van Jaarsveld HJ, Houterman S et al. Psychotropic drug prescription and the risk of falls in nursing home residents. *J Am Med Dir Assoc.* 2016;17:1089-1093.

18. Bennett A, Gnjidic D, Gillett M et al. Prevalence and impact of fall-risk-increasing drugs, polypharmacy, and drug-drug interactions in robust versus frail hospitalized falls patients: a prospective cohort study. *Drugs Aging.* 2014;31:225-232.

19. Akazawa M, Imai H, Igarashi A, Tsutani K. Potentially inappropriate medication use in elderly Japanese patients. *Am J Geriatr Pharmacother.* 2010;8:146-160.

20. Rollason V, Vogt N. Reduction of polypharmacy in the elderly: a systematic review of the role of the pharmacist. *Drugs Aging.* 2003;20:817-832.

21. Holt S, Schmiedl S, Thürmann PA. Potentially inappropriate medications in the elderly: the PRISCUS list. *Dtsch Arztebl Int.* 2010;107:543-551.

22. Beers MH, Ouslander JG, Rollingher I, Reuben DB, Brooks J, Beck JC. Explicit criteria for determining inappropriate medication use in nursing home residents. *Arch Intern Med.* 1991;151: 1825-1832.

23. The American Geriatrics Society 2015 Beers Criteria Update Expert Panel. American Geriatrics Society 2015 updated Beers criteria for potentially inappropriate medication use in older adults. J Am Geriatr Soc. 2015;63:2227-2246.

24. Hanlon JT, Semla TP, Schmader KE. Alternative medications for medications in the use of high-risk medications in the elderly and potentially harmful drug-disease interactions in the elderly quality measures. *J Am Geriatr Soc.* 2015;63:e8-e18.

25. Steinman MA, Beizer JL, DuBeau CE, Laird RD, Lundebjerg NE, Mulhausen P. How to use the American Geriatrics Society 2015 Beers Criteria—a guide for patients, clinicians, health systems, and payors. *J Am Geriatr Soc.* 2015;63:e1-e7.

26. American Geriatrics Society. AGS Clinical Guidelines and Recommendations. 2017. http://geriatrics-careonline.org/toc/american-geriatrics-societyupdated-beers-criteria-for-potentially-inappropriate-medication-use-in-older-adults/CL001.

27. Barry P, Gallagher P, Ryan C, O'mahony D. START (screening tool to alert doctors to the right treatment)—an evidence based screening tool to detect prescribing omissions in elderly patients. *Age Ageing.* 2007;36:632-638.

28. Gallagher P, O'Mahony D. STOPP (Screening Tool of Older Persons' potentially inappropriate Prescriptions): application to acutely ill elderly patients and comparison with Beers' criteria. *Age Ageing.* 2008;37:673-679.

29. O'Mahony D, O'Sullivan D, Byrne S, O'Connor MN, Ryan C, Gallagher P. STOPP/START criteria for potentially inappropriate prescribing in older people: version 2. *Age Ageing.* 2015;44:213-218.

30. Anrys P, Boland B, Degryse J, et al. STOPP/START version 2—development of software applications: easier said than done? *Age Ageing.* 2016;45:589-592.

31. Bain K, Holmes H, Beers M, Maio V, Handler SM, Pauker SG. Discontinuing medications: a novel approach for revising the prescribing stage of the medication-use process. *J Am Geriatr Soc.* 2008;56:1946-1952.

32. Garfinkel D, Zur-Gil S, Ben-Israel J. The war against polypharmacy: a new cost-effective geriatric-palliative approach for improving drug therapy in disabled elderly people. *Isr Med Assoc J.* 2007;9: 430-434.

33. Starner CI, Norman SA, Reynolds RG, Gleason PP. Effect of a retrospective drug utilization review on potentially inappropriate prescribing in the elderly. *Am J Geriatr Pharmacother.* 2009;7:11-19.

34. Graves T, Hanlon JT, Schmader KE, et al. Adverse events after discontinuing medications in elderly outpatients. *Arch Intern Med.* 1997;157:2205-2210.

35. Institute for Healthcare Improvement. How-to Guide: Prevent Adverse Drug Events by Implementing Medication Reconciliation. Cambridge, MA: Institute for Healthcare Improvement; 2011. www.ihi. org. Accessed January 9, 2017.

36. Joint Commission. National hospital patient safety goals. 2017. https://www.jointcommission.org/ assets/1/6/2017_NPSG_HAP_ER.pdf. Accessed January 26, 2017.

37. Whittington J, Cohen H. OSF healthcare's journey in patient safety. *Qual Manag Health Care.* 2004;13:53-59.

38. Agency for Healthcare Research and Quality. Educating patients before they leave the hospital reduces readmissions, emergency department visits and saves money. 2009. http://www.ahrq.gov/news/press/ pr2009/redpr.htm. Accessed January 4, 2017.

39. Jack BW, Chetty VK, Anthony D, Greenwald JL, Sanchez GM, et al. A reengineered hospital discharge program to decrease rehospitalization: a randomized trial. *Ann. Intern. Med.* 2009;150:178–187.

40. Pellegrin KL, Krenk L, Oakes SJ et al. Reductions in medication-related hospitalizations in older adults with medication management by hospital and community pharmacists: a Quasi-Experimental Study. *J Am Geriatr Soc.* 2017;65:212-219.

41. Use the Teach-Back Method: Tool #5. Rockville, MD: Agency for Healthcare Research and Quality. Content Last Reviewed February 2015. http://www.ahrq.gov/professionals/quality-patient-safety/ quality-resources/tools/literacy-toolkit/healthlittoolkit2-tool5.html. Accessed January 4, 2017.

# CHAPTER 2

# Reversal of Anticoagulation: Therapeutic Advances and Clinical Guidelines

Mark Goldin, MD, Gregory J. Hughes, PharmD, Zunaira Choudhary, MD, Sara Tariq, MD, Hira Shafeeq, PharmD, and Jessica Cohen, MD

## BACKGROUND

Anticoagulants save lives by preventing strokes in patients with atrial fibrillation (AF) and treating patients with thromboembolic disease. Their use will only increase as the incidence and prevalence of these disease processes continue to rise.[1,2] Although these drugs are integral parts of many treatment plans, the Agency for Healthcare Research and Quality labels them high risk for adverse drug events, and the elderly population is particularly vulnerable to such events.[3,4] Given this dichotomy of efficacy and harm, it is essential to be aware of new advances in emergency reversal strategies for oral anticoagulants.

This chapter focuses on areas of uncertainty, including the provider's dilemma on deciding to anticoagulate, the use of individual risk assessment tools in helping overcome this dilemma, and the importance of shared decision making with the patient. We then provide data on the novel antidotes available for oral anticoagulants, along with new agents that are currently being evaluated by the U.S. Food and Drug Administration (FDA). In discussing reversal strategies, it is important to first understand the approved uses, pharmacology, and bleed rates of the oral anticoagulants available for patients and providers. Refer to Table 2.1 for details of the agents.

The **anticoagulation** of elderly patients with AF exemplifies familiar themes of risk–benefit decision making encountered in medicine. The reservations surrounding **anticoagulation** in the elderly despite its ability to reduce the risk of debilitating strokes center around a few general points: an apparently unfavorable, general perception of the use of anticoagulants in the senior population; an unsettled debate positing

| | Mechanism of Action | FDA Indications | Half-Life (Hours) | Bleeding Rates | Source |
|---|---|---|---|---|---|
| **Warfarin** | Vitamin K antagonist | AF VTE treatment secondary prevention prophylaxis Valve replacement MI | 40 | See the given rates for oral anticoagulants | Ref. 40 |
| **Rivaroxaban** | Factor Xa inhibitor | Non–valvular AF VTE treatment secondary prevention prophylaxis post hip/knee surgery | 5-9 | ROCKET AF[41]: Rivaroxaban vs warfarin 3.6%/y vs 3.5%/y HR: 1.04 (NS) EINSTEIN-DVT[42]: rivaroxaban vs enoxaparin→warfarin 0.8% vs 1.2% (NS) EINSTEIN-PE[43]: rivaroxaban vs enoxaparin→warfarin 1.1% vs 2.2% ($P = 0.003$) | https://www.xareltohcp.com/shared/product/xarelto/prescribing-information.pdf |
| **Apixaban** ("pi_eliquis.pdf," n.d.) | Factor Xa inhibitor | Non–valvular AF VTE treatment secondary prevention prophylaxis post hip/knee surgery | 12 | AMPLIFY[44]: Apixaban vs enoxaparin→warfarin 0.6% vs 1.8% RR = 0.31 ($P < 0.0001$) ARISTOTLE[45]: apixaban vs warfarin 2.13%/y vs 3.09%/y HR = 0.69, RR 31% ($P < 0.0001$) | http://packageinserts.bms.com/pi/pi_eliquis.pdf |
| **Dabigatran** | Direct thrombin inhibitor | Non–valvular AF VTE treatment secondary prevention prophylaxis post hip surgery | 12-17 | RE-COVER & RE-COVER II: Parenteral→dabigatran vs parenteral→warfarin 1.4% vs 2% HR = 0.73 (NS) | Ref. 27 |
| **Edoxaban** | Factor Xa inhibitor | Non–valvular AF VTE treatment | 10-14 | ENGAGE AF-TIMI 48 Study[46]: Edoxaban high dose vs low dose vs warfarin 2.75% (HR 0.8, $P < 0.001$) vs 1.61% (HR 0.47, $P < 0.001$) vs 3.43% HOKUSAI-VTE[47]: heparin→edoxaban vs heparin→warfarin 1.4% vs 1.6% (NS) | https://www.accessdata.fda.gov/drugsatfda_docs/label/2015/206316lbl.pdf |

**TABLE 2.1 • FDA-Approved Indications, Half-Lives, and Bleeding Rates in Trials**

Abbreviations: AF, atrial fibrillation; DVT, deep vein thrombosis; FDA, U.S. Food and Drug Administration; HR, hazard ratio; MI, myocardial infarction; NS, nonsignificant; PE, pulmonary embolism; RR, relative ratio; VTE, venous thromboembolism.

the use of alternative, seemingly safer agents such as antiplatelet therapy to mitigate the consequences of potential falls; and the mentality that "fall risk" may serve as an informal exclusionary criterion for the prescription of anticoagulants. Current evidence suggests that some of these concerns may be disproportionate.

A systematic review attempted to characterize physician attitudes toward the use of anticoagulation for AF.[5] Patients at risk for falls or with histories of bleeding made the use of **anticoagulation** prohibitive in providers' minds. This study highlights the possibility that while some of the uncertainty in this area is tangible, the simple perception or reputation of these medications influences prescribers' behaviors. In overestimating the harms of anticoagulant therapy and underappreciating the benefits, physicians may be selectively narrowing the pool of patients they perceive as candidates for antithrombotic therapy. Among the elderly population, providers prescribed antithrombotic therapy in only half of eligible cases.[6] One decision analytic model found that an elderly person with AF carrying a moderate fall risk characterization would need to fall hundreds of times annually to warrant elimination of warfarin from his/her medication regimen, concluding that fall risk should not be considered in the decision-making process.[7] It may be preferable to focus on alleviating other risks of intracranial hemorrhage, such as reaching goals for hypertension management, especially in patients on antithrombotic therapy.[8]

In addition, the dilemma in balancing bleeding and thrombotic risks when viewing intracranial hemorrhage as the worst scenario in anticoagulated patients who fall may be looked at through different lenses and lead to differing recommendations. The gray area emerges from how patients are classified into stroke risk categories. Furthermore, although the use of full-dose aspirin has been promoted as a warfarin substitute for stroke risk reduction in fall-prone seniors, the literature does not support such a claim. Data have suggested that elderly patients with AF with high risk for stroke cannot achieve sufficient stroke risk reduction with aspirin monotherapy.[9] Two recent meta-analyses comparing antithrombotic and anticoagulant regimens have shown reduction in stroke with aspirin monotherapy: however, in one,[10] after adjusting for CHADS2 score and other study population characteristics, the effect of aspirin missed statistical significance; in the other,[11] relatively few of the included studies on aspirin reported CHADS2 scores, and those that did had mean scores near 2. As such, data on aspirin monotherapy in high-risk elderly populations are lacking.

As evident from the preceding discussion, the decision to anticoagulate in elderly patients is challenging and depends on a variety of factors related to both patients and providers. Informed decisions therefore require careful, individualized assessments of both patients' stroke and bleeding risks. AF increases the risk of stroke 5-fold and can be associated with an annual stroke risk of greater than 4%.[12] Because **anticoagulation** can reduce this risk, various risk assessment tools have been developed to help determine which patients would benefit from **anticoagulation**.

The aforementioned and commonly used CHADS2 score, based on risk factors identified in a registry of patients with AF not prescribed warfarin, identifies patients as low, moderate, or high risk for stroke to determine the need for aspirin alone versus **anticoagulation**.[13] However, because other risk factors, such as female sex, age 65 to 74, and the presence of vascular disease or previous myocardial infarction, have been validated as stroke risk factors,[14] and considering that patients who have a CHADS2 score of 0 have a stroke rate of 1.9%,[13] the new CHA2DS2-VASc score was promoted

### TABLE 2.2 • CHA$_2$DS$_2$-VASc Score

| Risk Factors | Points |
| --- | --- |
| Congestive heart failure | 1 |
| Hypertension | 1 |
| Age ≥75 y | 2 |
| Diabetes mellitus | 1 |
| Stroke/TIA | 2 |
| Vascular disease$^a$ | 1 |
| Age 65–74 y | 1 |
| Sex category (female) | 1 |

$^a$Vascular disease: prior myocardial infarction, peripheral arterial disease, or aortic plaque.
Abbreviation: TIA, transient ischemic attack.

by the 2010 European Society of Cardiology guidelines (Tables 2.2 and 2.3). This score accounts for these risk factors, minimizing the number of patients placed in the "intermediate risk" category, and providing clearer recommendations regarding aspirin and warfarin use.[13]

Bleeding risk must be evaluated concurrently with thrombosis risk. The HAS-BLED risk score was developed from a large cohort of European patients with AF,[15] and assigned points for hypertension, abnormal liver/renal function, stroke, previous bleeding, labile international normalized ratios, older age, and drug/alcohol use, with a total score ≥3 suggesting high bleeding risk (Tables 2.4 and 2.5). The older

### TABLE 2.3 • CHA$_2$DS$_2$-VASc Score and Stroke Risk

| CHA$_2$DS$_2$-VASc Score | Annual Stoke Risk (%) |
| --- | --- |
| 0 | 0 |
| 1 | 1.3 |
| 2 | 2.2 |
| 3 | 3.2 |
| 4 | 4.0 |
| 5 | 6.7 |
| 6 | 9.8 |
| 7 | 9.6 |
| 8 | 6.7 |
| 9 | 15.2 |

From Gage BF, Waterman AD, Shannon W, Boechler M, Rich MW, Radford MJ. Validation of clinical classification schemes for predicting stroke: results from the National Registry of Atrial Fibrillation. JAMA.2001;285:2864-2870.

**TABLE 2.4 • HAS-BLED Score**

| Risk factors | Points |
|---|---|
| Hypertension | 1 |
| Abnormal liver/renal function | 1 point each |
| Stroke | 1 |
| Bleeding history | 1 |
| Labile INRs | 1 |
| Elderly (>65 y) | 1 |
| Drugs or ETOH | 1 point each |

Abbreviations: INR, international normalized ratio; ETOH, ethanol.

HEMORR$_2$HAGES[16] score is based on a variety of risk factors including the presence of hepatic or renal disease, malignancy, thrombocytopenia, previous bleeding, anemia, excessive fall risk, uncontrolled hypertension, and genetic factors (CYP 2C9 polymorphisms). HAS-BLED was equally accurate in predicting bleeding risk in the overall population, slightly more accurate at predicting this risk in patients not on **anticoagulation** and in those on antiplatelet agents alone, and overall simpler to use in determining bleeding risk.

Given the complexity of balancing the risks and benefits of **anticoagulation**, patients eligible for anticoagulant therapy may benefit from shared decision making with their physicians. This treatment decision model proposes that providers have open discussions with patients about the risks and benefits of treatment options and arrive at decisions that the patient makes on the basis of the clinical knowledge they have acquired.[17] Such decisions could promote increased adherence to therapy. Although there are various areas of uncertainty regarding the decision to start **anticoagulation**

**TABLE 2.5 • HAS-BLED Score and Bleeding Risk**

| HAS-BLED Score | Annual Bleeding Risk (%) |
|---|---|
| 0 | 0.9 |
| 1 | 3.4 |
| 2 | 4.1 |
| 3 | 5.8 |
| 4 | 8.9 |
| 5 | 9.1 |
| 6-9 | Insufficient data |

From Pisters R, Lane DA, Nieuwlaat R, de Vos CB, Crijns HJ, Lip GY. A novel user-friendly score (HAS-BLED) to assess 1-year risk of major bleeding in patients with atrial fibrillation: the Euro Heart Survey. Chest.2010;138:1093-1100.

in elderly patients, this decision is ultimately guided by careful examination of risk factors for stroke and bleeding, and consideration of the patient's preferences and goals for their care.

# AREAS OF UNCERTAINTY

Once the decision to anticoagulate has been made, there still remains the challenge of choosing an anticoagulant. Enoxaparin remains the preferred therapy for cancer-related venous thromboembolism, in particular for having shown better safety than warfarin.[18] In other patients, choice of therapy has become more complex with the advent of **direct oral anticoagulants** (DOACs). Considering the metabolism and elimination of DOACs, these medications should be avoided in patients with significantly reduced renal function, those at the extremes of weight or advanced age, and those concomitantly treated with strong P-glycoprotein and/or CYP3A4 inducers/inhibitors.[19] Excluding these populations, DOACs offer clear benefits over warfarin with the convenience of oral formulations and without the need for serial blood monitoring. Patient-specific considerations may guide choice of DOAC. For instance, patients at particularly high risk for ischemic stroke may benefit most from dabigatran; those at high bleeding risk may benefit most from apixaban.[20]

As summarized in Table 2.1, in large trials all four FDA-approved DOACs have shown efficacy similar to that of warfarin in reducing risk of stroke in AF or recurrent venous thromboembolism, with comparable or superior bleeding profiles. Despite these data, the absence of FDA-approved **reversal agents** has historically served as a deterrent in prescribing DOACs. For this reason, it is important for physicians to be aware of existing and forthcoming reversal strategies that may assuage concerns (Table 2.6).

# DATA ON NEW ANTICOAGULATION REVERSAL THERAPEUTICS

## Prothrombin Complex Concentrates

Prothrombin complex concentrates (PCCs) contain variable quantities of endogenous clotting factors along with antithrombotics: protein C, protein S, and heparin. PCCs can be divided into three major categories: 3 factor PCCs (3FPCCs), 4 factor PCCs (4FPCCs), and activated PCCs (aPCCs). Factor VII is the differentiating feature among them. 3FPCCs contain negligible factor VII, 4FPCCs contain factor VII comparable to physiologic ratio, and aPCCs contain factor VII in an activated form. Kcentra is the only available 4FPCC in the United States currently approved for reversal of acquired coagulation factor deficiency by warfarin in adult patients with acute major bleeding or need for urgent surgery or invasive procedure.[21] 4FPCC contains the four vitamin K–dependent clotting factors (II, VII, IX, and X) along with antithrombotic proteins C and S. Administration of 4FPCC essentially replaces the vitamin K–dependent

**TABLE 2.6  •  Reversal Strategies for Oral Anticoagulants**

| Therapeutic Reversal Agent | Target Oral Anticoagulant | Mechanism of Reversal | Thrombogenic Potential | FDA Approval |
| --- | --- | --- | --- | --- |
| **Prothrombin complex concentrates (Kcentra)** | Warfarin | Replenishes vitamin K–dependent clotting factors (factors II, IX, X, and varying concentrations of VII). May also contain protein C and S | Yes[21] | Yes |
| **Idarucizumab (Praxbind)** | Direct thrombin inhibitors (dabigatran) | Irreversibly binds to dabigatran, thereby preventing it from binding to thrombin | Possible | Yes |
| **Andexanet alfa** | Factor Xa inhibitors (studied in apixaban and rivaroxaban) | Recombinant human factor Xa that binds active site of factor Xa inhibitors, preventing these from binding to endogenous factor Xa | Possible | Yes |
| **Ciraparantag** | Various agents including heparinoids, both direct and indirect factor Xa inhibitors, as well as the direct thrombin inhibitor dabigatran | Limited understanding of mechanism of action; binds to various agents and may render them ineffective | No, but data are limited | No |

clotting factors in a prompt manner. A therapeutic effect can be seen within 30 minutes of administration. However, the reversal effect starts to wear off within 12 to 24 hours, likely because of factor VII's short half-life. Therefore, 4FPCC must be administered with intravenous vitamin K to avoid rebound coagulopathy 12 to 24 hours after administration.[21,22] Use of 4FPCC is contraindicated in patients with active disseminated intravascular coagulopathy and a recent history of heparin-induced thrombocytopenia. Caution should be exercised in patients with recent thrombosis because PCCs can be associated with prothrombotic complications.[21]

The safety and efficacy of 4FPCC was tested prospectively in two randomized, phase IIIb studies.[23,24] The first trial examined its utility in urgent reversal due to life-threatening bleeding in nonsurgical patients and the latter tested its feasibility for urgent reversal before invasive surgery or procedure. 4FPCC was noninferior when compared with fresh frozen plasma (FFP) for reversal of warfarin-associated coagulopathy for acute major bleeding in nonsurgical patients and superior for treatment before an invasive surgery or procedure.[23,24] Independent, blinded investigators determined the efficacy of hemostasis at 24 hours as excellent, good, or poor on the basis of laboratory data and clinical judgment in 202 nonsurgical patients presenting with life-threatening major bleeding. Hemostatic efficacy was established in 72.4% patients in the 4FPCC treatment arm versus 65.4% patients in the FFP arm, proving noninferiority.[23] The parallel phase IIIb trial tested efficacy of 4FPCC in 168 patients for urgent reversal of warfarin before an invasive surgery or procedure. Effective hemostasis was achieved in 90% of patients in the 4FPCC treatment arm versus 75% in the FFP arm, establishing superiority when compared with FFP.[24]

A significant portion of patients in both phase IIIb trials were aged 65 years and older,[23,24] seeming to reflect that elderly patients are at a higher risk of bleeding on anticoagulants. 4FPCC offers several advantages in elderly patients including rapid reversal, significantly lower infusion volume, and reduced incidence of transfusion-associated reactions and infection when compared with FFP. Although 4FPCC demonstrated higher incidence of hemostatic efficacy in these patients depending on the international normalized ratio (INR), its effect on improving mortality and quality of life for those patients who survive major bleeding episodes remains unknown. 4FPCC has not been compared with 3FPCCs or activated PCCs for reversal of acquired coagulopathy due to warfarin. Nevertheless, 4FPCC is the preferred treatment for management of acute coagulopathy reversal associated with warfarin for major bleeding.[22,25] 4FPCC can also be considered for patients presenting with life-threatening acute coagulopathy because of oral anti-Xa inhibitors.[22]

### Idarucizumab

Idarucizumab is the first reversal agent approved by the FDA for any of the non–vitamin K antagonist oral anticoagulants ("Press Announcements—FDA approves Praxbind, the first reversal agent for the anticoagulant Pradaxa," n.d.). Idarucizumab is a humanized monoclonal antibody fragment that specifically binds to dabigatran. The binding affinity of dabigatran for idarucizumab is 350-fold higher than the binding affinity for thrombin. Once bound, this 1:1 complex is essentially irreversible because of a slow dissociation of dabigatran from idarucizumab.[26] This complex is then eliminated by protein catabolism, mainly in the kidney.[27] Idarucizumab only reverses the anticoagulant effects of dabigatran with no impact on other anticoagulants or antithrombotic therapies. In addition, because idarucizumab does not affect thrombin in any direct way, its use does not affect the coagulation cascade and therefore does not place the patient in a hypercoagulable state.

Idarucizumab was studied and approved on the basis of its reduction of unbound dabigatran, normalization of coagulation parameters in healthy volunteers, and an interim analysis of a multicenter, prospective, nonrandomized phase 3 trial.[28] This analysis was of 90 patients who were taking dabigatran and experiencing an overt, uncontrollable, or life-threatening bleed or who were undergoing a surgery or an invasive procedure that required normal hemostasis. In this study, coagulation parameters (dilute thrombin time [dTT] and ecarin clotting time [ECT]) had a median reversal of 100% immediately after idarucizumab infusion. dTT and ECT normalized immediately in more than 93% and 88% of patients, respectively. At 12 and 24 hours, dTT remained normal in >81% of patients and ECT remained normal in 54% of patients. Unbound serum concentrations of dabigatran were <20 ng/mL immediately after infusion and remained this low in 93% of patients at 12 hours and 79% of patients at 24 hours. Regarding clinical outcomes, in the patient group who had an overt, uncontrollable, or life-threatening bleed, the median time to bleeding cessation was 11.4 hours. In the patient group undergoing surgery or an invasive procedure, normal intraoperative hemostasis was reported in 92% of patients.[28] Five of 90 patients experienced a thrombotic event within 90 days of idarucizumab infusion and only one of these events occurred within 72 hours. Limitations of this evidence include the absence of a control group and a relatively small sample size.

Idarucizumab is given as a one-time 5-g intravenous dose. It is supplied as two 2.5-g vials that should be given immediately following one another. Coagulation parameters, such as activated partial thromboplastin time (aPTT), can again become elevated because of dabigatran 12 to 24 hours after idarucizumab use. In these circumstances, if clinically relevant bleeding occurs (or recurs), an additional 5-g dose can be administered.[27]

## Andexanet

Andexanet alfa is a recombinant molecule that was designed by introducing three modifications to native factor X: deletion of a critical membrane-binding domain; replacement of the linkage between heavy chain and light chain components; and mutation of the active-site serine residue, which renders the molecule enzymatically inactive. A series of experiments ex vivo demonstrated effective reversal of betrixaban, rivaroxaban, and apixaban inhibition of factor Xa in a dose-dependent manner. The group also demonstrated reversal of prolongation of prothrombin time produced by rivaroxaban. A thrombin generation assay showed that andexanet did not have significant procoagulant activity. Subsequently, in animal models, andexanet restored hemostasis after treatment with rivaroxaban as well as indirect factor Xa inhibitors enoxaparin and fondaparinux.[29]

The first human trial of andexanet studied reversal of factor Xa inhibition by apixaban and rivaroxaban in 101 healthy volunteers in a randomized, blinded manner.[30] In ANNEXA-A, 48 subjects received apixaban 5 mg twice daily for 3.5 days, which was followed by an andexanet 400 mg intravenous bolus (30 mg/min) alone, or the same bolus plus a 480-mg infusion over 2 hours. Similarly, in ANNEXA-R, 53 subjects received rivaroxaban 20 mg once daily for 4 days, followed by an andexanet 800-mg intravenous bolus (30 mg/min) alone, or the same bolus plus a 960-mg infusion over 2 hours. In both substudies, the bolus arms and bolus-plus-infusion arms were placebo controlled. Siegal et al showed rapid reduction in antifactor Xa activity after administration of andexanet, both for patients treated with apixaban (94% vs 21% with placebo; $P < 0.001$) and rivaroxaban (92% vs 18% with placebo; $P < 0.001$). In patients treated with bolus alone, this effect persisted for approximately 2 hours. In patients treated with bolus plus infusion, reduction in antifactor Xa activity was sustained for the duration of the infusion plus an additional 1 to 2 hours.[30] Furthermore, ≥80% reversal of antifactor Xa activity was seen in 100% of subjects receiving the full dose of andexanet, compared with 0% of subjects who received placebo ($P < 0.001$). Thrombin generation was rapidly restored within 2 to 5 minutes of andexanet administration and increased to above the lower limit of normal within 2 to 10 minutes in 100% patients in the apixaban substudy (vs 11% placebo) and 96% in the rivaroxaban substudy (vs 7% placebo) ($P < 0.001$).[30]

Authors addressed the potential for thrombogenesis in two assays. First, they noted that across both substudies, peak thrombin generation after andexanet administration was significantly higher than baseline. However, thrombin generation returned to within 2 standard deviations of the mean within 30 minutes. Second, levels of D-dimer and prothrombin fragments 1 and 2 also increased after andexanet administration. However, these levels returned to normal within 24 to 72 hours.[30]

These encouraging findings led to the later-phase ANNEXA-4 study, a prospective cohort study, which recruited patients aged 18 years and older who presented with major bleeding. This study is ongoing, although interim data for 67 patients were released.[31] Subjects received a bolus plus infusion of andexanet, dosed according to the timing of the most recent Xa inhibitor administration. Of 47 subjects in the efficacy analysis, 37 (79%) achieved either excellent or good hemostasis (defined by the time to cessation of visible bleeding, percent decline in hemoglobin for nonvisible bleeding, or increase in size of hematoma volume for intracranial bleeding). There were no observed infusion reactions and no neutralizing antibodies detected. There were 12 thrombotic events, 4 of which occurred within 3 days of andexanet administration; only one subject had resumed therapeutic **anticoagulation**. Although the study involved only a single cohort, authors concluded that andexanet had demonstrated acceptable efficacy and safety to continue recruitment.

There remain several limitations of andexanet, including the need to match dosing to specific factor Xa inhibitors, the inconvenience of bolus-plus-infusion administration, the possibility of decreased efficacy from nonneutralizing antibodies on subsequent dosing, and thrombogenic potential. Nevertheless, andexanet represents a promising class-specific anticoagulant antidote.[32-34]

## Ciraparantag

Ciraparantag, also not yet FDA approved, is a novel, water-soluble, small molecule that many believe holds promise as a universal antidote. Targets are bound by noncovalent hydrogen bonding and charge–charge interactions. In pharmacologic studies, ciraparantag has demonstrated binding affinity for heparinoids, both direct and indirect factor Xa inhibitors, as well as the direct thrombin inhibitor dabigatran.[35] Thromboelastography has demonstrated the ability of ciraparantag to reverse **anticoagulation**, and rat-tail transaction models have shown reduced bleeding.[35,36] Edoxaban was identified in preclinical studies as perhaps the most responsive target for ciraparantag.[36] In the first human phase 1/2 study, with 7 cohorts of 10 patients, subjects receiving edoxaban 60 mg showed a mean increase in whole blood clotting time (WBCT) of 37% within 3 hours. A single-dose ciraparantag infusion reduced WBCT to within 10% of baseline value in <10 minutes (compared with 12 to 15 hours with placebo) and remained at that level for 24 hours. No serious adverse events were reported. Notably, D-dimer and prothrombin fragments 1 and 2 remained at baseline levels, showing no suggestion of thrombogenic potential.[37,38]

A subsequent phase 1/2 study with 4 cohorts of 10 patients treated with enoxaparin showed similar results: enoxaparin 1.5 mg/kg increased mean WBCT 30%; ciraparantag reduced WBCT to within 20% of baseline in 2 to 5 minutes; there was no reversal with placebo; WBCT levels remained stable for the ensuing 12 to 24 hours; and there were no serious adverse events and no evidence of thrombogenic potential.[35]

Despite these early data, along with ciraparantag's stability and relatively straightforward dosing, there are several outstanding concerns. Notably, WBCT is rarely used in the clinical setting and is not validated as a measure of reversal. In addition, there is still a need for studies on drug–drug interactions, as well as late-phase trials in patients with acute bleeding or other indication for rapid reversal.[39]

# SUMMARY

Anticoagulants are life-saving medications that prevent and treat thromboembolic disease and are of particular importance in the elderly population for prevention of stroke in AF. The advent of **direct oral anticoagulants** and **reversal agents** has yielded more options for patients, although complicating clinical decision making. The decision to anticoagulate in AF depends on the risks of stroke versus bleeding. The accompanying HAS-BLED score for predicting bleeding allows an estimation of net clinical benefit. Despite these tools, uncertainty remains. Notably, **anticoagulation** has traditionally been avoided in patients with recurrent falls. Yet, decision analytic modeling has shown that patients on warfarin would need hundreds of falls annually to warrant discontinuation. At the same time, **direct oral anticoagulants**, while theoretically simpler to dose than warfarin, should be dose reduced or avoided in cases of renal impairment, extreme age or weight, or concomitant use of strong P-glycoprotein and/or CYP3A4 inducers/inhibitors.

Prothrombin complex concentrates consist of endogenous coagulation factors and anticoagulants. One 4-factor prothrombin complex concentrates (factors II, VII, IX, X, proteins C, and S), when administered with intravenous vitamin K, effectively reversed warfarin in cases of life-threatening bleeding or need for urgent surgery/procedure in two-phase IIIb trials, although it may be associated with thrombogenesis. Idaruci-zumab, a humanized monoclonal antibody, reversed dabigatran-associated bleeding in 11.4 hours in a late-stage trial and had no effect on thrombin in pharmacodynamic studies. Andexanet alfa, a recombinant molecule derived from factor X, is a class-spe-cific reversal agent for factor Xa inhibitors. In trials of healthy individuals (AN-NEXA-A, ANNEXA-R), andexanet alfa reversed apixaban and rivaroxaban, although increased levels of D-dimer and prothrombin fragments 1 and 2, suggesting potential thrombogenesis; the late-stage ANNEXA-4 trial is ongoing. Finally, ciraparantag, a small water-soluble molecule, reversed edoxaban and enoxaparin in phase 1/2 trials (by WBCT) and holds promise as a potential universal reversal agent.

## References

1. Colilla S, Crow A, Petkun W, Singer DE, Simon T, Liu X. Estimates of current and future incidence and prevalence of atrial fibrillation in the U.S. adult population. *Am J Cardiol*. 2013;112:1142-1147.

2. Deitelzweig SB, Lin J, Lin G. Preventing venous thromboembolism following orthopedic surgery in the United States: impact of special populations on clinical outcomes. *Clin Appl Thromb Hemost*. 2011;17:640-650.

3. Classen DC, Jaser L, Budnitz DS. Adverse drug events among hospitalized medicare patients: epi-demiology and national estimates from a new approach to surveillance. *Jt Comm J Qual Patient Saf*. 2010;36:12-21.

4. Budnitz DS, Lovegrove MC, Shehab N, Richards CL. Emergency hospitalizations for adverse drug events in older Americans. *N Engl J Med*. 2011;365:2002-2012.

5. Pugh D, Pugh J, Mead GE. Attitudes of physicians regarding anticoagulation for atrial fibrillation: a systematic review. *Age Ageing*. 2011;40:675-683.

6. Ezekowitz MD, Falk RH. The increasing need for anticoagulant therapy to prevent stroke in patients with atrial fibrillation. *Mayo Clin Proc*. 2004;79:904-913.

7. Man-Son-Hing M, Nichol G, Lau A, Laupacis A. Choosing antithrombotic therapy for elderly patients with atrial fibrillation who are at risk for falls. *Arch Intern Med*. 1999;159:677-685.

8. Chapman N, Huxley R, Anderson C, et al. Effects of a perindopril-based blood pressure-lowering regi-men on the risk of recurrent stroke according to stroke sub-type and medical history: the PROGRESS Trial. *Stroke*. 2004;35:116-121.

9. EAFT (European Atrial Fibrillation Trial) Study Group. Secondary prevention in non-rheumatic atri-al fibrillation after transient ischaemic attack or minor stroke. *Lancet*. 1993;342:1255-1262.

10. Tereshchenko LG, Henrikson CA, Cigarroa J, Steinberg JS. Comparative effectiveness of interventions for stroke prevention in atrial fibrillation: a network meta-analysis. *J Am Heart Assoc*. 2016;5:1-17.

11. Tawfik A, Bielecki JM, Krahn M, et al. Systematic review and network metaanalysis of stroke preven-tion treatments in patients with atrial fibrillation. *Clin Pharmacol*. 2016;8:93-107.

12. Fernández CS, Formiga F, Camafort M, et al. Antithrombotic treatment in elderly patients with atrial fibrillation: a practical approach. *BMC Cardiovasc Disord*. 2015;15:143.

13. Gage BF, Waterman AD, Shannon W, Boechler M, Rich MW, Radford MJ. Validation of clinical classi-fication schemes for predicting stroke: results from the National Registry of Atrial Fibrillation. *JAMA*. 2001;285:2864-2870.

14. Friberg L, Rosenqvist M, Lip GYH. Evaluation of risk stratification schemes for ischaemic stroke and bleeding in 182 678 patients with atrial fibrillation: the Swedish Atrial Fibrillation cohort study. *Eur Heart J*. 2012;33:1500-1510.

15. Pisters R, Lane DA, Nieuwlaat R, de Vos CB, Crijns HJ, Lip GY. A novel user-friendly score (HAS-BLED) to assess 1-year risk of major bleeding in patients with atrial fibrillation: the Euro Heart Survey. *Chest*. 2010;138:1093-1100.

16. Gage BF, Yan Y, Milligan PE, et al. Clinical classification schemes for predicting hemorrhage: results from the National Registry of Atrial Fibrillation (NRAF). *Am Heart J*. 2006;151:713-719.

17. Seaburg L, Hess EP, Coylewright M, Ting HH, McLeod CJ, Montori VM. Shared decision making in atrial fibrillation: where we are and where we should be going. *Circulation*. 2014;129:704-710.
18. Meyer G, Marjanovic Z, Valcke J, et al. Comparison of low-molecular-weight heparin and warfarin for the secondary prevention of venous thromboembolism in patients with cancer: a randomized controlled study. *Arch Intern Med*. 2002;162:1729-1735.
19. Burnett AE, Mahan CE, Vazquez SR, Oertel LB, Garcia DA, Ansell J. Guidance for the practical management of the direct oral anticoagulants (DOACs) in VTE treatment. *J Thromb Thrombolysis*. 2016;41:206-232.
20. Schaefer JK, McBane RD, Wysokinski WE. How to choose appropriate direct oral anticoagulant for patient with nonvalvular atrial fibrillation. *Ann Hematol*. 2016;95:437-449.
21. Kcentra Product Labeling. http://www.fda.gov/ucm/groups/fdagov-public/@fdagov-bio-gen/documents/document/ucm350239.pdf. Accessed August 8, 2017.
22. Frontera JA, Lewin JJ III, Rabinstein AA, et al. Guideline for reversal of antithrombotics in intracranial hemorrhage: a statement for healthcare professionals from the neurocritical care society and society of critical care medicine. *Neurocrit Care*. 2016;24:6-46.
23. Sarode R, Milling TJ, Refaai MA, et al. Efficacy and safety of a 4-factor prothrombin complex concentrate in patients on vitamin K antagonists presenting with major bleeding: a randomized, plasma-controlled, phase IIIb study. *Circulation*. 2013;128:1234-1243.
24. Goldstein JN, Refaai MA, Milling TJ, et al. Four-factor prothrombin complex concentrate versus plasma for rapid vitamin K antagonist reversal in patients needing urgent surgical or invasive interventions: a phase 3b, open-label, non-inferiority, randomised trial. *Lancet*. 2015;385:2077-2087.
25. Ageno W, Gallus AS, Wittkowsky A, Crowther M, Hylek EM, Palareti G. Oral anticoagulant therapy: antithrombotic therapy and prevention of thrombosis, 9th ed: American College of Chest Physicians Evidence-Based Clinical Practice Guidelines. *Chest*. 2012;141:e44S-e88S.
26. Schiele F, van Ryn J, Canada K, et al. A specific anti-dote for dabigatran: functional and structural characterization. *Blood*. 2013;121:3554-3562.
27. Pradaxa. Prescribing Information. https://www.pradaxa.com/pradaxa-vs-warfarin?utm_source-5bing&utm_medium5cpc&utm_campaign5SN%20%7C%20BR%20%7C%20Pradaxa&utm_term-5pradax a&utm_content5_pradaxa. Accessed July 11, 2017.
28. Pollack CV, Reilly PA, Eikelboom J, et al. Idarucizumab for dabigatran reversal. *N Engl J Med*. 2015;373:511-520.
29. Lu G, DeGuzman FR, Hollenbach SJ, et al. A specific antidote for reversal of anticoagulation by direct and indirect inhibitors of coagulation factor Xa. *Nat Med*. 2013;19:446-451.
30. Siegal DM, Curnutte JT, Connolly SJ, et al. Andexanet alfa for the reversal of factor Xa inhibitor activity. *N Engl J Med*. 2015;373:2413-2424.
31. Connolly SJ, Milling JR TJ, Eikelboom JW, et al. Andexanet alfa for acute major bleeding associated with factor Xa inhibitors. *N Engl J Med*. 2016;375:1131-1141.
32. Ansell JE. Reversing the effect of oral anticoagulant drugs: established and newer options. *Am J Cardiovasc Drugs*. 2016;16:163-170.
33. Connors JM. Antidote for factor Xa anticoagulants. *N Engl J Med*. 2015;373:2471-2472.
34. Ansell JE, Laulicht BE, Bakhru SH, Hoffman M, Steiner SS, Costin JC. Ciraparantag safely and completely reverses the anticoagulant effects of low molecular weight heparin. *Thromb Res*. 2016;146:113-118.
35. Kaatz S, Bhansali H, Gibbs J, Lavender R, Mahan CE, Paje DG. Reversing factor Xa inhibitors – clinical utility of andexanet alfa. *J Blood Med*. 2017;8:141-149.
36. Laulicht B, Bakhru S, Jiang X, et al. Antidote for new oral anticoagulants: mechanism of action and binding specificity of PER977. *N Engl J Med*. 2014;371:2141-2142.
37. Ansell JE, Bakhru Sh, Laulicht BE, et al. Use of PER977 to reverse the anticoagulant effect of edoxaban. *N Engl J Med*. 2014;371;2141-2142.
38. Ansell JE, Bakhru SH, Laulicht BE, et al. Single-dose ciraparantag safely and completely reverses anticoagulant effects of edoxaban. *Thromb Haemost*. 2017;117(2):238-245.
39. Weitz JI, Eikelboom JW. Ciraparantag for enoxaparin reversal: adding to the evidence. *Thromb Res*. 2016;146:106-107.

40. U.S. Food & Drug Administration. Coumadin (warfarin sodium) tablets. http://www.accessdata.fda.gov/drugsatfda_docs/label/2011/009218s107lbl.pdf. Accessed August 8, 2017.

41. Halperin JL, Halperin JL, Hankey GJ, et al. Efficacy and safety of rivaroxaban compared with warfarin among elderly patients with nonvalvular atrial fibrillation in the rivaroxaban once daily, oral, direct factor Xa inhibition compared with vitamin K antagonism for prevention of stroke and embolism trial in atrial fibrillation (ROCKET AF). *Circulation*. 2014;30:138-146.

42. EINSTEIN Investigators. Oral rivaroxaban for symptomatic venous thromboembolism. *N Engl J Med*. 2010;363:2499-2510.

43. EINSTEIN–PE Investigators. Oral rivaroxaban for the treatment of symptomatic pulmonary embolism. *N Engl J Med*. 2012;366:1287-1297.

44. Agnelli G, Buller HR, Cohen M, et al; AMPLIFY Investigators. Oral apixaban for the treatment of acute venous thromboembolism. *N Engl J Med*. 2013;369:799-808.

45. Granger CB, Alexander JH, McMurray JJV, et al; ARISTOTLE Committees and Investigators. Apixaban versus warfarin in patients with atrial fibrillation. *N Engl J Med*. 2011;365:981-992.

46. Giugliano RP, Ruff CT, Braunwald E, et al. Edoxaban versus warfarin in patients with atrial fibrillation. *N Engl J Med*. 2013;369:2093-2104.

47. Hokusai-VTE Investigators. Edoxaban versus warfarin for the treatment of symptomatic venous thromboembolism. *N Engl J Med*. 2013;369:1406-1415.

# CHAPTER 3

# Advances in Managing Type 2 Diabetes in the Elderly: A Focus on Inpatient Care and Transitions of Care

Alyson Myers, MD, Patricia Garnica, ANP-BC, and Jason Ling, MD

## BACKGROUND

As the population ages, the rates of **type 2 diabetes** mellitus (T2DM) have increased in those older than 75 years. Approximately 30.3 million (9.4%) of the U.S. population has diabetes, and 25.2% of these cases are in persons older than 65 years.[1] Although the prevalence continues to increase, the rate of new cases of diabetes has begun to decline.[2] Despite this, diabetes is the seventh leading cause of death, with mortality rates greatest in those aged 65 and over.[3] This population is also vulnerable to complications such as end-stage renal disease or limb amputation. These complications can even be seen in **elderly** patients with newly diagnosed T2DM.[4, 5]

In **elderly** patients diagnosed with T2DM, obesity is not as prevalent as it is in younger diagnosed patients. Older persons develop more hepatic and muscle fat, as opposed to the increased central adiposity seen with younger patients.[6] Comorbid depression also has also been inconsistently associated with poor glycemic control in **elderly** patients.[7,8] There are other issues unique to **elderly** patients with T2DM, such as frailty, malnutrition, worsening renal and/or hepatic function, and cognitive impairment, all of which can affect management decisions.[6] Poor nutrition in the **elderly** must also be considered in diabetes care. As a part of the aging process, **elderly** patients have a decreased sense of both smell and taste.[7] Poor dentition or swallowing difficulties can impair adequate oral intake.[7] As a result, timing of meals and amount of meal consumption need to be taken into account in treatment decisions for diabetes management in this population. These physical and psychosocial factors must be considered in the treatment and glycemic targets of **elderly** patients because they are susceptible to hypoglycemia, which can have detrimental effects in this population.[8]

Hypoglycemia in the inpatient and postdischarge setting has been associated with increased mortality,[9,10] cardiac decompensation,[11] and cognitive impairment. Both the American Diabetes Association (ADA) and American Geriatrics Society have encouraged a hemoglobin $A_{1c}$ (HbA$_{1c}$) target of 7% to 8% for most **elderly** patients and a target of 8% to 8.5% for those with a limited life expectancy.[8] For those with an HbA$_{1c}$ of less than 7%, there is concern about increased rates of hypoglycemia.[12] However, some studies have demonstrated that those with HbA$_{1c}$ >9% can have frequent episodes of hypoglycemia alternating with a rebound hyperglycemia as well.[13] Caution must be taken in **elderly** patients using medications such as insulin and/or sulfonylureas because they are most associated with hypoglycemia.[14]

Hypoglycemia as an admitting diagnosis is greatest for **elderly** patients older than 75.[15] In a Medicare sample of persons with T2DM, there were more admissions for those with hypoglycemia than with hyperglycemia, especially in patients who were black or older than 75.[14] In the Action in Diabetes and Vascular Disease: Preterax and Diamicron Modified Release Controlled Evaluation study, older age, increased creatinine, low body mass index (BMI), and longer duration of diabetes were some of the factors associated with increased risk of severe hypoglycemia (<40 mg/dL).[9] The risk for hypoglycemia is not limited to the use of insulin or sulfonylureas. Low HbA$_{1c}$, comorbid heart disease, and drug-drug interactions or certain genotypes of CYP2C9 are also associated with increased rates of hypoglycemia in the **elderly**.[16]

# AREAS OF UNCERTAINTY

## Inpatient Admission of Elderly Patients with Diabetes

On admission, it is crucial for the admitting provider to reconcile a patient's medications because polypharmacy occurs frequently in **elderly** patients.[8] In a cohort of older adults admitted to the medicine service, those with diabetes on average took 12.6 medications, in comparison with 9.4 medications for those without diabetes.[17] Many patients with diabetes also concomitantly take medications for dyslipidemia, hypertension, renal protection, and/or cardiovascular disease. This can lead to drug-drug interactions or changes in the drug metabolism. Using insulin or oral hypoglycemic agents with insulin sensitizers such as metformin, thiazolidinediones (TDZs), or glucagon-like peptide 1 (GLP-1) agonists can lead to hypoglycemia if the insulin dose is not adjusted.[18] Caution must also be taken when using multiple agents that lead to insulin release, such as the outpatient use of a sulfonylurea with the meglitinide class of drugs: repaglinide or nateglinide. Another example includes the use of repaglinide with the fibrate gemfibrozil, leading to increased duration of repaglinide.[18]

## Inpatient Monitoring and Glycemic Targets

In non–critically ill persons, the target for glycemic control is <140 mg/dL for fasting blood sugars and <180 mg/dL for random blood sugars; however, it has not been clearly defined for the **elderly**.[19] If the patient is eating, blood sugar monitoring should occur before meals and at bedtime. For those who are nil per os (NPO), or receiving tube feeds, monitoring of blood sugar should occur every 6 hours. In patients with hypoglycemia unawareness, checking blood sugar at 2 or 3 AM may also be useful.

## Treatment of Inpatient Hyperglycemia

Hyperglycemia is defined as a serum or finger-stick (FS) glucose >180 mg/dL in non–critically ill inpatients. Infection, stress hormones, immobility, medications, and alternate forms of nutrition can lead to hyperglycemia.[19] **Inpatient management** of diabetes has changed with the introduction of the 2004 inpatient hyperglycemia guidelines.[20] These guidelines suggest that subcutaneous (sq) basal and bolus insulin is the preferred therapy; thus oral or non–insulin sq agents are discontinued on admission.[21] During hospital admission, oral intake status can vary because of illness, surgery, or NPO status for testing; so use of sulfonylureas can lead to hypoglycemia. Hypoxia or acute kidney injury from dehydration, infection, or other causes could potentially lead to metformin-associated lactic acidosis (MALA) if metformin is used.[22] Newer agents such as sodium-glucose cotransporter 2 inhibitors (SGT2is) should be avoided because they are associated with volume depletion, especially in the **elderly** or in those treated with diuretics.[16] The added advantage of using insulin instead of oral agents is that insulin has anti-inflammatory and anti-counterregulatory hormonal properties.[7]

Basal insulins can differ in the risk of nocturnal hypoglycemia. Neutral protamine hagedorn (NPH) an intermediate-acting insulin, peaks after 4 to 6 hours; thus, it is most likely to cause nocturnal hypoglycemia. Premixed insulin with NPH and short or rapid insulin should be avoided while inpatient; they are associated with greater rates of hypoglycemia because of fixed dosing,[23] especially if they are dosed at bedtime as opposed to with dinner.[7] There are five long-acting basal insulins currently on the market: glargine 100 or 300 U/mL, levemir, and degludec 200 U/mL. These basal insulins vary in their duration of action and insulin concentration per milliliter. In a meta-analysis of seven randomized phase IIIa trials, degludec has been associated with less overnight hypoglycemia in **elderly** patients when compared with glargine.[24] There have been no studies indicating that any of these insulins have any increased improvement in $HbA_{1c}$. The same can be said for the three rapid insulins on the market: glulisine 100 U/mL, lispro 100 or 200 U/mL, and aspart 100 U/mL.

Starting a basal-bolus regimen is based on the patient's home dosing and/or weight. The suggested technique is to calculate the total daily dose (TDD). The TDD is divided as 50% basal and 50% bolus. The dose used for those with type 1 diabetes mellitus (T1DM) is generally between 0.2 and 0.4 U/kg, whereas it is greater for those with T2DM: 0.4 to 0.8 U/kg. In a retrospective review of patients with diabetes treated with a dose greater than 0.8 U/kg, there was a 3-fold increased risk of hypoglycemia as compared to those who got 0.2 U/kg.[25] It has been suggested that the $HbA_{1c}$ level should also be used when determining the weight-based level because those with higher $HbA_{1c}$ on admission tend to have worse glycemic control when hospitalized.[26]

For those who use basal-bolus insulin therapy at home, only 50% to 80% of their TDD should be given while hospitalized.[22]

In addition to basal-bolus therapy, correctional scale insulin is often a part of inpatient diabetes management. It is not recommended to be a standalone therapy[21] except in certain cases, in which the patient maintains glycemic control without the use of basal therapy.[27] Basal insulin with correctional scale is a better option and can allow for glycemic control similar to that of basal-bolus therapy.[28] Basal-bolus or basal with correctional scale is associated with less hyperglycemia.[28] Correctional scale is generally given every 6 hours if a patient is not eating or is on tube feeds. If the patient is eating, it should be administered before meals and at bedtime. The addition of the bedtime scale has not been associated with any improvements in mean fasting blood sugars in patients who receive it as compared to those who do not.[29] There was also no difference seen in the glycemic control of those who received bedtime correctional scale at 3 AM or before breakfast.[29]

## Inpatient Hyperglycemia Secondary to Enteral and Parenteral Nutrition

Glucose management during enteral feeds depends on the frequency of feeds: bolus versus continuous. Diabetic feeds have lower carbohydrate composition, higher fiber content, and slowly digested carbohydrates that decrease postprandial excursions.[30] For continuous feeds, basal insulin with short-acting insulin is the preferred therapy. NPH insulin administered sq every 6 hours or long-acting agents; both glargine or levemir sq every 12 hours are options for basal therapy.[31] The newer basal agents such as degludec or glargine U300 are only delivered as pens, so their use is limited in the inpatient setting. NPH is often the basal insulin of choice for those on tube feeds because of its shorter duration of time.[30] For patients receiving bolus tube feeds, regular insulin every 6 hours or rapid insulin every 4 hours can be used as a standalone therapy.[31] If the tube feeds are stopped for any reason, then a D5 or D10 infusion at a rate up to 50 mL/h should be initiated to prevent hypoglycemia.[30] The choice of hourly rate or concentration of glucose is based on the patient's renal function, cardiopulmonary status, and glucose levels because infusing high levels of glucose would stimulate release of endogenous insulin, thus worsening hypoglycemia.

Total parenteral nutrition (TPN) is indicated for persons with conditions such as severe malnutrition or gastrointestinal problems that impede enteral feeding such as short gut syndrome or inflammatory bowel disease.[32] TPN can lead to hyperglycemia, often requiring a modification of the carbohydrate content to 150 to 200 g/d[30] or adding regular insulin to the TPN solution.[33] Poor glycemic control (blood sugar >180 mg/dL) in persons requiring TPN is associated with increased inpatient death in non–critically ill patients.[34] Factors such as older age, comorbid malignancy, severe malnutrition, and high carbohydrate load in TPN also increases the risk of inpatient death.[34] The diagnosis of diabetes itself was not implicated in this increased risk of death. A randomized controlled trial (RCT) examining the best treatment options for enteral and TPN therapy is warranted because none have been conducted thus far in elderly or nonelderly populations.[35]

## Inpatient Hyperglycemia Secondary to Corticosteroid Therapy

Steroids induce hyperglycemia by precipitating insulin resistance and disrupting the signaling of glucose transport 4, thereby increasing gluconeogenesis in the liver.[36] Randomized studies have been lacking in the area of hyperglycemia management in persons receiving supraphysiologic doses of corticosteroid therapy.[22] Patient age and BMI (>26 kg/m$^2$) can both increase the risk of onset of **type 2 diabetes** in those treated with steroids.[36] In addition, steroid dose and frequency must be used to determine whether hyperglycemia will ensue. In a study of **elderly** patients treated with oral corticosteroids, the incidence of T2DM after 1 year of therapy was 4.3%, increasing to 11% after 3 years.[37] For patients who are being treated with supraphysiologic steroid therapy (Table 3.1), blood sugars increase most in the postprandial period; thus, the severity of hyperglycemia can be missed if only fasting blood sugars are tested.[38] As a result, the basal-bolus regimen should be heavier on the bolus dosing than on the basal dosing, where 60% to 70% of the TDD is bolus insulin and the remaining 30% to 40% is basal. For patients on short-acting once-daily steroids, which peak in 4 to 8 hours as does prednisone or prednisolone, a dose of NPH can be used.[23] It is recommended that the dose of NPH be based on the prednisone dosing—over 40 mg/day: 0.4 U/kg; 30 mg/day: 0.3 U/kg; 20 mg/day: 0.2 U/kg; and 10 mg/day: 0.1 U/kg.[38] Those using longer-acting steroids such as dexamethasone or methylprednisolone require a longer-acting basal insulin with bolus therapy.[22]

## Inpatient Hypoglycemia

Hypoglycemia is defined as glucose of <70 mg/dL; it is deemed severe if it is <40 mg/dL.[40] Hypoglycemia can be caused by oral diabetes agents or insulin, but can be also be caused by non–medication factors. Provider factors such as reduction in steroid dosing without reduction of the insulin dose or a mismatch in the timing of insulin with meals can be causes for hypoglycemia.[41] In addition, sepsis, renal or hepatic failure, malnourishment, or malignancy can precipitate hypoglycemia.[40] Patient factors such as HbA$_{1c}$ <7%, low BMI, outpatient insulin therapy, high albumin to creatinine ratio, and longer duration of diabetes have been associated with a greater risk of hypoglycemia.[41] Longer duration of diabetes can also lead to impairment of counterregulatory responses from glucagon or stress hormones. Inpatient hypoglycemia has been associated with a longer length of stay[25] as well as increased inpatient mortality.[42] Hypoglycemia induces a sympathoadrenal response that leads to increased cardiac demand

| TABLE 3.1 • Physiologic Doses of Steroids[39] | |
| --- | --- |
| **Name of Steroid** | **Physiologic Dose, mg** |
| Betamethasone | 0.6 |
| Dexamethasone | 0.75 |
| Methylprednisolone/triamcinolone | 4 |
| Prednisone/prednisolone | 5 |
| Hydrocortisone | 20 |

Data from Liu D, Ahmet A, Ward L, et al. A practical guide to the monitoring and management of the complications of systemic corticosteroid therapy. *Allergy Asthma Clin Immunol.* 2013;9:30.

as well as release of inflammatory markers, which can induce endothelial damage and a prothrombotic state.[41] This cascade of events can lead to myocardial infarction (MI) or even death.

Standardized protocols should be developed and implemented in which those with hypoglycemia receive immediate treatment with glucose gel, juice, or soda. If unable to have oral intake, intramuscular glucagon or intravenous (IV) dextrose can also be used.

# ELEMENTS TO ADDRESS TRANSITION OF CARE IN THE OLDER PATIENT WITH DIABETES UPON DISCHARGE

Once the patient is ready for discharge, **transition of care** (TOC) becomes important. TOC is defined as the movement of patients between healthcare locations, providers, or different levels of care within the same locations because their condition and care need change.[43] Because of the complexity of care required by **elderly** patients on discharge from the hospital, the TOC must be efficiently coordinated among healthcare providers, patients, family members, caregivers, insurance plans, and administrators to minimize harm and to avoid wasteful loss of healthcare resources.[44]

Transitional care has to be effective, efficient, timeless, safe, and fair.[45] The Affordable Care Act, a Hospital Readmissions Reduction Program, requires the Centers for Medicare & Medicaid Services to reduce payments to hospitals with excess of 30-day readmissions.[46] Older patients are usually discharged with complex medical problems, high stress, and vulnerability.[47] Identifying and addressing potential barriers of care will promote outpatient recovery.

## Medical Nutrition Therapy

Dietary habits play an important role in glycemic control; however, it is well known that changing eating habits at an older age is difficult. Also, some older patients depend on others for food shopping and meal preparation, whereas others might have decreased appetite secondary to age, acute illness, chronic health problems, and side effects from medications as well as have financial limitations for food acquisition.[48] It is important to evaluate the nutritional status and food habits for these patients during hospitalization.[49] Furthermore, in long-term care facilities, liberal diet plans have been associated with improvement in food and beverage intake in the **elderly**.[50]

## Physical Activity

Activity in the **elderly** population with diabetes is as important as it is for their younger counterparts.[51] However, physical limitations can greatly decrease activity levels. Patients with diabetes complications such as neuropathy, peripheral vascular disease, amputations, stroke, depression, retinopathy, or blindness are increasingly challenged to keep up with activity levels.

Diabetes is also associated with lower skeletal muscle strength and quality in the aging population.[52] Evaluating activity levels before admission and at time of discharge will assist providers in determining patients' needs during TOC. Programs to enhance mobility, endurance, gait, balance, and overall strength are important for patients in long-term care facilities.[50]

## Diabetes Medications

Pharmacologic recommendations in this age group are the same as those for younger patients with diabetes, with modifications. The process of medication reconciliation on discharge might be cumbersome; thus, the assistance of an endocrinologist or an inpatient diabetes team might be beneficial. A patient-centered approach should include assessing the $HbA_{1c}$ goal, medication efficacy, hypoglycemia risk, impact on weight, potential side effects, cost, and patient preferences.[23]

# THERAPEUTIC ADVANCES

## Oral Diabetes Medications

### Biguanides

Metformin is still the first line of therapy for all patients with **type 2 diabetes**. Its efficacy, low hypoglycemia risk, few side effects, ease of use, low cost, and beneficial effects on weight loss make it a safe choice for select **elderly** patients.[53] It can also be given to patients with mild to moderate renal dysfunction. In the past, metformin was discontinued if creatinine was above 1.4 in women and 1.5 in men; however, in 2016, the U.S. Food and Drug Administration (FDA) recommended the use of metformin in patients with a glomerular filtration rate (GFR) >30 mL/min/1.73 m².[54] For those not previously on metformin, it should not be started on patients with a GFR < 45 mL/min/1.73 m² and lower doses (such as 500 mg daily or twice daily) should be given to patients with moderate renal dysfunction.[53,55]

Metformin is found in multiple diabetes medication combination tablets reducing polypharmacy, which might increase adherence. It is also found in liquid form for patients who cannot swallow tablets. Metformin is contraindicated in advanced or worsening renal disease, liver disease, hypoxia, or hypoperfusion states including acute or recurrent congestive heart failure (HF), low ejection fraction, and acute MI. It is also contraindicated in patients with alcohol abuse because of the rare but potentially fatal risk of MALA.[56] Treatment should not be initiated in someone ≥80 years of age unless renal function is >45 mL/min/1.73 m². Metformin might increase the risk of vitamin $B_{12}$ deficiency, requiring the discontinuation of the medication and $B_{12}$ supplementation.[57] Side effects of metformin include diarrhea, nausea, or abdominal pain (Table 3.2). To decrease these side effects, it is recommended to start at 500 mg daily or twice daily and titrate weekly to 1000 mg per os (PO) twice daily with meals. Using the extended-release form can decrease the risk of these side effects as well.[58] It

**TABLE 3.2 •** Oral Diabetes Medications: Mechanism of Action, Side Effects

*Oral Diabetes Medications*

| Medication Classification | Names Generic (Commercial) | Mechanism of Action | Side Effects |
|---|---|---|---|
| Biguanides | Metformin, metformin XR or ER (Glucophage, Glucophage XR or ER, Glumetza, Fortamet) | Decrease hepatic glucose production, intestinal absorption of glucose, and improve insulin sensitivity by increasing peripheral glucose uptake and utilization | Lactic acidosis (rare), diarrhea, nausea, vomiting, flatulence, asthenia, and vitamin $B_{12}$ deficiency |
| Sulfonylureas (SUs) | Glyburide (DiaBeta, Glynase PresTab, Micronase) Glimepiride (Amaryl) Glipizide (Glucotrol) | Stimulate insulin secretion from the pancreatic beta-cell (insulin secretagogues) | Hypoglycemia, hunger, weight gain, skin reactions, gastrointestinal upset, and dark-colored urine |
| Meglitinides | Nateglinide (Starlix) Repaglinide (Prandin) | Stimulate insulin secretion from the pancreatic beta-cell Shorter duration of action than SUs | Hypoglycemia and weight gain; less common: gastrointestinal upset, flulike symptoms, joint pain, and temporary hair loss |
| Thiazolidinediones | Rosiglitazone (Avandia) Pioglitazone (Actos) | Improve insulin sensitivity and decrease insulin resistance by binding to peroxisome proliferator-activated receptor gamma in adipocytes to promote adipogenesis and fatty acid uptake | Edema/exacerbation of heart failure, weight gain, macular edema, decreased hematocrit and hemoglobin levels, increased bone fracture risk, and increased bladder cancer risk in smokers (pioglitazone only) |
| Alpha-glucosidase inhibitors (AGIs) | Acarbose (Precose) | Inhibit enzymes (glycoside hydrolases) needed to digest carbohydrates improving postprandial hyperglycemia by decreasing the rate of digestion of complex carbohydrates | Flatulence, diarrhea, and abdominal pain; less frequent: nausea, vomiting, dyspepsia and liver dysfunction |
| Sodium-glucose cotransporter 2 inhibitors (SGLT2i) | Canagliflozin (Invokana) Dapagliflozin (Farxiga) Empagliflozin (Jardiance) Ertugliflozin (Steglatro) | Block the SGLT2 protein involved in 90% of glucose reabsorption in the proximal renal tubule, increase renal glucose excretion (glucosuria) | Dehydration, hyperkalemia, genital mycotic infections, urinary tract infection, bone fractures, increased risk of lower limb amputations, increase low density lipoprotein. Serious side effects include ketoacidosis, urinary tract infection with sepsis or pyelonephritis, requiring hospitalization |

**TABLE 3.2 • Oral Diabetes Medications: Mechanism of Action, Side Effects** (*continued*)

*Oral Diabetes Medications*

| Medication Classification | Names Generic (Commercial) | Mechanism of Action | Side Effects |
|---|---|---|---|
| Dipeptidyl peptidase(DPP-4) inhibitors | Sitagliptin (Januvia) Saxagliptin (Onglyza) Alogliptin (Nesina) Linagliptin (Tradjenta) | Block the action of DPP-4, an enzyme that destroys a group of gastrointestinal hormones called incretins. Incretins enhance the production of insulin after eating and reduce the production of glucagon by the liver when it is not needed. They also slow down digestion and decrease appetite | Angioedema, skin reactions, increased risk for acute pancreatitis, nausea, vomiting, headache, exacerbation of heart failure, flulike symptoms and severe joint pain |

is important to note that most older adults with renal impairment have normal serum creatinine values. Obtaining GFR levels to assess kidney function is recommended to evaluate kidney function before starting a new medication.[59]

## Sulfonylureas

This group of diabetic medications contains long-acting insulin secretagogues that are inexpensive and commonly used in the outpatient setting. However, they pose a high risk of hypoglycemia in the **elderly** population, especially in those with decreased oral intake and impaired renal function (Table 3.2). According to the Beers Criteria of Potentially Inappropriate Drugs for older adults, glyburide is found to be especially dangerous because of its prolonged hypoglycemic effect. Alternatives in this group of medications are glimepiride and glipizide because they are less associated with prolonged hypoglycemia.[60] Glimepiride dose should be reduced for GFR of 30 mL/min and avoided in lower GFR levels. Glipizide doses do not have to be adjusted for renal disease, but starting at lower doses is recommended because it still carries hypoglycemia risk.[61]

Old age (over 75 years), renal impairment, and liver disease are conditions in which sulfonylureas should not be used as first-line therapy, but as second- or third-line agents in T2DM. Sulfonylureas should be discontinued in older patients with worsening renal or liver function and patients with autonomic failure due to aging and longer duration of diabetes because of increased risk of hypoglycemia unawareness.[62]

## Meglitinides

Shorter-acting insulin secretagogues, such as meglitinides are a safer option in the **elderly** population because of their short half-life.[63] Their benefit is that they can be taken right before a meal and held if the patient does not eat. In addition, doses can be adjusted for patients with variable food intake. These secretagogues should be taken with each meal, so adherence may decrease, especially for patients with polypharmacy. Side effects include cold or flulike symptoms, back pain, headache, dizziness, blurred vision, joint pain, and temporary hair loss[64,65] (Table 3.2). There are two medications in this class of drugs: nateglinide, which is eliminated renally, and repaglinide, which is eliminated through the liver. The cost of repaglinide is less than that of nateglinide because it is generic, which can also help when choosing between these medications.[64,65]

## Thiazolidinediones

According to the Beers Criteria of Potentially Inappropriate Drugs for older adults, all other diabetes medication classes should be considered before TZDs.[60] This is mainly due to the increased risk of fractures and HF noted for those taking TZD medications.[66] Several safety alerts regarding the cardiotoxicity of TZDs have been launched by regulatory agencies starting from May 2007. Rosiglitazone use was suspended in the United States and European Union in 2010, leaving pioglitazone as the only choice in this class of drugs.[67] However, in 2013, the FDA removed prescribing restrictions on rosiglitazone because new data no longer showed increased risk of MI.[68] Clinical trials data suggest an increased risk of bladder cancer in patients exposed to pioglitazone; the risk may be increased with tobacco use or duration of use (Table 3.2).[69]

## Alpha-Glucosidase Inhibitors

A high percentage of patients have sustained elevated $HbA_{1c}$ because of persistent elevation of postprandial plasma glucose. Alpha-glucosidase inhibitors (AGIs) specifically target postprandial plasma glucose. They are designed to specifically delay the digestion of complex carbohydrates, thus significantly reducing postprandial hyperglycemia and insulin excursions. Acarbose is the most studied and prescribed medication in this group and is not associated with weight gain, but in fact with small but consistent weight loss. When administered as monotherapy, acarbose should not cause hypoglycemia.[70] Flatulence (74%), diarrhea (31%), and abdominal pain (19%) are the most common side effects of acarbose (Table 3.2).[71] There are no known differences in side effects between age groups.

## Sodium-Glucose Cotransporter 2 Inhibitors

This group of medications prevents the reabsorption of renal-filtered glucose levels, resulting in decreased serum glucose levels.[72] The drug causes the kidneys to remove glucose from the body through the urine, demonstrating an improvement in $HbA_{1c}$ levels by 0.5% to 1.0%.[73] Benefits of this drug class include weight loss and improved blood pressure.[74] In December 2016, the FDA approved a new indication for Jardiance (empagliflozin) to reduce the risk of cardiovascular death in adult patients with T2DM and cardiovascular disease.[75] However, the FDA also confirmed increased risk of leg and foot amputations with the use of canagliflozin. People with risk factors such as prior amputation, peripheral vascular disease, neuropathy, and diabetic foot ulcers should not be started on this medication and the medication should be discontinued on anyone receiving canagliflozin with any of the noted risk factors.[76]

In the **elderly** population, risks and benefits of use must be determined on a case-by-case basis. Side effects may include dehydration, hyperkalemia, genital mycotic infections (especially in patients with a history of these infections and uncircumcised males), bone fractures, and increased levels of low-density lipoprotein cholesterol.[77] Studies done by the drug maker of canagliflozin indicated that patients aged 65 and older had a higher incidence of adverse reactions related to reduced intravascular volume. These effects were even greater in those older than 75 years and at the expense of a smaller reduction in $HbA_{1c}$.[78] Use of these drugs in the **elderly** also potentiates the risk of euglycemic ketoacidosis and serious urinary tract infections such as urosepsis or pyelonephritis requiring hospitalization. Patients with a history of pancreatic insulin deficiency, caloric restriction, and alcohol abuse may also be predisposed to euglycemic ketoacidosis (Table 3.2).[79]

## The Dipeptidyl Peptidase 4 Inhibitors

This group of diabetes medications enhances glucose-dependent insulin secretion from pancreatic β cells, by preventing dipeptidyl peptidase 4 (DPP-4)–mediated degradation of endogenously released incretin hormones.[80] There have only been a few reports about the use of DPP-4 inhibitors in **elderly** patients with T2DM. In 2015, a comparative review of the efficacy and safety of sitagliptin was conducted in Japanese patients with T2DM. They concluded that $HbA_{1c}$ improved after 2 years of sitagliptin therapy, and age did not seem to influence the incidence of hypoglycemic events. These results confirm the efficacy and safety of sitagliptin in patients 75 years and older. Angioedema, urticaria, and other immune-mediated dermatologic effects have been reported as well as increased risk of acute pancreatitis, and HF.[81] The potential increased risk of HF with DPP-4 inhibitors was reported in a study of saxagliptin, but was not observed in subsequent trials. Therefore, there needs to be caution among patients with a previous history of HF.[82] In 2015, the FDA warned that DPP-4 inhibitors may cause joint pain that can be severe and disabling, which resolved once the medication was discontinued (Table 3.2).[83]

## Injectable/Inhaled Diabetes Medications

### GLP-1 Agonists

Aging is characterized by a progressive impairment in carbohydrate tolerance, possibly related to disorderly insulin release, reduced insulin production, and reduced GLP-1 secretion.[84] Furthermore, the relative contribution of postprandial glucose is higher than that of fasting glucose in older adults.[85] GLP-1 receptor agonists are effective in glycemic control and are well tolerated without increasing the risk of hypoglycemia in older patients.[86] Because GLP-1 receptor agonists delay gastric emptying and increase satiety leading to weight loss, they may be a good option for overweight and obese patients.[87] However, this class of medications should be avoided in frail, underweight, or malnourished older patients. Liraglutide is not affected by renal impairment and end-stage renal disease.[88] In 2017, the FDA approved a new indication for Victoza (liraglutide) to reduce the risk of major adverse cardiovascular (CV) events, heart attack, stroke, and CV death in adults with **type 2 diabetes** and established CV disease.[89]

Exenatide, however, is excreted through the kidney and is not recommended for use in severe renal impairment or end-stage renal disease.[90]

Some GLP-1 agonists can be administered once weekly, reducing the number of injections, side effects, and potentially improving adherence. Compared with other once-weekly GLP-1 agonists, dulaglutide showed a greater reduction in $HbA_{1c}$, fasting plasma glucose, and body weight.[91] The risk of hypoglycemia among once-weekly GLP-1 agonists was similar. GLP-1 agonists are contraindicated in patients with personal or family history of medullary thyroid carcinoma and in patients with multiple endocrine neoplasia syndrome type 2 because of an increase in the incidence of thyroid C-cell tumors seen in rodents.[92,93] There is also a risk of acute pancreatitis in this medication group.

Patients should be counseled on the signs and symptoms of acute pancreatitis, such as persistent, severe abdominal pain with or without vomiting, which must be immediately reported. A recent study conducted on patients aged 70 years or older using lixisenatide for 24 weeks demonstrated a substantial decrease in $HbA_{1c}$ and 2-hour postprandial blood sugars without statistically significant hypoglycemia versus placebo. It also showed greater decrease in weight.[94]

## Insulin

As the elderly population is extremely heterogeneous, the risks and benefits of insulin therapy must be carefully and individually considered. As people get older, insulin resistance increases and pancreatic islet cell function decreases.[95] The development of insulin deficiency in some patients with long-standing **type 2 diabetes** might make insulin therapy not a choice but a necessity in the older adult. The risk of hypoglycemia is the biggest concern because of the fact that the risk increases with age, presence of comorbidities, and diabetes complications especially if renal insufficiency is present (Table 2.3). In addition, the patient's ability to prepare and inject insulin must be addressed.[55]

The use of insulin analogs, instead of human insulins, represents a safer choice for older adults. The pharmacokinetics and stability of analogs decrease the risk of hypoglycemia. Insulin detemir and insulin glargine may be used instead of NPH or human 70/30 mixed insulin to lower the frequency of hypoglycemic events.[66] If insulins need to be mixed, then the use of premixed insulin vials or pens is recommended to prevent errors when mixing two insulins in a syringe.[66]

The newest insulin analog approved by the FDA is Fiasp, a rapid-acting aspart insulin with added niacinamide (vitamin $B_3$) that helps increase the speed of the initial insulin absorption, resulting in an onset of appearance in the blood in approximately

*Injectable/Inhaled Diabetes Medications*

| | | |
|---|---|---|
| Glucagon-Like Peptide 1 (GLP-1)Agonists | Exenatide (Byetta)<br>Liraglutide (Victoza)<br>Semaglutide (Ozempic)<br>Lixisenatide (Adlyxin)<br>Exenatide (Bydureon) weekly<br>Dulaglutide (Trulicity) (Daily or weekly injections) | Enhance glucose-dependent insulin secretion release from the pancreatic islets, inhibit inappropriate postmeal glucagon release, reduce food intake, and slow gastric emptying. | Nausea, vomiting, diarrhea, headache, urticaria; more serious effects include pancreatitis; at risk for thyroid C-cell tumors in persons with a family history |
| Basal insulins | • Intermediate NPH recombinant insulin<br>(Novolin N)<br>(Humulin N)<br>• Insulin analogs<br>Detemir (Levemir)<br>Glargine U100 (Lantus)<br>Glargine U300 (Toujeo)<br>Degludec (Tresiba)<br>Glargine (Basaglar) | NPH is a recombinant human insulin that has a peak of action and day-to-day variability. It is usually given 2 times a day to maintain glucose control for 24 h.<br><br>Insulin analogs are synthetic insulins that mimic the body's natural pattern of insulin release for 24 h without a peak and very little day-to-day variability. Usually given once a day. | Hypoglycemia (less risk with insulin analogs than with intermediate NPH recombinant insulin)<br>All insulin products can cause hypokalemia, weight gain, and lipodystrophy may occur at the injection site and delay insulin absorption.<br>Injection site reactions include redness, pain, itching, hives, swelling, inflammation.<br>Beta-blockers, diuretics, clonidine, and lithium salts can weaken the effects of basal insulins.<br>Dose adjustments might be necessary in those with renal or liver disease. |
| Bolus insulins | • Regular recombinant insulin<br>(Novolin R)<br>(Humulin R)<br>• Insulin analogs<br>Aspart (Novolog or Fiasp)<br>Glulisine (Apidra)<br>Lispro (Humalog)<br>lispro follow-on insulin (Admelog) | Bolus insulins (mealtime or correction insulins) are rapid-acting insulins that keep blood glucose levels under control following a meal or to correct hyperglycemic excursions. | Hypoglycemia (lesser risk with insulin analogs than with regular recombinant insulin). Timing of hypoglycemia usually reflects the time–action profile of administered insulin. Other factors such as changes in food intake, injection site, and exercise may increase the risk of hypoglycemia. |

*(continued)*

**TABLE 3.3** • Injected/Inhaled Diabetes Medications: Mechanism of Action, Side Effects (*continued*)

*Injectable/Inhaled Diabetes Medications*

| Mixed insulins | • NPH/regular recombinant mix insulin (Novolin 70/30) (Humulin 70/30)<br>• NPH recombinant and rapid-acting analog mix insulin (Humalog Mix 75/25) (Humalog Mix 50/50) (Novolog Mix 70/30)<br>• Basal insulin analog and GLP-I analog Degludec plus liraglutide (Xultophy 100/3.6)<br>Glargine plus lixisenatide (Soliqua 100/30) | Action, onset, duration of mixed insulins are based on the combination profile and percentage of insulin or GLP-I agonist preparation.<br>The numbers next to the names indicate the percentage of insulin/GLP-I agonist found in each mix. | Side effects are directly related to each preparation combination and include hypoglycemia, weight gain, hypokalemia, injection site reactions, lipodystrophy, drugs interaction, dose adjustments for insulin-based mix preparations. GLP-I agonists (see preceding text)<br>Patient awareness of the timing of injection, food intake, dosing, and side effects are particularly important to prevent side effects and adverse reactions with mixed insulins. |
|---|---|---|---|
| Concentrated insulin U-500 | Recombinant regular insulin U-500 (Humulin R U-500) | Regular insulin U-500 is five times more concentrated than U-100 insulin.<br>The subcutaneous administration of this insulin has shown mean time of onset of action of less than 15 min with a mean duration of action of 21 h (range 13–24 h). The time–action characteristics reflect both prandial and basal activity. This effect has been attributed to the high concentration of the preparation.<br>Usually administered two or three times a day, 30 min before a meal. | Owing to its high concentration, hypoglycemia is the most commonly observed side effect.<br>Overdosing effects can be catastrophic or fatal. The use of this insulin is limited to patients with severe insulin resistance requiring 200 or more units of insulin per day.<br>All other side effects are similar to those in any other insulin preparation. |
| Bolus inhaled insulin | Human insulin (Afrezza) | Inhaled insulin is human insulin pulmonary absorbed into the systemic circulation. The action, metabolism, and elimination are comparable to a rapid-acting human insulin analog. | Inhaled insulin can cause a decline in lung function; therefore, lung function needs to be evaluated before the initiation of treatment, at 6 mo, and a year after.<br>Cough, sore throat, and all other side effects are similar to those in any other insulin preparation. |

2.5 minutes. Owing to this accelerated absorption, caution should be exercised when administered to geriatric patients. The initial dosing, dose increments, and maintenance dosage should be conservative to avoid hypoglycemia.[96]

The use of basal insulin plus GLP-1 receptor agonists is associated with less hypoglycemia and with weight loss instead of weight gain, but may be less tolerable and have a greater cost. In November 2016, the FDA approved two different once-daily combination products containing basal insulin plus a GLP-1 receptor agonist: insulin glargine plus lixisenatide and insulin degludec plus liraglutide (Table 3.3).

## Concentrated Insulin Products

Several concentrated insulin preparations are currently available. These might be particularly useful in people with significant insulin resistance and high insulin requirements.[97] U-500 regular insulin, by definition, is five times as concentrated as U-100 regular insulin and has a delayed onset and longer duration of action than U-100 regular, possessing both prandial and basal properties. U-500 regular insulin is available in both prefilled pens and vials (a dedicated syringe was FDA approved in July 2016).[53] It is important for the prescriber and the older patient starting this type of insulin to understand the potential devastating and/or fatal effects of dose medication errors while using this insulin (Table 3.3).

U-200 degludec and U-300 glargine are two and three times as concentrated as their U-100 formulations, have longer durations of action, and allow for higher doses of basal insulin administration per volume to be used.[53] U-200 insulin has low variability and lower (nocturnal) or similar risk of hypoglycemia compared with U-100 insulin. U-300 glargine insulin has low variability, less weight gain, and lower nocturnal hypoglycemia in some studies in comparison with U-100 glargine.[97] Caution with initial dosing, dose titration, and maintenance doses is recommended to avoid hypoglycemia. If accidental overdose occurs, the hypoglycemic effect will be longer than that of other basal insulins and more detrimental to older adults.[98] Concentrated preparations may be more comfortable for the patient and may improve adherence for patients with insulin resistance who require large doses of insulin. Concentrated insulins are available only in prefilled pens to minimize the risk of dosing errors.[53] In clinical trials conducted by the makers of U-300 and U-200, no differences were found in the safety and effectiveness of these insulins in individuals 65 years or older when compared with younger subjects. However, caution was recommended in the **elderly** population with insulin sensitivity.[99,100] Patients who can potentially benefit from this group of insulins are the ones with increasing insulin resistance and insulin requirements (Table 3.3).

## Biosimilars: "Follow-up" Insulins

A biosimilar product is a biologic product that is approved if it is very similar to an FDA-approved biologic product, known as a reference product, and has no clinically meaningful differences in terms of safety and effectiveness from the reference product.[101] Basaglar was approved as a biosimilar in Europe. However, in December of 2015, the FDA approved Basaglar (U-100 insulin glargine injection), as a "follow-up" not a "biosimilar" long-acting human insulin analog to improve glycemic control in adult and pediatric patients with T1DM and in adults with T2DM.[102] The most common adverse reactions associated with Basaglar or Lantus in clinical trials were hypoglycemia, allergic reactions, injection site reactions, pitting at the injection site (lipodystrophy), itching, rash, edema (fluid retention), and weight gain (Table 3.3).[103] In clinical studies conducted in **elderly** patients using this preparation, there was no difference in safety or efficacy when compared with younger subjects.[104]

In December 2017, the first "follow-up" rapid-acting insulin was approved under the name of Admelog, which is the same as lispro insulin (reference product).[105]

Other insulins are in development including the U-500 short-acting analog (Fluorolog) and U-400 premix such as insulin BIOD-531, among others.[97] One of the benefits of producing biosimilar insulins for this age group is that they are less expensive than their reference counterparts while still providing equivalent action profile. Basaglar is 15% to 20% less expensive than Lantus. Pharmacy Benefit Managers (PBMs), which provide pharmaceutical coverage for 266 million Americans, had indicated that they favored Basaglar on 2017 formularies. America's second- and third-biggest PBMs—CVS Caremark and UnitedHealth stated that Basaglar preferred formulary status in 2017.[106]

## Inhaled Insulin

In 2014, the FDA approved Afrezza (insulin human) Inhalation Powder, a rapid-acting inhaled insulin that is administered at the beginning of each meal.[107] No overall differences in safety or effectiveness were observed between patients over 65 and younger patients. However, Afrezza is contraindicated in patients with chronic lung disease, such as asthma, or chronic obstructive pulmonary disease because of the increased risk of acute bronchospasm (Table 3.3). It also should not be used in patients with a history of lung cancer or are at risk of lung cancer. Spirometry is necessary to evaluate lung function in all candidates before starting therapy, at 6 months, and a year because Afrezza can cause a decline in lung function. Because Afrezza is a rapid-acting insulin, it also carries the risk of hypoglycemia; and careful monitoring, and dose adjustments need to be made especially in patients with renal and liver disease.[108] Inhaled insulin use is limited in the **elderly** population because there is a decline in lung function with age and a continued adverse effect of smoking.

## Insulin Through Subcutaneous Insulin Infusion Therapy

In addition to inhaled insulin, there have been several advances in sq insulin delivery: continuous subcutaneous insulin infusion (CSII) or **insulin pump** therapy. **Insulin pumps** work by delivering both basal and bolus insulin. Basal insulin is rapid, short-acting, or highly concentrated insulin released in small pulses every few minutes 24 hours a day through a catheter placed under the skin.[109] Boluses are given to correct for an elevated blood sugar and/or to cover for a meal. Currently, there are a variety of **insulin pumps** in the market, including the Tandem t:slim and t:flex, the Insulet Omnipod, the SOILL Development Dana Diabecare IIS, the Valeritas V-Go, the Medtronic MiniMed 530 G with Enlite, the Medtronic Minimed Paradigm Revel, and the Medtronic Minimed 630G and 670G. In 2017, both Roche and Animas decided to discontinue the production of **insulin pumps** and exit the **insulin pump** market.[110,111]

There are two options for pump attachment—the catheter can be directly attached to the skin as a pod or attached to the skin with tubing connected to the device. Devices with tubing offer different choices of infusion sets (ie, different tubing lengths and capacity of fill amount of cannulas) and the opportunity to disconnect from the pump at the infusion site. Each device can hold a different amount of insulin in the reservoir, so patients who are insulin resistant may require devices with larger reservoirs such as the t:flex. They all allow users to assess how long an insulin bolus is active in the body, or "insulin on board," and each are able to set temporary rates of basal insulin for different lengths of time (between 12 and 72 hours) if patients require more or less insulin, for example, if he/she is sick or is exercising. Devices vary in the increment amounts of insulin it can give; for example, Tandem pumps offer hourly basal dosing in increments of 0.001 U and boluses in increments of 0.01 U, whereas both Animas and Medtronic pumps have hourly basal dosing in 0.025 U increments and Medtronic allows boluses in increments of 0.025 units (Table 3.4). Another distinguishing feature is that some can be integrated with continuous glucose monitors (CGMs) or devices that track glucose levels continuously throughout the day, which eliminates the need to carry a separate CGM receiver by displaying the data on the pump screen.[112]

One of the innovative advances of integrating CSII and CGMs together is allowing for automation of insulin delivery by the pump. For example, the MiniMed 530 G with Enlite has a "threshold suspend pump" feature, which allows for automatic cessation of insulin delivery from the pump when a preset low blood glucose threshold is detected by the CGM.[113] Another breakthrough is the ability to share data with others. Dexcom has a SHARE component enabled by Bluetooth and cloud technology, which allows caregivers to track data in real time on their smartphones to be alerted of any potential problems.[114] Together, CSII and CGM have changed the landscape of how patients are managed with diabetes; however, the success of these devices is directly correlated to the type of patients who use them and how providers introduce it. Patients need to be educated, capable, and willing to use the devices correctly. It is important that they receive the proper education, training, and support to be able to maintain their individualized glycemic goals.[115]

## Continuous Glucose Monitoring

CGMs were developed to improve glucose monitoring and are continuously evolving to improve its accuracy and ease of use. They work by placing a sensor under the skin in the interstitial fluid space that measures the glucose every 5 to 15 minutes and sends the information to the transmitter device. There are several CGMs in the

**TABLE 3.4** • Insulin Pumps

| Insulin Pump | Tubing (Y/N) | Size and Weight | Reservoir | Basal Range | Bolus Range |
|---|---|---|---|---|---|
| Animas OneTouch Ping (discontinued, taken off market) | Y | Pump: 3.25 × 2 × 0.86 inches 3.74 oz Meter remote: 3.8 × 2.4 × 1.1 inches 3.88 oz | 200-unit cartridge | From 0.025 to 25 units per hour in 0.025 unit increments | 0.05 to 35 units in 0.05 unit increments |
| Animas Vibe (discontinued, taken off market) | Y | 3.25 × 2 × 0.86 inches 3.7 oz | 200-unit cartridge | From 0.025 to 25 units per hour in 0.025 unit increments | From 0.05 to 35 units in 0.05 unit increments |
| Insulet OmniPod | N | Pod: 1.5 × 2.0 × 0.57 inches 0.88 oz | Reservoir holds 200 units | From 0.05 to 30 units per hour in 0.05 unit increments | From 0.05 to 30 units. Increments of 0.05, 0.1, 0.5, or 1 unit |
| Medtronic Diabetes MiniMed 530G with Enlite | Y | 2 × 3.3 × 0.81 inches 3.4 oz | Model 551: 180-unit reservoir | From 0.025 to 35 units per hour in 0.025 unit increments for up to 0.975 units. Increments of 0.05 units for between 1 and 9.95 units. Increments of 0.1 units for 10 units or more | From 0.025 to 25 units. Increments of 0.025 units up to 0.975 units. Increments of 0.05 units for 0.975 units or more |

| Device | | Dimensions / Weight | Reservoir | Basal | Bolus |
|---|---|---|---|---|---|
| Medtronic Diabetes MiniMed Paradigm Revel | Y | Model 523: 2 × 3.3 × 0.82 inches 3.4 oz | 180-unit reservoir | From 0.025 to 35 units per hour in 0.025 unit increments for up to 0.975 units. Increments of 0.05 units for between 1 and 9.5 units. Increments of 0.1 units for 10 units or more | From 0.025 to 25 units. Increments of 0.025 units up to 0.975 units. Increments of 0.05 units for 0.975 units or more |
| Medtronic MiniMed 670G | Y | Pump: 2.1 × 3.78 × 0.96 inches 3.0 oz | 300-unit cartridge | From 0 to 35 units per hour or the max basal rate amount, whichever is lower | From 0.025, 0.05, to 0.1 unit increments |
| Roche Insulin Delivery System Accu-Chek Combo (discontinued, taken off market) | Y | Pump: 3.2 × 2.2 × 0.8 inches 3.9 oz | 315-unit cartridge | From 0.05 to 25 units per hour. Deliver in 0.01 unit increments for up to 1 unit per hour, in 0.05 unit increments for up to 10 units per hour, and in 0.1 unit increments for up to 25 units per hour | From 0.1 to 25 units in increments of 0.1, 0.2, 0.5, 1, and 2 units for standard boluses. |
| Tandem T:flex | Y | 3.13 × 2 × 0.84 inches 4.05 oz | 480 unit cartridge | From 0.5 to 15 units per hour in 0.001 unit increments | From 0.5 to 60 units in 0.01 unit increments |
| Tandem t:slim G4 pump | Y | 3.13 × 2 × 0.6 inches 3.95 oz | 300 unit cartridge | From 0.1 to 15 units per hour in 0.001 unit increments | From 0.05 to 25 units in 0.01 unit increments with an option for up to an additional 25 units |

market, including the Dexcom G4 and G5, the Medtronic Enlite, the Abbott Freestyle Navigator II, and the Abbott Freestyle Libre. Patients are typically required to calibrate the device every 12 hours by comparing the sensor glucose reading with that of an FS. In September 2017, the FDA approved the first continuous glucose monitoring system—the Freestyle Libre Flash—that can be used for adults without calibration using a blood sample.[116] Some of the differences between the CGMs include sensor longevity (approved for use between 6 and 7 days), alert settings (high and low alerts as well as rate of change alerts), alert volume, transmitters (some with radio and Bluetooth capability), model display, and accuracy, which is best measured by looking at the mean absolute relative difference, signifying the difference between FS and sensor values.[117]

Several advances in the technology of CGMs have made them much more appealing. Senseonics' Eversense has developed a 90-day implantable CGM that has been approved in Europe; it provides ease of use because no sensor is inserted under the skin.[118,119] There have been improvements in CGM calibration algorithms, resulting in improved sensor performance.[120] Also, most companies now have platforms that make data from devices available to the patient and clinician through a universal portal or smartphone application that permits easier data access.[121]

There are still many barriers that prohibit CGMs from being used widely. These include the following: (1) cost and variable reimbursement, (2) the need for recalibrations, (3) periodic replacement of sensors, (4) day-to-day variability in glycemic patterns, (5) lack of training and inexperience among physicians interpreting CGM results, (6) lack of FDA approval for insulin dosing and for use in hospital and intensive care unit (ICU) settings, (7) lack of standardization for analysis of CGM data, and (8) time, cost, and inconvenience for uploading data for analysis.[122] However, many of these barriers are being addressed with continued development of technology and further research.

## Use of Continuous Subcutaneous Insulin Infusion With or Without Continuous Glucose Monitor Therapy in Elderly Patients With Type 2 Diabetes Mellitus

According to the 2016 Endocrine Society guidelines, it is suggested that CSII be used in patients with T2DM when they have poor glycemic control, despite intensive insulin therapy, oral agents, and other injectable medications and lifestyle modifications.[123] It does not, however, specify the role of CSII in elderly patients. There are very few studies that assess the role of CSII and whether CSII is superior to multiple daily injections (MDIs) for this patient population. In systematic reviews and meta-analyses that compare CSII and MDIs in adult patients with T2DM, there was no difference in HbA$_{1c}$ or reduction in hypoglycemia.[122]

This conclusion was reinforced by the results of a 12-month randomized clinical trial involving older patients (≥60 years old) in which glucose variability was improved equally with CSII and MDI treatment. Fifty-three patients underwent CSII therapy and 54 patients underwent MDI therapy for 12 months and were asked to complete monthly eight-point self-monitored glucose profiles and CGMs for up to 72 hours at months 0, 6, and 12. There was no difference in the eight-point profiles with respect to mean glucose, mean preprandial and postprandial glucose, standard deviation, or range of glucose values. With the CGM data, there was no significant difference between the mean glucose, range, or area under the curve high (>180 mg/dL), and area under the curve low (<70 mg/dL).[124]

Another study looked at 107 older patients (patients ≥60 years of age) with **type 2 diabetes** who were randomized to CSII with insulin lispro or MDI with insulin glargine and insulin lispro. Subjects received titration of insulin dosing for 4 weeks, after which things were maintained unless there was a medical necessity. The subjects in the CSII and MDI groups had mean $HbA_{1c}$ of 8.4% and 8.1%, respectively. The results of the study showed no significant difference of $HbA_{1c}$ between both treatment groups. The mean $HbA_{1c}$ fell by 1.7% in the CSII group and 1.6% in the MDI group.[125] Treatment satisfaction for both groups improved from baseline and was statistically significant individually; however, the change in treatment satisfaction was not statistically significant comparatively.

These two studies demonstrated that there were no consistent data on the benefit of CSII over MDI. The available clinical evidence we have so far is still not consistent, and the study populations were generally heterogeneous. More studies are necessary to further evaluate the role of CSII in the **elderly** population.

## Continuous Subcutaneous Insulin Infusion Therapy in the Hospital

According to the 2016 Endocrine Society guidelines, patients on CSII should continue CSII in the hospital with either type of diabetes as long as there are clear protocols in the hospital to evaluate patients as suitable candidates and there are appropriate monitoring and safety protocols.[123] There are no RCTs that have evaluated the benefit of continuing CSII versus transitioning to MDI or intravenous insulin infusion therapy in the **elderly**. There are studies that have shown that hospitals with well-developed protocols for diabetes care can effectively manage safe and effective CSII therapy.[126] A review of 136 patients with **insulin pumps** who had 253 hospitalizations demonstrated that most patients using an **insulin pump** can continue their therapy in the inpatient setting with appropriate patient selection and usage guidelines. The appropriate measures included endocrinology consultation, **insulin pump** order sets, and a signed agreement specifying patient responsibility for continued pump use and documentation of an **insulin pump** flow sheet.[127] Both the ADA and the American Association of Clinical Endocrinologists support these findings, assuming the patients have the physical and mental capacity for continued CSII use.[123]

If a hospital institution is unable to guarantee appropriate evaluation and support, it may decide against the use of CSII within the hospital. It is recommended that an endocrinologist evaluate the patient to determine whether CSII should be continued. Factors such as medical illness, co-medications, and mental status changes strongly influence whether the patient can continue **insulin pump** therapy. If the endocrinologist decides it is not safe for the patient to continue CSII, it is imperative that the patient be appropriately transitioned to MDI. To do this, one can calculate the TDD of insulin on the **insulin pump** by adding up the daily set basal rate and bolus doses together to calculate the TDD. Then divide this into two equal parts: 50% will be basal insulin (ie, insulin glargine) and 50% will be given as premeal insulin (ie, insulin lispro, aspart, or glulisine).

CSII can also be continued in patients undergoing same-day or outpatient surgery, which may involve fasting and/or conscious sedation. The physician who is managing the **insulin pump** patient should give recommendations for **insulin pump** setting adjustments in preparation for the surgery. Often, the temporary basal feature can be used so a patient can receive less basal insulin during the time they are NPO. Patients should also be encouraged to bring extra tubing, reservoirs, and/or pod supplies because hospitals cannot provide CSII supplies.

There are, however, other considerations to take into account for the patient's safety. One is patient movement that could inadvertently disconnect the **insulin pump** catheter, making it important to inspect the insertion site and its connection to the device before, during, and after any procedures.[128] Second is exposure to radiography, wherein pump manufacturers recommend that pumps and/or CGMs be placed out of range of radiation or magnetic fields. If radiography is needed, it is recommended that the devices be disconnected or removed beforehand with a proper transition to MDI insulin.[129]

## Use of Continuous Glucose Monitors in Patients With Type 2 Diabetes Mellitus

The 2016 Endocrine Society guidelines recommend short-term, intermittent CGM in adult patients with T2DM who have $HbA_{1c}$ levels >7% and are willing and able to use the device.[123] There were, however, insufficient studies on the role of CGM use in the **elderly** population. This recommendation is based on data from a well-performed RCT by Vigersky et al.[130] The trial involved 100 adults with T2DM on therapies including diet, exercise, and various combinations of antihyperglycemic medications including oral medications only, the GLP-1 agonist exenatide, and basal but not prandial insulin. Half of the subjects were randomly assigned to self-monitoring of blood glucose (SMBG) before meals and at bedtime and the other half were assigned to real-time continuous glucose monitors (RT-CGM). The mean ages of the SMBG and RT-CGM groups were only 60 and 55 years, respectively. The results showed that intermittent CGM use for 12 weeks resulted in significant reductions in $HbA_{1c}$, which was sustained during a 40-week follow-up period. The mean, unadjusted $A_{1c}$ decreased by 1.0%, 1.2%, 0.8%, and 0.8% in the RT-CGM group versus 0.5%, 0.5%, 0.5%, and 0.2% in the SMBG group at 12, 24, 38, and 52 weeks, respectively ($P = 0.04$). This improvement occurred without a greater intensification of medication compared with the control group, which reflects improvement of self-care prompted by CGM use.[130] Although there are a few publications that focus on CGMs with older patients, most of these studied patients had T1DM and not T2DM.

Another recent study evaluated two groups of seniors with T1DM or T2DM who were using RT-CGM (n = 210) and were RT-CGM "hopefuls" ($n = 75$), who could not get RT-CGM because of lack of insurance coverage.[131] As of January 12, 2017, patients at the age of 65 who switch to Medicare can have RT-CGMs as a covered benefit. The mean age of study participants was 70.7 years, and mean diabetes duration was 36 years. Only 25 patients (8.8%) of the total patients who were studied had T2DM. They were given online surveys about history of hypoglycemia and quality of life, and found that patients who used RT-CGM had fewer moderate ($P < 0.01$) and severe ($P < 0.01$) hypoglycemic episodes over 6 months than RT-CGM "hopefuls." Also RT-CGM users reported significantly better quality of life, less hypoglycemic fear ($P < 0.05$), and less diabetes distress ($P < 0.05$) than RT-CGM "hopefuls."

Overall, there is still a need for more consistent data from well-performed RCTs to confirm that these results are generalizable to the **elderly** T2DM population. There is an ongoing Daily Injections and Continuous Glucose Monitoring in Diabetes study that could provide conclusive data regarding the potential benefits of CGMs in the diabetes mellitus population; however, the eligible age for study was 25 years old, and it is unclear how many of these patients are **elderly**.[132]

## Use of Continuous Glucose Monitoring in the Hospital

Because CGM technology can detect early warning alarms against hyper/hypoglycemia, there has been increased interest in the possible use of CGMs in the hospital setting. It is important to be aware that that various agents (ie, acetaminophen, alcohol, and vitamin C) may lead to false interpretations of glucose levels by the CGM.[133] Several studies have evaluated the use of CGM in hospitalized patients. One such study looked at 124 patients on mechanical ventilation who were randomly assigned to RT-CGM versus control (selective arterial glucose measurements according to an algorithm). The results showed that the percentage of time patients in the RT-CGM group had a glucose level <110 was 59% ± 20%, whereas those in the control group had 55% ± 18%. The rate of severe hypoglycemia was lower in the real-time CGM group (1.6% vs 11.5% in the control group, $P = 0.031$). Although the real-time CGM reduced hypoglycemic events by 9.9%, there was no improved glycemic control.[134]

Recently, the FDA expanded the approved use of Dexcom's G5 Mobile CGM to allow for replacement of FS blood glucose for diabetes treatment decisions in those aged 2 or older. They evaluated data from two clinical studies of the G5 mobile system, which included 130 adults and children aged 2 years and older and compared the blood glucose values with the values from the CGM device. They noticed improved accuracy from other systems in the past, with the mean absolute relative difference of 9% in adults and 10% in pediatric patients. This is the first FDA-approved CGM that can be used to make diabetes treatment decisions without confirmation with a traditional FS test. This does not eliminate the need to do FS testing because the system still requires calibration with two daily FS every 12 hours. This does, however, allow some patients to manage their disease more comfortably.[135]

# ADVANCES IN THE FUTURE: THE CLOSED-LOOP SYSTEM AND ITS POTENTIAL IN THE INPATIENT SETTING

There has been development of an artificial pancreas, otherwise known as a closed-loop system, which has been researched in the field of diabetes technology over the past 10 years. The closed-loop system consists of three components: a CGM device to measure glucose concentrations, CSII, and an algorithm that calculates the amount of insulin to be delivered on the basis of real-time glucose measurements.[136,137] These components communicate or "talk" with one another, and the results thus far have been encouraging. Recently, the FDA approved the first hybrid closed-loop system, the Medtronic Minimed 670 G system, which is able to decrease or stop insulin delivery when it detects low sugars and increase the insulin delivery when the system detects high sugars, without any input from the user. This device, however, is currently only approved for patients with T1DM.[138]

There are a few studies that have tested the closed-loop system in the inpatient hospital setting. Brief use of the closed-loop system during the postoperative period in the surgical ICU has been studied.[139] One group had glucose levels controlled using the correctional scale method with insulin lispro ($n = 44$), and the second group had a programmed infusion using the closed-loop system ($n = 44$). Postoperative glucose values were checked every 2 hours up to 18 hours after the operation, and patients were assessed for length of stay and incidence of surgical site infections. The study showed that patients achieving moderate (FS 140) and tight control (FS 80–110) were higher in the closed-loop group compared with the correctional scale method, and that the closed-loop group had significantly lower surgical site infections, length of hospitalization, and cost.

Another study of 24 critically ill patients (predominantly trauma and neurosurgical patients) randomized to either closed-loop therapy or IV insulin infusion protocol. Both treatment groups received actrapid (regular) insulin. The mean age of the closed-loop therapy and IV insulin infusion group was 62 and 58 years, respectively. Their primary end point was to assess the percentage of time the FS was between 106 and 145. The study showed that the time period in which glucose was in the target range was significantly increased in the closed-loop system compared with the IV insulin protocol group.[140]

Another recent study looked at the safety using closed-loop insulin delivery in the inpatient units. The study evaluated patients 18 years and older with T2DM and divided the patients into two groups, one with closed-loop delivery using insulin lispro ($n = 20$) and the other with conventional sq insulin delivery using local insulin practice guidelines ($n = 20$). The mean age of the closed-loop and control group was 67 and 69 years, respectively. The study showed that the proportion of patients in the target glucose range (FS 100-180) in the closed-loop group was higher than that in the control group (59.8% vs 38.1%, respectively), and that the closed-loop insulin delivery was safe and significantly more effective in glycemic control compared with the control group.[141]

Although the closed-loop system seems promising, there are still a number of limitations before it can be used in the hospital. Most of the published studies have been small and limited to the ICU.[136] There is a need for larger studies assessing the outcomes of closed-loop systems and the feasibility of using them in the inpatient hospital setting without much technical support. Although the data are limited, the closed-loop system may provide healthcare providers with a valuable clinical tool to manage inpatient hyperglycemia, and the outlook is promising.

# SUMMARY

As the population ages, so does the frequency of chronic illness such as coronary artery disease, hypertension, or diabetes. T2DM has nearly tripled in prevalence among those older than 75 years.

Renal/hepatic failure, poor nutritional status, limited mobility, and cognitive impairment are some of the factors that can predispose **elderly** patients to hypoglycemia or hyperglycemia. As a result, the diabetes guidelines have been modified to recommend less stringent glycemic control for this vulnerable population.

In this review, the authors address the **inpatient management** of **type 2 diabetes**, in which patients are transitioned off of their oral antihyperglycemic agents and started on insulin therapy. Insulin dosing has to be adjusted in those with changes in renal function, concomitant steroid use, decreased oral intake, or utilization non–enteral nutrition. In addition, there is a discussion of the transition of inpatient insulin therapy to outpatient care. Medication reconciliation is crucial and has a significant impact on the outcome and quality of care. This review examines established and newer agents such as SGT2is and concentrated insulin. Creatinine clearance is an important factor in the dosing of these agents because **elderly** patients can have a normal creatinine with a compromised creatinine clearance. Lastly, this review examines the use of the evolving diabetes therapeutic technology: **insulin pumps** and sensors. These devices are no longer limited to the outpatient settings because hospitals are devising **insulin pump** policies that allow patients to continue to use their device. Its role in the **elderly** population, however, is poorly understood and requires further research for its applicability.

As the prevalence of T2DM continues to rise and population continues to age, inpatient care and care transitions remains an essential key in management of **elderly** persons with T2DM.

## References

1. National Center for Chronic Disease Prevention and Health Promotion Division of Diabetes Translation. National Diabetes Statistics Report, 2017. Estimates of Diabetes and Its Burden in the United States. https://www.cdc.gov/diabetes/pdfs/data/statistics/national-diabetes-statistics-report.pdf. Accessed September 18, 2018.

2. Centers for Disease Control and Prevention. Diabetes Report Card 2017. https://www.cdc.gov/diabetes/pdfs/library/diabetesreportcard2017-508.pdf. Accessed September 18, 2018. Last Updated March 1, 2018.

3. Murphy SL, Xu JQ, Kochanek KD, Curtin SC, Arias E. Deaths: final data for 2015. *National Vital Statistics Reports*. 2017;66(6).

4. Huang ES, Laiteerapong N, Liu JY, John PM, Moffet HH, Karter AJ. Rates of complications and mortality in older patients with diabetes mellitus: the diabetes and aging study. *JAMA Intern Med*. 2014;174:251.

5. Bethel MA. Longitudinal incidence and prevalence of adverse outcomes of diabetes mellitus in elderly patients. *Arch Intern Med*. 2007;167:921.

6. Sinclair A, Dunning T, Rodriguez-Mañas L. Diabetes in older people: new insights and remaining challenges. *Lancet Diabetes Endocrinol*. 2015;3:275-285.

7. Gilden JL, Gupta A. Non-ICU hospital care of diabetes mellitus in the elderly population. *Curr Diab Rep*. 2015;15:26.

8. American Diabetes Association. Older Adults: Standards of Medical Care in Diabetes—2018. *Diabetes Care*. 2018;41(suppl 1):S119-S125.

9. Zoungas S, Patel A, Chalmers J, et al. Severe hypoglycemia and risks of vascular events and death. *N Engl J Med*. 2010;363:1410-1418.

10. Majumdar SR, Hemmelgarn BR, Lin M, et al. Hypoglycemia associated with hospitalization and adverse events in older people: population-based cohort study. *Diabetes Care*. 2013;36:3585-3590.

11. Clement S. Upcoming trends for inpatient diabetes management. *Diabetes Technol Ther*. 2016;18:4-6.

12. Lipska KJ, Ross JS, Miao Y, et al. Potential overtreatment of diabetes mellitus in older adults with tight glycemic control. *JAMA Intern Med*. 2015;175:356.

13. Lipska KJ, Warton EM, Huang ES, et al. HbA1c and risk of severe hypoglycemia in type 2 diabetes: the diabetes and aging study. *Diabetes Care*. 2013;36:3535-3542.

14. Lipska KJ, Ross JS, Wang Y, et al. National trends in US hospital admissions for hyperglycemia and hypoglycemia among Medicare beneficiaries, 1999 to 2011. *JAMA Intern Med*. 2014;174:1116.

15. Centers for Disease Control and Prevention. Emergency department visit rates for hypoglycemia as first-listed diagnosis per 1,000 diabetic adults aged 18 years or older, by age, United States, 2006-2009. 2016. https://www.cdc.gov/diabetes/statistics/hypoglycemia/fig5byage.htm. Accessed December 27, 2016.

16. Holstein A, Hahn M, Patzer O, et al. Impact of clinical factors and CYP2C9 variants for the risk of severe sulfonylurea-induced hypoglycemia. *Eur J Clin Pharmacol*. 2011;67:471-476.

17. Formiga F, Vidal X, Agustí A, et al. Inappropriate prescribing in elderly people with diabetes admitted to hospital. *Diabet Med*. 2016;33:655-662.

18. Freeman JS, Gross B. Potential drug interactions associated with treatments for type 2 diabetes and its comorbidities: a clinical pharmacology review. *Expert Rev Clin Pharmacol*. 2012;5:31-42.

19. Inzucchi SE. Management of hyperglycemia in the hospital setting. *N Engl J Med*. 2006;355:1903-1911.

20. American College of Endocrinology Task Force on Inpatient Diabetes Metabolic Control. American college of endocrinology position statement on inpatient diabetes and metabolic control. *Endocr Pract*. 2004;10(suppl 2):4-9.

21. The ACE/ADA Task Force on Inpatient Diabetes. American college of endocrinology and American diabetes association consensus statement on inpatient diabetes and glycemic control: a call to action. *Diabetes Care.* 2006;29:1955-1962.

22. Khazai NB, Hamdy O. Inpatient diabetes management in the twenty-first century. *Endocrinol Metab Clin North Am.* 2016;45:875-894.

23. American Diabetes Association. Diabetes care in the hospital: Standards of Medical Care in Diabetes—2018. *Diabetes Care.* 2018;41(suppl 1):S144-S151.

24. Sorli C, Warren M, Oyer D, et al. Elderly patients with diabetes experience a lower rate of nocturnal hypoglycaemia with insulin degludec than with insulin glargine: a meta-analysis of Phase IIIa trials. *Drugs Aging.* 2013;30:1009-1018.

25. Rubin DJ, Rybin D, Doros G, et al. Weight-based, insulin dose–related hypoglycemia in hospitalized patients with diabetes. *Diabetes Care.* 2011;34:1723-1728.

26. Pasquel FJ, Gomez-Huelgas R, Anzola I, et al. Predictive value of admission Hemoglobin $A_{1c}$ on inpatient glycemic control and response to insulin therapy in medicine and surgery patients with type 2 diabetes: table 1. *Diabetes Care.* 2015;38:e202-e203.

27. Umpierrez GE, Smiley D, Zisman A, et al. Randomized study of basal-bolus insulin therapy in the inpatient management of patients with type 2 diabetes (RABBIT 2 trial). *Diabetes Care.* 2007;30:2181-2186.

28. Umpierrez GE, Smiley D, Hermayer K, et al. Randomized study comparing a basal-bolus with a basal plus correction insulin regimen for the hospital management of medical and surgical patients with type 2 diabetes: basal plus trial. *Diabetes Care.* 2013;36:2169-2174.

29. Vellanki P, Bean R, Oyedokun FA, et al. Randomized controlled trial of insulin supplementation for correction of bedtime hyperglycemia in hospitalized patients with type 2 diabetes. *Diabetes Care.* 2015;38:568-574.

30. Gosmanov AR, Umpierrez GE. Management of hyperglycemia during enteral and parenteral nutrition therapy. *Curr Diab Rep.* 2013;13:155-162.

31. Umpierrez GE, Hellman R, Korytkowski MT, et al. Management of hyperglycemia in hospitalized patients in non-critical care setting: an endocrine society clinical practice guideline. *J Clin Endocrinol Metab.* 2012;97:16-38.

32. Van Gossum A, Cabre E, Hebuterne X, et al. ESPEN guidelines on parenteral nutrition: gastroenterology. *Clin Nutr.* 2009;28:415-427.

33. Cheng AYY. Achieving glycemic control in special populations in hospital: perspectives in practice. *Can J Diabetes.* 2014;38:134-138.

34. Olveira G, Tapia MJ, Ocon J, et al. Parenteral nutrition-associated hyperglycemia in non-critically ill inpatients increases the risk of in-hospital mortality (multicenter study). *Diabetes Care.* 2013;36:1061-1066.

35. Draznin B, Gilden J, Golden SH, et al. Pathways to quality inpatient management of hyperglycemia and diabetes: a call to action. *Diabetes Care.* 2013;36:1807-1814.

36. Kwon S, Hermayer KL, Hermayer K. Glucocorticoidinduced hyperglycemia. *Am J Med Sci.* 2013;345:274-277.

37. Blackburn D, Hux J, Mamdani M. Quantification of the risk of corticosteroid-induced diabetes mellitus among the elderly. *J Gen Intern Med.* 2002;17:717-720.

38. Clore J, Thurby-Hay L. Glucocorticoid-induced hyperglycemia. *Endocr Pract.* 2009;15:469-474.

39. Liu D, Ahmet A, Ward L, et al. A practical guide to the monitoring and management of the complications of systemic corticosteroid therapy. *Allergy Asthma Clin Immunol.* 2013;9:30.

40. Brutsaert E, Carey M, Zonszein J. The clinical impact of inpatient hypoglycemia. *J Diabetes Complications.* 2014; 28:565–572.

41. Eiland L, Goldner W, Drincic A, Desouza C. Inpatient hypoglycemia: a challenge that must be addressed. *Curr Diab Rep.* 2014;14:445. doi:10.1007/s11892-013-0445-1

42. Turchin A, Matheny ME, Shubina M, et al. Hypoglycemia and clinical outcomes in patients with diabetes hospitalized in the general ward. *Diabetes Care.* 2009;32:1153-1157.

43. Naylor MD, Aiken LH, Kurtzman ET, et al. The importance of transitional care in achieving health reform. *Health Aff (Millwood).* 2011;30:746-754.

44. Families USA. The promise of care coordination: transforming health care delivery. 2017. http://familiesusa.org/sites/default/files/product_documents/Care-Coordination.pdf. Accessed January 31, 2017.

45. Allen J, Hutchinson AM, Brown R, et al. Quality care outcomes following transitional care interventions for older people from hospital to home: a systematic review. *BMC Health Serv Res.* 2014; 14:346.

46. Centers for Medicare & Medicaid Services. Readmissions Reduction Program (HRRP). 2016. https://www.cms.gov/medicare/medicare-fee-for-service-payment/acuteinpatientpps/readmissions-reduction-program.html

47. Daly J, Elliott D, Cameron-Traub E, et al. Health status, perceptions of coping, and social support immediately after discharge of survivors of acute myocardial infarction. *Am J Crit Care.* 2000;9:62.

48. Donini LM, Poggiogalle E, Piredda M, et al. Anorexia and eating patterns in the elderly. *PLoS One.* 2013;8:e63539.

49. Persson MD, Brismar KE, Katzarski KS, et al. Nutritional status using mini nutritional assessment and subjective global assessment predict mortality in geriatric patients. *J Am Geriatr Soc.* 2002;50:1996-2002.

50. Munshi MN, Florez H, Huang ES, et al. Management of diabetes in long-term care and skilled nursing facilities: a position statement of the American diabetes association. *Diabetes Care.* 2016;39:308-318.

51. Umpierrez GE, ed. *Therapy for Diabetes Mellitus and Related Disorders.* Alexandria, VA: American Diabetes Association; 2014:1093.

52. Park SW, Goodpaster BH, Strotmeyer ES, et al. Accelerated loss of skeletal muscle strength in older adults with type 2 diabetes: the health, aging, and body composition study. *Diabetes Care.* 2007;30:1507-1512.

53. American Diabetes Association. 8. Pharmacologic approaches to glycemic treatment. *Diabetes Care.* 2017;40(suppl 1):S64-S74.

54. U.S. Food and Drug Administration, Drug Safety Communications. FDA revises warnings regarding use of the diabetes medicine metformin in certain patients with reduced kidney function. 2017. http://www.fda.gov/downloads/drugs/drugsafety/ucm494140.pdf

55. American Geriatrics Society. Diabetes in older adults: A consensus report. 2017. http://www.americangeriatrics.org/files/documents/ADA_Consensus_Report.pdf. Accessed January 31, 2017.

56. Crowley MJ, Diamantidis CJ, McDuffie JR, et al. Clinical outcomes of metformin use in populations with chronic kidney disease, congestive heart failure, or chronic liver disease: a systematic review. *Ann Intern Med.* 2017;166:191-200.

57. Drugs.com. Metformin. 2017. https://www.drugs.com/pro/metformin.html. Accessed January 31, 2017.

58. GLUCOPHAGE (metformin hydrochloride) Tablets. GLUCOPHAGE XR (metformin hydrochloride) Extended-Release Tablets. https://www.accessdata.fda.gov/drugsatfda_docs/label/2017/020357. Accessed October 8, 2018.

59. Medscape. Impaired kidney function in older adults with normal serum creatinine. 2017. http://www.medscape.com/viewarticle/558225. Accessed January 31, 2017.

60. American Pharmacists Association. Updated beers criteria: a more comprehensive guide to medication safety in older adults . 2017. https://www.pharmacist.com/updated-beers-criteria-more-comprehensive-guide-medication-safety-older-adults. Accessed January 31, 2017.

61. Ioannidis I. Diabetes treatment in patients with renal disease: is the landscape clear enough? *World J Diabetes.* 2014;5:651-658.

62. Sola D, Rossi L, Schianca GPC, et al. Sulfonylureas and their use in clinical practice. *Arch Med Sci.* 2015;11:840-848.

63. Bajwa SS, Baruah M, Kalra S, et al. Management of diabetes mellitus type-2 in the geriatric population: current perspectives. *J Pharm Bioallied Sci.* 2014;6:151.

64. Novo Nordisk. PI—Prandin. 2017. http://www.novo-pi.com/prandin.pdf. Accessed January 31, 2017.

65. Novartis. Starlix. 2017. https://www.pharma.us.novartis.com/sites/www.pharma.us.novartis.com/files/Starlix.pdf. Accessed January 31, 2017.

66. Pharmacologic Glycemic Management of Type 2 Diabetes in Adults. *Canadian Journal of diabetes.* 2018;42:S88-S103. https://www.sciencedirect.com/science/article/pii/S1499267117308456. Accessed October 8,2018.

67. Leal I, Romio SA, Schuemie M, et al. Prescribing pattern of glucose lowering drugs in the United Kingdom in the last decade: a focus on the effects of safety warnings about rosiglitazone: effect of safety warnings on prescribing of glucose lowering drugs in UK. *Br J Clin Pharmacol*. 2013;75:861-868.

68. U.S. Food & Drug Administration: Drug Safety and Availability. FDA drug safety communication: FDA requires removal of some prescribing and dispensing restrictions for rosiglitazone-containing diabetes medicines. 2017. http://www.fda.gov/Drugs/DrugSafety/ucm376389.htm. Accessed February 7, 2017.

69. Mark Ruscin J, Linnebir SA. Drug-related problems in the elderly. Merck Manuals Professional Version. 2017. http://www.merckmanuals.com/professional/geriatrics/drug-therapy-in-the-elderly/drug-related-problems-in-the-elderly. Accessed January 31, 2017.

70. Godbout A, Chiasson JL. Who should benefit from the use of alpha-glucosidase inhibitors? *Curr Diab Rep*. 2007;7:333-339.

71. RxList. Precose (Acarbose). 2017. http://www.rxlist.com/precose-drug.htm. Accessed January 31, 2017.

72. Clar C, Gill JA, Court R, Waugh, N. Systematic review of SGLT2 receptor inhibitors in dual or triple therapy in type 2 diabetes. *BMJ Open*. 2017;2.

73. Davis CS, Fleming JW, Warrington LE. Sodium glucose co-transporter 2 inhibitors: a novel approach to the management of type 2 diabetes mellitus. *J Am Assoc Nurse Pract*. 2014;26(7):356-363. 2017. https://rap.northshorelij.com/ehost/pdfviewer/DanaInfo5web.b.ebscohost.com+pdfviewer?vid54&sid55f990a34-d648-45b9-9248-6dc428f1e27a%40sessionmgr103&hid5116. Accessed February 1, 2017.

74. Riser Taylor S, Harris KB. The clinical efficacy and safety of sodium glucose cotransporter-2 inhibitors in adults with type 2 diabetes mellitus. *Pharmacotherapy*. 2013;33:984-999.

75. U.S. Food & Drug Administration. FDA approves Jardiance to reduce cardiovascular death in adults with type 2 diabetes. 2016. https://www.fda.gov/NewsEvents/Newsroom/PressAnnouncements/ucm531517.htm

76. FDA Drug Safety Communication. FDA confirms increased risk of leg and foot amputations with the diabetes medicine canagliflozin (Invokana, Invokamet, Invokamet XR) [Internet]. 2016. https://www.fda.gov/downloads/Drugs/DrugSafety/UCM558427.pdf

77. Elmore LK, Baggett S, Kyle JA, et al. A review of the efficacy and safety of canagliflozin in elderly patients with type 2 diabetes. *Consult Pharm*. 2014;29:335-346.

78. Invokana. Impact long-term patient outlook with consistent A1C, body weight, and systolic blood pressure (BP) reductions: Invokana (Canagliflozin). 2017. https://www.invokanahcp.com/clinical-trial-results/a1c-change-in-older-patients

79. U.S. Food & Drug Administration. FDA Drug Safety Communication: FDA revises labels of SGLT2 inhibitors for diabetes to include warnings about too much acid in the blood and serious urinary tract infections. 2017. http://www.fda.gov/Drugs/DrugSafety/ucm475463.htm

80. Baetta R, Corsini A. Pharmacology of dipeptidyl peptidase-4 inhibitors: similarities and differences. *Drugs*. 2011;71(1):1441-1467. https://rap. northshorelij.com/ps/DanaInfo5go.galegroup.com+retrieve.do?tabID5T002&resultListType5RESULT_LIST&searchResultsType5SingleTab&searchType5AdvancedSearchForm&currentPosition56&docId5GALE%7CA264271708&docType5Drug+overview&sort5Relevance&contentSegment5&prodId5HRCA&contentSet5GALE%7CA264271708&searchId5R3&userGroupName5nysl_me_lijm&inPS5true

81. Karagiannis T, Boura P, Tsapas A. Safety of dipeptidyl peptidase 4 inhibitors: a perspective review. *Ther Adv Drug Saf*. 2014;5:138-146.

82. Filion KB, Suissa S. DPP-4 inhibitors and heart failure: some reassurance, some uncertainty. *Diabetes Care*. 2016;39:735-737.

83. U.S. Food & Drug Administration. FDA Drug Safety Communication: FDA warns that DPP-4 inhibitors for type 2 diabetes may cause severe joint pain. 2017. http://www.fda.gov/Drugs/DrugSafety/ucm459579.htm

84. Chiu CJ, Du YF, Ou HY, et al. Achieving glycemic control in elderly patients with type 2 diabetes: a critical comparison of current options. *Clin Interv Aging*. 2014;9:1963-1980.

85. Munshi MN, Pandya N, Umpierrez GE, et al. Contributions of basal and prandial hyperglycemia to total hyperglycemia in older and younger adults with type 2 diabetes mellitus. *J Am Geriatr Soc*. 2013;61:535-541.

86. Linnebjerg H, Kothare PA, Seger M, et al. Exenatide—pharmacokinetics, pharmacodynamics, safety and tolerability in patients ≥75 years of age with type 2 diabetes. *Int J Clin Pharmacol Ther*. 2011;49:99-108.

87. Suzuki D, Toyoda M, Kimura M, et al. Effects of liraglutide, a human glucagon-like peptide-1 analogue, on body weight, body fat area and body fat-related markers in patients with type 2 diabetes mellitus. *Intern Med*. 2013;52(10):1029-1034.

88. Malm-Erjefalt M, Bjornsdottir I, Vanggaard J, et al. Metabolism and excretion of the once-daily human glucagon-like peptide-1 analog liraglutide in healthy male subjects and its in vitro degradation by dipeptidyl peptidase IV and neutral endopeptidase. *Drug Metab Dispos*. 2010;38:1944-1953.

89. U.S. Food & Drug Administration. Victoza. https://www.accessdata.fda.gov/drugsatfda_docs/label/2017/022341s027lbl.pdf#page=40

90. Giorda CB, Nada E, Tartaglino B. Erratum to: pharmacokinetics, safety, and efficacy of DPP-4 inhibitors and GLP-1 receptor agonists in patients with type 2 diabetes mellitus and renal or hepatic impairment. A systematic review of the literature. *Endocrine*. 2014;46:420-422.

91. Drucker DJ, Sherman SI, Gorelick FS, et al. Incretin-based therapies for the treatment of type 2 diabetes: evaluation of the risks and benefits. *Diabetes Care*. 2010;33:428-433.

92. Singh S, Chang H, Richards TM, et al. Glucagonlike Peptide 1–Based Therapies and Risk of Hospitalization for Acute Pancreatitis in Type 2 Diabetes Mellitus: A Population-Based Matched Case-Control Study. *JAMA Intern Med*. 2013;173(7):534-539.

93. REMS_Factsheet.pdf. 2017. http://www.tanzeumrems.com/assets/pdf/REMS_Factsheet.pdf

94. Meneilly GS, Roy-Duval C, Alawi H, et al. Lixisenatide therapy in older patients with type 2 diabetes inadequately controlled on their current antidiabetic treatment: the GetGoal-O randomized trial. *Diabetes Care*. 2017;40:485-493.

95. American Diabetes Association. American Diabetes Association and American Geriatrics Society Publish consensus report on diabetes in older adults. 2012. http://www.diabetes.org/newsroom/press-releases/2012/consensus-report-diabetes-in-older-adults.html

96. Novo Nordisk. FIASP. http://www.novo-pi.com/fiasp.pdf

97. Dashora, U, Castro, E. Insulin U100, 200, 300, or 500?. *Br J Diabetes*. 2016;16:10-15.

98. Atkin SL, Aye M. Patient safety and minimizing risk with insulin administration – role of insulin degludec. *Drug Healthc Patient Saf*. 2014;6:55-67.

99. Sanofi. Toujeo. http://products.sanofi.us/toujeo/toujeo.pdf

100. Novo Nordisk. Tresiba. http://www.novo-pi.com/tresiba.pdf

101. U.S. Food & Drug Administration. Biosimilars. 2017. http://www.fda.gov/Drugs/DevelopmentApprovalProcess/HowDrugsareDevelopedandApproved/ApprovalApplications/TherapeuticBiologicApplications/Biosimilars/default.htm

102. U.S. Food & Drug Administration. FDA approves Basaglar, the first "follow-on" insulin glargine product to treat diabetes. Press Announcements. 2017. http://www.fda.gov/NewsEvents/Newsroom/PressAnnouncements/ucm477734.htm

103. Basaglar. Identical amino acid sequence to Lantus (insulin glargine injection). 2017. https://www.basaglar.com/hcp/about-basaglar

104. Basaglar. Beginsulin. [cited 2017 Feb 2]. https://www.basaglar.com/en/

105. U.S. Food & Drug Administration. FDA approves Admelog, the first short-acting "follow-on" insulin product to treat diabetes. 2017. https://www.fda.gov/NewsEvents/Newsroom/PressAnnouncements/ucm588466.htm

106. Ault A. Rising insulin costs in us get pushback as basaglar launches. Medscape; 2016. http://www.medscape.com/viewarticle/873353. Accessed March 11, 2017.

107. U.S. Food & Drug Administration. FDA approves Afrezza to treat diabetes . Press Announcements. 2017. https://www.fda.gov/NewsEvents/Newsroom/PressAnnouncements/ucm403122.htm. Accessed March 11, 2017.

108. Sanofi. Afrezza. http://products.sanofi.us/afrezza/afrezza.pdf. Accessed March 11, 2017.

109. McAdams BH, Rizvi AA. An overview of insulin pumps and glucose sensors for the generalist. *J Clin Med*. 2016;5:e5.

110. Hoskins M. NEWSFLASH: Roche stops selling Accu-Chek insulin pumps in U.S. January 17, 2017. https://www.healthline.com/diabetesmine/newsflash-roche-discontinues-insulin-pumps

111. Animas stop making insulin pumps. January 24, 2018. https://www.diabetes.org.uk/About_us/News/animas-stop-making-insulin-pumps

112. Scheiner G. Product guide: insulin pumps. *Diabetes Forecast*. March 2016. http://www.diabetesforecast.org/2016/mar-apr/product-guide-insulin-pumps.html. Accessed January 7, 2017.

113. Hawbaker, K. How to: use the threshold suspend feature. *The LOOP Blog*. March 17, 2014. https://www.medtronicdiabetes.com/loop-blog/how-to-use-the-threshold-suspend-feature/. Accessed January 7, 2017.

114. Dexcom. Dexcom G4 PLATINUM Receiver with Share (Pediatric). 2015. http://www.dexcom.com/dexcom-share. Accessed January 7, 2017.

115. Yeh HC, Brown TT, Maruthur N, et al. Comparative effectiveness and safety of methods of insulin delivery and glucose monitoring for diabetes mellitus: a systematic review and meta-analysis. *Ann Intern Med*. 2012;157:336.

116. U.S. Food & Drug Administration. FDA approves first continuous glucose monitoring system for adults not requiring blood sample calibration. September 27, 2017. https://www.fda.gov/newsevents/newsroom/pressannouncements/ucm577890.htm. Accessed February 12, 2018.

117. Scheiner G. Continuous Glucose Monitoring Systems (CGM) Medtronic and Dexcom review and comparison. *Integrated Diabetes Services*. March 3, 2016. http://integrateddiabetes.com/continuous-glucosemonitoring-systems-cgm-medtronic-dexcom-reviewcomparison/. Accessed January 7, 2017.

118. Attvall S. Senseonics reveals topline CGM data Eversense 90 day CGM sensor MARD 8.8%. PRECISE II Study. Dagensdiabetes.se—Det senaste inom diabetologi. 2016. http://dagensdiabetes.info/index.php/alla-senaste-nyheter/2294-senseonics-reveals-topline-cgmdata-eversense-90-day-cgm-sensor-mard-8-8-precise-iistudy. Accessed January 7, 2017.

119. Dehennis A, Mortellaro MA, Ioacara S. Multisite study of an implanted continuous glucose sensor over 90 days in patients with diabetes mellitus. *J Diabetes Sci Technol*. 2015;9:951-956.

120. Facchinetti A, Sparacino G, Guerra S, et al. Real-time improvement of continuous glucose monitoring accuracy: the smart sensor concept. *Diabetes Care*. 2013;36:793-800.

121. Kropff J, DeVries JH. Continuous glucose monitoring, future products, and update on worldwide artificial pancreas projects. *Diabetes Technol Ther*. 2016;18:S2-S53.

122. Rodbard D. Continuous glucose monitoring: a review of successes, challenges, and opportunities. *Diabetes Technol Ther*. 2016;18:S2-S3.

123. Peters AL, Ahmann AJ, Battelino T, et al. Diabetes technology-continuous subcutaneous insulin infusion therapy and continuous glucose monitoring in adults: an endocrine society clinical practice guideline. *J Clin Endocrinol Metab*. 2016;101:3922-3937.

124. Johnson SL, McEwen LN, Newton CA, et al. The impact of continuous subcutaneous insulin infusion and multiple daily injections of insulin on glucose variability in older adults with type 2 diabetes. *J Diabetes Complications*. 2011;25:211-215.

125. Herman WH, Ilag LL, Johnson SL, et al. A clinical trial of continuous subcutaneous insulin infusion versus multiple daily injections in older adults with type 2 diabetes. *Diabetes Care*. 2005;28:1568-1573.

126. Houlden RL, Moore S. In-hospital management of adults using insulin pump therapy. *Can J Diabetes*. 2014;38:126-133.

127. Cook CB, Beer KA, Seifert KM, et al. Transitioning insulin pump therapy from the outpatient to the inpatient setting: a review of 6 Years' experience with 253 cases. *J Diabetes Sci Technol*. 2012;6:995-1002.

128. Boyle ME, Seifert KM, Beer KA, et al. Guidelines for application of continuous subcutaneous insulin infusion (insulin pump) therapy in the perioperative period. *J Diabetes Sci Technol*. 2012;6:184-190.

129. Medtronic. Important safety information. 2017. https://www.medtronicdiabetes.com/important-safety-information. Accessed January 7, 2017.

130. Vigersky RA, Fonda SJ, Chellappa M, et al. Short-and long-term effects of real-time continuous glucose monitoring in patients with type 2 diabetes. *Diabetes Care*. 2012;35:32-38.

131. Polonsky WH, Peters AL, Hessler D. The impact of real-time continuous glucose monitoring in patients 65 Years and older. *J Diabetes Sci Technol*. 2016;10:892-897.

132. ClinicalTrials.gov. Multiple Daily Injections and Continuous Glucose Monitoring in Diabetes (DIaMonD). 2017. https://clinicaltrials.gov/ct2/show/NCT02282397. Accessed January 17, 2017.

133. Garg SK. The future of glucose monitoring. *Diabetes Technol Ther*. 2016;18(suppl 2):S2-iv-S2-2.

134. Holzinger U, Warszawska J, Kitzberger R, et al. Realtime continuous glucose monitoring in critically ill patients. *Diabetes Care*. 2010;33:467-472.

135. U.S. Food & Drug Administration. FDA expands indication for continuous glucose monitoring system, first to replace fingerstick testing for diabetes treatment decisions. 2017. http://www.fda.gov/NewsEvents/Newsroom/PressAnnouncements/ucm534056.htm. Accessed January 7, 2017.

136. Hovorka R. Closed-loop insulin delivery: from bench to clinical practice. *Nat Rev Endocrinol.* 2011;7:385-395.

137. Thabit H, Hovorka R. Glucose control in non-critically ill inpatients with diabetes: towards closed-loop. *Diabetes Obes Metab.* 2014;16:500-509.

138. Tilleskjor S. Breaking News: FDA approves the MiniMed 670G system, world's first hybrid closed loop system. *Between The Lines Blog Medtronic Diabetes.* September 29, 2016. https://www.medtronicdiabetes.com/blog/introducing-the-minimed-670g-system/. Accessed January 7, 2017.

139. Okabayashi T, Nishimori I, Maeda H, et al. Effect of intensive insulin therapy using a closed-loop glycemic control system in hepatic resection patients. *Diabetes Care.* 2009;32:1425-1427.

140. Leelarathna L, English SW, Thabit H, et al. Feasibility of fully automated closed-loop glucose control using continuous subcutaneous glucose measurements in critical illness: a randomized controlled trial. *Crit Care.* 2013;17:R159.

141. Thabit H, Hartnell S, Allen JM, et al. Closed-loop insulin delivery in inpatients with type 2 diabetes: a randomised, parallel-group trial. *Lancet Diabetes Endocrinol.* 2017;5:117-125.

# Vitamins and Dietary Supplements for the Older Adult: What Works and Why?

CHAPTER 4

Maha Saad, PharmD, Nicolas Fausto, PharmD, and Nicole Maisch, PharmD

## BACKGROUND

**Dietary supplements (DSs)**, defined under the Dietary Supplement Health and Education Act (DSHEA) of 1994, include **vitamins**, minerals, botanicals, and amino acids, among others.[1] **DSs** are classified by the U.S. Food and Drug Administration (FDA) under the food umbrella and can therefore bypass premarket review and approval before marketing. Unlike pharmaceutical products, manufacturers of **DSs** are not required to provide rigorous clinical evidence. The only update to DSHEA has been that "new dietary ingredients" introduced after 1994 must notify the FDA 75 days before release and provide information that the new dietary ingredient is "reasonably expected to be safe" when used for the recommended condition.[2,3]

Supplements are frequently used. On the basis of the 2007 to 2010 National Health and Nutrition Examination Survey (NHANES), older adults were more likely to use supplements for site-specific health reasons (ie, bone, joint, heart, eye). A significant inverse trend between age and higher prevalence of use of **DSs** to "improve overall health," "supplement the diet," "boost immunity or prevent colds," and to "get more energy" was reported.[4] Updated NHANES 1999 to 2012 monitors trends in DS use among US adults. Over seven cycles of the survey, supplement use remained stable, with 52% of adults using **DSs** in the previous month. Consistent with previous data, supplement use increased as a function of age, with 72% of adults older than 65 years reporting use compared with only 40% aged 20 to 39 years.[5,6]

This chapter provides an overview of existing evidence, reasons for use, and safety concerns of DS. We also present the often conflicting evidence regarding the use of select **DSs**, focusing on the elderly population.

61

## Dietary Supplement Labeling Statements

DS manufacturers may make three types of labeling statements and claims: nutrient content, health claim, and structure-function (S-F). The nutrient claim describes the level of a nutrient in **DSs**. The health claims describe a link between a DS's ingredients and effects on a disease. The FDA typically applies a substantiation standard for health claims of "competent and reliable scientific evidence." Examples of such claims include calcium or calcium with vitamin D and the reduced risk of osteoporosis or sodium and high blood pressure (BP). The S-F claims describe the intended benefit of the DS on the structure or function of the body. Examples include "promotes vitality" or "maintains a healthy circulatory system." The FDA requires that all DS advertisements using S-F claims carry a disclaimer stating "This statement has not been evaluated by the FDA. This product is not intended to diagnose, treat, cure, or prevent any disease."[7] The S-F claims, at times indistinguishable from health claims, are not regulated by the FDA and do not require premarket approval. Unfortunately, this allows companies to make claims and market their supplements depending on unsubstantiated benefits and has led to increased consumption.[2,3]

# AREAS OF UNCERTAINTY

## General Safety Concerns

Adulteration occurs when supplements present significant or unreasonable risk of illness or injury when used in accordance with the suggested labeling or, if unlabeled, under ordinary conditions of use. In addition, adulteration occurs when the supplement is a new ingredient or entity lacking adequate evidence or information to ensure its safety of use, or it has been declared an imminent hazard by the Secretary of the Department of Health and Human Services, or contains a dietary ingredient that is present in sufficient quantity to render the product poisonous or deleterious to human health.[8] Such ingredients are usually undeclared, rendering them unrecognizable by patients or healthcare providers. Consumers may unknowingly take products contaminated with varying quantities of approved prescription drug ingredients, controlled substances, or untested pharmacologically active ingredients leading to harm. As part of the FDA's targeted effort to reduce adulteration, it periodically publishes Public Notifications advising consumers against using specific products confirmed to contain approved or unapproved drug.[9] Manufacturers of **DSs** must comply with specific current Good Manufacturing Practices. The FDA, the Federal Trade Commission, and Department of Justice Consumer Protection Branch are responsible for all regulatory investigations and actions against noncompliant manufacturers.[10] Some manufacturers voluntarily submit their supplements to more rigorous testing by the United States Pharmacopeial Convention (USP), a nonprofit organization that sets standards for identity, potency, quality, and purity of medicines, food ingredients, and **DSs**. If the product meets USP's quality standards, use of the "USP Verified" mark is granted (Table 4.1).[11,12]

The identification of adverse events related to supplements depends primarily on postmarketing data and surveillance. Patients often take supplements unbeknown to their healthcare providers, resulting in significant patient harm. Many patients perceive supplements as safe, unaware that serious side effects and interactions with prescription medications can occur. As is the case with prescription medications, it is mandatory for manufacturers of DSs to collect and report serious adverse events to the FDA MedWatch program.[13] Approximately 60 000 vitamin toxicity exposures were submitted in 2015.[14]

## Increasing Use at a Cost?

Controversy remains as to whether DSs cause more harm than benefit. Many supplements are essential and have demonstrated efficacy, especially when treating deficiencies. However, conflicting, even harmful data exist for many indications. For example, the Iowa Women's Health Study (IWHS), an observational trial of approximately 40 000, primarily white women aged 55 to 69 years who completed questionnaires regarding their DS use over 30 years, found an increased risk of total mortality associated with several DSs including multivitamins, iron, folic acid, vitamin $B_6$, magnesium, zinc, and copper.[15]

Sales, and in turn use, of DSs have increased tremendously over the past 20 years. The number of products on the market is estimated to have reached more than 55 000 in 2012.[16] In 2014, total sales of all DSs in the United States was approximately $36.7 billion, multivitamins accounting for $14.3 billion.[17]

Because, in part, of these factors, the National Institutes of Health (NIH) is committed to expanding the evidence base on the efficacy and safety of DSs. They have invested $250 to 300 million per year in DS research through the scientific peer-review process. The National Center for Complementary and Integrative Health, an NIH institute, funded clinical studies that have examined the safety and efficacy of commonly

| TABLE 4.1 • Reputable Dietary Supplement Resources | |
|---|---|
| **Resources** | **Website** |
| NIH DS fact sheets | https://ods.od.nih.gov/factsheets/list-all/ |
| The USP Dietary Supplement Verification Program for manufacturers | http://www.usp.org/verification-services/manufacturers#processincludes |
| USP-verified products listing | http://www.quality-supplements.org/verified-products/verified-products-listings |
| National Center for Complementary and Integrative Health | https://nccih.nih.gov/ |

Abbreviations: DS, dietary supplement; NIH, National Institutes of Health; USP, the United States Pharmacopeial Convention.

used **DSs** for a number of health outcomes. The NIH-supported Age-Related Eye Disease Studies investigated combinations of **vitamins** C and E, zinc, and the carotenoids beta-carotene, lutein, and zeaxanthin, and demonstrated that a specific formulation could safely and effectively reduce the progression of age-related macular degeneration.[18] However, most of the larger NIH-supported clinical trials have failed to demonstrate significant benefit compared with controls.[10,16,19-21]

Many patients using supplements do so in addition to conventional medical treatment, but many of them either do not disclose such use[22] or are not asked about DS use by their physician on hospital admission.[23] This could lead to inaccurate medication reconciliation and documentation, place patients at a greater risk of adverse drug reactions or interactions, and delay appropriate medical treatments. Physician awareness of DS use is particularly important, especially at discharge, to ensure that patients are treated safely and appropriately.[22] This presents a great opportunity to evaluate the patients' medication list and conduct a comprehensive review with the objective of deprescribing to minimize risk of harm.

# THERAPEUTIC ADVANCES

## Specific Supplement Reviews

### Multivitamins

There is no standard or regulatory definition available for multivitamin (MVI) or mineral supplements; the term can refer to products of widely varied compositions and characteristics. The types and levels of **vitamins**, minerals, and other ingredients available in products are determined by the manufacturer and frequently in much higher amounts than the recommended intake and even surpassing upper levels (ULs).[17] A better strategy may be to target high-risk populations and the nutrients that are of public health concern rather than including many **vitamins** that are unnecessary and potentially harmful.[24]

The 2015 Dietary Guidelines for Americans recommends that nutritional needs and requirements should be met primarily from foods; only in some cases, fortified foods. DSs may be useful in providing one or more nutrients that otherwise may be consumed in less-than-recommended amounts.[24] Experts conclude that evidence is insufficient to recommend MVI use to prevent chronic diseases, including cancer and cognitive and cardiovascular diseases (CVDs).[25-30]

Dietary Reference Intakes (DRIs) are nutrient reference values developed by Health and Medicine Division (HMD), formerly known as the Institute of Medicine of the National Academies. DRIs are specified on the basis of age, sex, and lifestage and cover more than 40 nutrient substances. DRIs replaced the Recommended Dietary Allowance in the United States and the Recommended Nutrient Intake in Canada. The DRIs are a set of several reference values related to both adequate intake and UL of intake.[31]

Because the elderly are the major consumers of DSs, they take MVIs mainly to improve or maintain their health. In 65-year-olds, NHANES data found that multivitamin use has remained stable when compared with 1999-2000 ($P < 0.05$).[5] The long-term safety of multivitamins is questionable. Of concern, the IWHS study found significant increases in all-cause, but not in cardiovascular (CV) or in cancer mortality in patients taking multivitamins (relative risk [RR] 95% confidence interval [CI], 1.06 [1.02-1.10], 1.03 [0.97-1.09], 1.00 [0.94-1.07], respectively).[15]

### Vitamin E

Vitamin E is a lipid-soluble antioxidant vitamin; it has been used to prevent and treat coronary heart disease (CHD), cancer, and cognitive decline.[31] In 2013, the U.S. Preventive Services Task Force recommended against the use of vitamin E for the prevention of CVD and cancer.[27] According to NHANES 2011-2012, vitamin E use in older adults decreased in both vitamin E–containing supplements and vitamin E–only supplements compared with 1999-2000 ($P < 0.001$).[5] The findings with respect to vitamin E and mortality are mixed: the IWHS study found no association between vitamin E and mortality, all-cause, CV, or cancer.[15] On the basis of a recent meta-analysis, there was a trend for a higher risk of all-cause mortality with vitamin E; however, the pooled effect of vitamin E compared with placebo showed a significant reduction in CV mortality (RR [95% CI], 1.02 [0.99-1.05]; 0.88 [0.80-0.96], respectively).[32]

The SELECT trial, a 7-year multinational randomized placebo-controlled trial of approximately 35 000 men, examined the association between vitamin E with or without selenium (Se) supplementation and prostate cancer risk. Although there was an increase for all groups compared with placebo, only the vitamin E–alone arm resulted in a significant increase in prostate cancer of 17%.[21]

A 2017 Cochrane Review assessed the efficacy of vitamin E in the treatment of mild cognitive impairment (MCI) and dementia due to Alzheimer disease (AD). There was no difference between the vitamin E and placebo groups in any clinically important effect on neuropsychiatric symptoms measured with the Neuropsychiatric Inventory and no effect on the probability of progression from MCI to probable dementia due to AD over 36 months. There was also no difference in the risk of experiencing at least one serious adverse event over 6 to 48 months or in the risk of death. Patients with AD receiving vitamin E showed less functional decline on the Alzheimer's Disease Cooperative Study/Activities of Daily Living Inventory than people receiving placebo at 6 to 48 months. The authors concluded that the results are based on small trials; therefore, further research will likely affect results.[33]

### Vitamin A

Vitamin A is a lipid-soluble vitamin with antioxidant properties found in sweet potatoes, carrots, spinach, and liver. Beta-carotene is the main precursor of vitamin A.[34] On the basis of the NHANES 2011-2012 survey, vitamin A use in those 65 years or older remained stable in both vitamin A–containing supplements and standalone supplements when compared with 1999-2000 survey data.[5]

Vitamin A has been linked to lung cancer, osteopenia, and increased mortality.[35,36] The IWHS study found trends toward increased mortality in patients taking vitamin A, with cancer mortality reaching significance, not all-cause or CV (RR [95% CI], 1.16 [1.04-1.29], 1.06 [0.99-1.13], 1.02 [0.92-1.13], respectively).[15] A recent meta-analysis showed a significant increased cancer risk with vitamin A, but not cancer mortality (RR [95% CI], RR: 1.16 [1.00-1.35]; 1.08 [0.82-1.43], respectively). Subgroup analyses showed that the excess cancer risk was more pronounced in those taking vitamin A alone ≥25 000 IU/d. Cancer mortality was only significantly increased in the high-dose subgroup as well (RR [95% CI], 1.24 [1.05-1.47]). Moreover, high-dose vitamin A significantly increased the risk of all-cause mortality [RR [95% CI], 1.12 [1.04-1.21]). Beta-carotene given as an individual supplement and at doses above 30 mg/d was significantly associated with all-cause mortality (RR [95% CI], 1.06 [1.02-1.10]; 1.10 [1.03-1.18], respectively).[32]

### Vitamin B(s)

Folic acid, a water-soluble B vitamin, is found in supplements and fortified foods. It is used alone or combined with other B **vitamins** in treatment or prevention of CVD, macrocytic anemia, and neural tube deficiency. According to the NHANES 2011–2012 survey, in patients 65 years or older, vitamin B use stayed stable for vitamin B–containing supplements and varied among vitamin B–only supplement with an increase with vitamin $B_{12}$.[5] The IWHS study found trends toward increased mortality in patients taking folic acid and vitamin $B_6$ with all-cause mortality reaching significance, not cancer or CV mortality.[15] In a meta-analysis, folic acid given as a single high dose above 5 mg/d was protective in terms of CV risk (RR [95% CI], 0.81 [0.70-0.94]). However, there was no effect on all-cause or CV mortality, regardless of dose.[32] Two meta-analyses showed that folic acid supplementation had no significant effect on cancer risk.[32,37] Another meta-analysis of 11 studies demonstrated that folic acid supplementation was associated with a significant benefit in reducing the risk of stroke in patients with CVD (RR[95%], 0.90 [0.84-0.97]; $P = 0.005$). Such a benefit was mainly seen in patients with a decrease in homocysteine concentrations of 25% or greater, those with a daily folate dose of >2 mg, and populations in regions with no or partly fortified grain.[38]

### Antioxidants

A double-blind, placebo-controlled clinical trial, evaluating a combination of antioxidants (vitamin E, C, alpha lipoic acid, coenzyme Q) resulted in a small reduction in cerebrospinal fluid markers that may represent a decrease in oxidative stress. However, the combination was associated with significant cognitive decline, characterized by lower scores on the Mini-Mental State Examination.[39] In a 2012 Cochrane Review, vitamin E, beta-carotene, and higher doses of vitamin A were associated with an increase in mortality.[40]

### Selenium

Se, an essential trace mineral and a cofactor for antioxidants, is found in soil, water, and foods such as liver and seafood.[41] Chronic dosing of 200 mg/d for a mean of 7.7 years and high serum Se levels have been associated with type 2 diabetes.[42-44] A recent Cochrane Review revealed an increased risk of diabetes that failed to reach statistical significance and an increase in alopecia and grade 1 to 2 dermatitis (RR [95% CI], 1.06 [0.97-1.15]; 1.28 [1.01-1.62]; 1.17 [1-1.35], respectively).[45]

Elderly patients use Se for primary prevention of CVD and various cancers. In those 65 years or older, NHANES survey data found its use as part of a multivitamin/mineral supplement has remained stable, but has declined as a standalone supplement ($P = 0.002$).[5] The IWHS study found no association between Se and mortality, all-cause, CV, or cancer.[15] A 2013 Cochrane Review concluded that the limited data do not support Se use, with no significant effect on all-cause mortality, CV mortality, or fatal/nonfatal CVD.[45] A recent meta-analysis of Se at a median dose of 100 mg/d for a median of 5 years showed no benefit on CVD, overall, alone, or in combination.[46] This was confirmed in a 2017 meta-analysis also finding no association between Se and all-cause mortality, CV mortality, or CVD.[32]

In 2003, the FDA allowed for a health claim for supplements containing Se stating that it "may reduce the risk of certain types of cancer; however, the FDA has determined that this evidence is limited and not conclusive."[47] A 2018 Cochrane Review determined that there is also no convincing evidence to support the use of Se in the prevention of any type of cancer. Overall, trials are inconsistent and poorly designed, with newer, more rigorous randomized controlled trials (RCTs) showing less benefit and even trending toward a higher risk of some cancers such as non–melanoma skin cancers.[48] A recent meta-analysis also showed no association between Se and cancer mortality or cancer.[32]

### Calcium

Calcium is necessary to maintain the bone, but is also crucial in mediating nerve transmission, vasoconstriction/dilation, hormonal regulation, and intracellular signaling. Calcium predominantly comes from dairy products.[49] The DRI is 1000 to 1300 mg. The UL is 2500 mg and 2000 mg/d for adults aged 19 to 50 years and older, respectively.[49,50] According to NHANES data, calcium use, not as part of multivitamins, has increased ($P = 0.02$).[5]

The IWHS found that calcium supplementation was associated with reduced cancer mortality (RR [95% CI], 0.89 [0.83-0.94]).[15] However, a more recent meta-analysis only found a reduced cancer risk, but not cancer mortality (RR [95% CI], 0.37 [0.22-0.63]; 2.88 [0.12-67.3], respectively).[32]

Calcium's effects on CV outcomes raise concern. A 2008 RCT was designed to identify a possible association between calcium supplementation and CV events in older women. Calcium supplementation was associated with an increased risk of MI and a nonsignificant increase in a composite of MI, stroke, or sudden death compared with placebo (RR [95% CI], 2.12 [1.01-4.47]; 1.47 [0.97-2.23], respectively).[51] A reanalysis of the Women's Health Initiative CaD study also found an increased risk of MI or revascularization and a nonsignificant increase of MI or stroke (hazard ratio [HR] [95% CI], 1.16 [1.01-1.34], $P = 0.04$; 1.16 [1.00-1.35], $P = 0.05$, respectively). A meta-analysis of trials using calcium or calcium plus vitamin D found an increased risk of MI and a composite of MI or stroke (RR [95% CI], 1.24 [1.07-1.45], $P = 0.004$; 1.15 [1.03-1.27], $P = 0.009$, respectively).[52] A subsequent meta-analysis showed nonsignificant trends toward increased MI with calcium alone or combined with vitamin D, but not vitamin D alone (RR [95% CI], 1.28 [0.97-1.68]; 1.06 [0.92-1.21]; 0.86 [0.54-1.37], respectively).[53] Some data suggest that this risk is highest for calcium intake above the median and in men.[54-56] The IWHS study found that self-reported calcium supplementation was associated with a reduction in total and CV mortality (HR [95% CI], 0.91 [0.88-0.94]; 0.87 [0.82-0.92], respectively). The authors state, however, that this was not consistent with previous studies.[15] A 2017 meta-analysis found no association between calcium supplementation and either CVD risk or CV mortality.[32] A meta-analysis commissioned by the National Osteoporosis Foundation and the American Society for Preventive Cardiology and subsequent guidelines conclude that calcium supplementation within normal limits provides neither CV benefit nor risk in generally healthy adults.[57,58]

## Vitamin D

Vitamin D is a lipid-soluble vitamin with broad biologic effects including maintenance of plasma calcium and phosphate required for bone mineralization.[49] It also reduces inflammation and modulates cell growth and neuromuscular and immune function. Vitamin D is naturally present in very few foods, with fatty fish and egg yolks being exceptions. Other sources of vitamin D include dermal synthesis and supplementation.[49,59] The DRI is 15 to 20 mg (600-800 IU) and the UL of vitamin D is 4000 IU daily.[49] Potential for adverse events has been linked to levels above 125 nmol/L.[49] Vitamin D deficiency is associated with serum levels <30 to 50 nmol/L.[49,60] Experts recommend that serum vitamin D levels be maintained above 5047 or 75 nmol/L.[50,60,61]

Older adults are at particular risk of vitamin D deficiency because of less efficient dermal synthesis of vitamin D and reduced sun exposure.[49] NHANES data reveals that vitamin D use has increased in people older than 65, both as part of multivitamin preparations and standalone products.[5] This data also reveal that the percentage of those patients taking higher than recommended doses, even into the UL level has increased significantly over time, especially in the elderly. Specifically, those aged 70 and older taking 1000 IU/d or more has increased from 0.4% in 1999 to 2000 to 38.5% in 2013 to 2014. Similarly, those taking 4000 IU/d or more has risen from 1.4% in 2009 to 2010 to 6.6% in 2013 to 2014, raising concern because these high doses are more likely to cause toxicity.[62]

Vitamin D increases the risk of nephrolithiasis (RR [95% CI], 1.17 [1.02-1.34]; $P = 0.02$).[63] Hypercalcemia is more common in those receiving vitamin D (RR (95%

CI), 2.28 [1.57-3.31]). Calcium plus vitamin D was also found to produce gastrointestinal adverse effects (RR [95% CI], 1.04 [1.00-1.08]) and renal disease (RR [95% CI], 1.16 [1.02-1.33]).[64]

The IWHS and two subsequent meta-analyses found that vitamin D had no significant effect on total, cancer, or CV mortality, or on CV risk.[15,32,64] As outlined subsequently, the data are conflicting for these outcomes.

A meta-analysis of RCTs revealed that vitamin D3 reduced risk of all-cause mortality, whereas D2 had no influence on all-cause mortality (RR [95% CI], 0.89 [0.80-0.99]; 1.04 [0.97-1.11], respectively). Low circulating vitamin D levels (<30 ng/mL) were associated with significantly increased risk of all-cause mortality when compared with higher levels.[65,66] Every 10 ng/mL decline in vitamin D was associated with 16% increase in risk of all-cause mortality.[65] Similarly, a 2014 Cochrane Review found that vitamin D3 decreased mortality in elderly people living independently or in institutional care (RR [95% CI], 0.94 [0.91-0.98]; $P = 0.002$).[63] Another Cochrane review also found a reduction in all-cause mortality (RR [95% CI], 0.93 [0.88-0.98]; $P = 0.009$).[67]

A meta-analysis found that the bottom tertile of baseline circulating vitamin D was associated with increased cancer mortality when compared with the top tertile (RR [95% CI], 1.14 [1.01-1.29]).[65] A similar increase in cancer mortality was seen in another meta-analysis, but only among those who already had cancer (RR [95% CI], 1.7 [1.00-2.88]).[66] Two Cochrane reviews found that D3 significantly reduced cancer mortality (RR [95% CI], 0.88 [0.78-0.98]; 0.88 [0.78-0.98], respectively). Although some of these values are statistically significant, the authors warned that there is substantial risk for error due to the number of participants examined and risk of attrition bias.[63,67]

Despite the finding that low levels of baseline circulating vitamin D are associated with increased CV mortality, most data have not shown a difference with vitamin D supplementation.[65,66] A 2011 meta-analysis was unable to identify a significant association between CV risk and vitamin D use when looking at MI and stroke.[68] More recently, a post hoc analysis of the RECORD trial revealed that vitamin D may actually protect against cardiac failure (HR [95% CI], 0.75 [0.58-0.97], $P = 0.027$). However, the associated meta-analysis did not confirm this finding. Furthermore, there were no significant associations between vitamin D and stroke or MI in either the post hoc analysis or meta-analysis.[69]

Vitamin D is likely to provide benefits in elderly patients at risk for falls and fractures when given in combination with calcium.[61,70] The U.S. Preventive Services Task Force (USPTF) found that vitamin D combined with calcium, but not alone, reduces fracture risk in older institutionalized adults (RR [95% CI], 0.71 [0.55-0.91]).[70,71] Fall risk was reduced by vitamin D supplementation in a meta-analysis of nine RCTs (RR [95% CI], 0.83 [0.77-0.89]).[72] However, a new meta-analysis showed a reduction in fall risk when combined with calcium, but not alone (OR [95% CI], 0.87[0.80-0.94]).[73] A Cochrane review investigated vitamin D with or without calcium for prevention of fractures in postmenopausal women and older men. Analysis revealed high-quality evidence that vitamin D alone is unlikely to be effective in reducing hip fractures or any other new fractures. Vitamin D plus calcium, however, was found to reduce hip fractures and any fractures (RR [95% CI], 0.84 [0.74-0.96]; 0.95 [0.90-0.99], respectively).[64] In contrast, not even the combination of calcium/vitamin D resulted in fracture benefit in a recent meta-analysis of 33 randomized clinical trials of community-dwelling older adults.[74] For the prevention of fractures, the American Geriatric Society recommends vitamin D (at least 1000 IU/d), along with calcium, in institutionalized and community-dwelling older adults, but not vitamin D alone.[61] The USPTF recommends calcium/vitamin D for prevention of fractures in adults at risk for falls or vitamin D deficiency.[75]

### Omega-3 Fatty Acids

Omega-3 (n-3s) fatty acids, namely, alpha-linolenic, eicosapentaenoic acid (EPA) and docosahexaenoic acid (DHA), are obtained in foods such as tofu, chia, flaxseed, soybean/canola oils, and fish. Omega-3 is widely available in both prescription and DS form (ie, fish oil). They are commonly used for the prevention and treatment of CVD, hypertriglyceridemia, dementia, depression, asthma, and inflammatory diseases. Omega-3 fatty acids are well tolerated but may cause gastrointestinal disturbances, headache, malodorous sweat, unpleasant taste, and bad breath. High doses may be associated with reduced immune function and reduced platelet aggregation.[76] Methylmercury toxicity is a concern with high consumption of contaminated fish such as shark, swordfish, king mackerel, tilefish, and farm-raised salmon but not **DSs**.[77-79] NHANES data indicate that n-3 use, in all exogenous forms, has increased in adults older than 65 ($P$ <0.001).[5] The American Heart Association (AHA) recommends eating at least two servings of fatty fish per week to acquire DHA/EPA. It also encourages tofu and plant oils that provide alphalinolenic.[80] The FDA allowed for a health claim for supplements containing EPA/DHA stating that "supportive, but not conclusive research shows that consumption of EPA and DHA omega-3 fatty acids may reduce the risk of coronary heart disease"; however, it must not recommend more than 2 g/d of EPA + DHA.[81]

Although the benefit of a diet rich in n-3s is clear, as first demonstrated in the Inuit and Japanese populations, the use of **DSs** is more controversial.[82] Several recent studies and meta-analyses have shown that n-3s from **DSs** may not be as protective as dietary sources.[83-90]

A 2016 systematic review of 61 RCTs and 37 observational trials, sponsored by the NIH/Office of Dietary Supplements, found that, statistically, marine oils significantly lower triglycerides and total:HDL-c ratio, and raise HDL-c and LDL-c (high strength of evidence). However, marine oils (EPA + DHA) have no effects on risk of major adverse CV events, all-cause death, sudden cardiac death, revascularization, or BP (high strength of evidence). There was also no effect of marine oils on risk of atrial fibrillation (AF) (moderate strength of evidence); and no effect of marine oil on risk of CVD death, CHD death, total CHD, MI, angina pectoris, heart failure (HF), total stroke, and hemorrhagic stroke (low strength of evidence).[91] In 2017, the AHA updated its recommendations regarding n-3 supplementation for the prevention of CVD

**TABLE 4.2 • 2017 American Heart Association Science Advisory on Omega-3 Supplementation and the Prevention of Clinical CV Disease**

| Recommendation | Indication |
| --- | --- |
| Treatment is reasonable | • Secondary prevention of CHD and sudden cardiac death among patients with prevalent CHD<br>• Secondary prevention of outcomes in patients with HF |
| Treatment is not indicated | • Prevention of CVD mortality in diabetes mellitus/prediabetes<br>• Prevention of CHD among patients at high risk for CVD<br>• Primary prevention of stroke (high CVD risk with or without prevalent CHD)<br>• Secondary prevention of AF in patients with previous AF<br>• AF after cardiac surgery |
| No recommendation can be made | • Primary prevention of CHD (general population)<br>• Primary prevention of AF<br>• Primary prevention of HF<br>• Secondary prevention of stroke |

Data from Siscovick DS, Barringer TA, Fretts AM, et al. Omega-3 polyunsaturated fatty acid (fish oil) supplementation and the prevention of clinical cardiovascular disease: a science advisory from the American heart association. *Circulation.* 2017;135:e867-e884.
Abbreviations: AF, atrial fibrillation; CHD, coronary heart disease; CVD, cardiovascular disease; HF, heart failure.

(Table 4.2). It only recommends that n-3s are reasonable for secondary prevention of CHD death and in those with reduced ejection fraction HF, given the low risk of treatment. No benefit of supplementation was found for primary prevention of stroke, primary prevention of CHD (in patients with high CVD risk), CVD prevention in patients with diabetes/prediabetes, secondary prevention of AF, or AF after cardiac surgery. Recommendations could not be made because of lack of data for secondary prevention of stroke, primary prevention of CHD (in the general population), HF, or AF.[92] Subsequently, a meta-analysis of 10 trials including over 77 000 patients at high risk for CVD, found no significant association between n-3 supplementation and risk of CHD, stroke, revascularization, or all-cause mortality.[93]

Further data are needed to clarify the role of n-3s in AD, dementia, age-related macular degeneration, cancer prevention, rheumatoid arthritis, depression, inflammatory bowel disease, and others. Results of VITAL, a large ongoing RCT in over 25 000 older adults, will shed light on the role of n-3s (with or without vitamin $D_3$) for the primary prevention of CHD, cancer, and stroke. VITAL uses the prescription product; therefore, the role of **DSs** may remain questionable.[94,95]

# SUMMARY

The consumption of **dietary supplements (DSs)**, including **vitamins** and **minerals**, is significant in older adults; this may be the result of current regulations and ease of introducing supplements into an ever-growing market.

The use of such supplements is not always effective and has been proved to be sometimes harmful.

Current evidence does not support the use of vitamin E, vitamin A, and Se supplements. The use of folic acid and vitamin B supplements is controversial and is only justified in cases of a deficiency. Calcium supplementation has been linked to an increase in CV events; however, supplementation within normal limits provides neither CV benefit nor risk in generally healthy adults. Vitamin D is likely to provide benefit in elderly patients at risk for falls and fractures when given in combination with calcium. The evidence with vitamin D supplements is conflicting regarding its effect on total, cancer, and CV mortality, or on CV risk. Omega-3 fatty acid supplementation is reasonable for secondary prevention of CHD death and in those with reduced ejection fraction HF.

Healthcare providers need to remain abreast of emerging evidence and recommendations regarding the use of DSs and counsel patients regarding the potential benefits and adverse effects related to vitamins and other supplements. The DSs' effectiveness in relationship to the cost burden to patients, and potential prescription drug supplement interactions need to be considered.

## References

1. National Institutes of Health Office of Dietary Supplements. Dietary supplement health and education Act of 1994. Public law 103-417. https://ods.od.nih.gov/About/DSHEA_Wording.aspx. Accessed March 10, 2017.
2. Zakaryan A, Irwin GM. Regulation of herbal dietary supplements: is there a better way? *Drug Info J.* 2012;46:532-544.
3. Avery RJ, Eisenberg MD, Cantor JH. An examination of structure-function claims in dietary supplement advertising in the U.S.: 2003-2009. *Prev Med.* 2017;97:86-92.
4. Bailey RL, Gahche JJ, Miller PE, et al. Why US adults use dietary supplements. *JAMA Intern Med.* 2013;173:355-361.
5. Kantor ED, Rehm CD, Du M, et al. Trends in dietary supplement use among US adults from 1999-2012. *JAMA.* 2016;316:1464-1474.
6. Cohen PA. The supplement paradox: negligible benefits, robust consumption. *JAMA.* 2016;316:1453-1454.
7. Brody T. Food and dietary supplement package labeling guidance from FDA's warning letters and Title 21 of the code of federal regulations. *Compr Rev Food Sci Food Saf.* 2016;15:92-129.
8. Cole MR, Fetrow CW. Adulteration of dietary supplements. *Am J Health Syst Pharm.* 2003;60:1576-1580.
9. Pawar RS, Grundel E. Overview of regulation of dietary supplements in the USA and issues of adulteration with phenethylamines (PEAs). *Drug Test Anal.* 2017;9:500-517.
10. Kuszak AJ, Hopp DC, Williamson JS, et al. Approaches by the US National Institutes of Health to support rigorous scientific research on dietary supplements and natural products. *Drug Test Anal.* 2016;8:413-417.
11. Srinivasan VS. Challenges and scientific issues in the standardization of botanicals and their preparations. United States Pharmacopeia's dietary supplement verification program–a public health program. *Life Sci.* 2006;78:2039-2043.
12. United States Pharmacopeial Convention. Dietary supplement verification program participants. http://www.usp.org/verification-services/manufacturers#processincludes. Accessed March 14, 2017.
13. United States Government Accountability Office. Report to Congressional Requesters. Dietary Supplements. FDA should take further actions to improve oversight and consumer understanding. GAO Highlights Report No. GAO-09-250. 2009. http://www.gao.gov/new.items/d09250.pdf. Accessed March 14, 2017.

14. Mowry JB, Spyker DA, Brooks DE, Zimmerman A, Schauben JL. 2015 annual report of the American association of poison control centers' national poison data system (NPDS): 33rd annual report. *Clin Toxicol (Phila)*. 2016;54:924-1109.

15. Mursu J, Robien K, Harnack LJ, et al. Dietary supplements and mortality rate in older women: the Iowa Women's Health Study. *Arch Intern Med*. 2011;171:1625-1633.

16. Garcia-Cazarin ML, Wambogo EA, Regan KS, et al. Dietary supplement research portfolio at the NIH, 2009-2011. *J Nutr*. 2014;144:414-418.

17. National Institutes of Health Office of Dietary Supplements. Multivitamin/mineral supplements. 2015. https://ods.od.nih.gov/factsheets/MVMS-HealthProfessional/. Accessed March 14, 2017.

18. Age-Related Eye Disease Study Research Group. A randomized, placebo-controlled, clinical trial of high dose supplementation with vitamins C and E, beta carotene, and zinc for age-related macular degeneration and vision loss. *Arch Ophthalmol*. 2001;119:1417-1436.

19. Neuhouser ML, Wassertheil-Smoller S, Thomson C, et al. Multivitamin use and risk of cancer and cardiovascular disease in the Women's Health Initiative cohorts. *Arch Intern Med*. 2009;169:294-304.

20. Shelton RC, Keller MB, Gelenberg A, et al. Effectiveness of St John's Wort in major depression: a randomized controlled trial. *JAMA*. 2001;285:1978-1986.

21. Klein EA, Thompson IM Jr, Tangen CM, et al. Vitamin E and the risk of prostate cancer: the selenium and vitamin E cancer prevention trial (select). *JAMA*. 2011;306:1549-1556.

22. Kennedy J, Wang CC, Wu CH. Patient disclosure about herb and supplement use among adults in the US. *Evid Based Complement Alternat Med*. 2008;5:451-456.

23. Gardiner P, Sadikova E, Filippelli AC, et al. Medical reconciliation of dietary supplements: don't ask, don't tell. *Patient Educ Couns*. 2015;98:512-517.

24. U.S. Department of Health and Human Services and U.S. Department of Agriculture. 2015–2020 dietary guidelines for Americans. 8th ed. 2015. Available at: http://health.gov/dietaryguidelines/2015/guidelines/. Accessed March 14, 2017.

25. Grodstein F, O'Brien J, Kang JH, et al. Long-term multivitamin supplementation and cognitive function in men: a randomized trial. *Ann Intern Med*. 2013;159:806-814.

26. Lamas GA, Boineau R, Goertz C, et al. Oral high-dose multivitamins and minerals after myocardial infarction: a randomized trial. *Ann Intern Med*. 2013;159:797-805.

27. Fortmann SP, Burda BU, Senger CA, et al. Vitamin and mineral supplements in the primary prevention of cardiovascular disease and cancer: an updated systematic evidence review for the U.S. Preventive Services Task Force. *Ann Intern Med*. 2013;159:824-834.

28. National Institutes of Health State-of-the-Science Panel. National Institutes of Health state-of-the-science conference statement: multivitamin/mineral supplements and chronic disease prevention. *Am J Clin Nutr*. 2007;85:257S-264S.

29. World Cancer Research Fund/American Institute for Cancer Research. *Food, Nutrition, Physical Activity, and the Prevention of Cancer: A Global Perspective*. Washington, DC: American Institute for Cancer Research; 2007.

30. Ólafsdóttir B, Gunnarsdóttir I, Nikulβsdóttir H, et al. Dietary supplement use in the older population of Iceland and association with mortality. *Br J Nutr*. 2017;117(10):1463-1469.

31. National Academies of Sciences Engineering Medicine. Dietary reference intakes tables and application. http://www.nationalacademies.org/hmd/Activities/Nutrition/SummaryDRIs/DRI-Tables.aspx. Accessed March 14, 2017.

32. Schwingshackl L, Boeing H, Stelmach-Mardas M, et al. Dietary supplements and risk of cause-specific death, cardiovascular disease, and cancer: a systematic review and meta-analysis of primary prevention trials. *Adv Nutr*. 2017;8:27-39.

33. Farina N, Llewellyn D, Isaac MG, et al. Vitamin E for Alzheimer's dementia and mild cognitive impairment. *Cochrane Database Syst Rev*. 2017;1:CD002854.

34. Institute of Medicine, Food and Nutrition Board. *Dietary Reference Intakes for Vitamin A, Vitamin K, Arsenic, Boron, Chromium, Copper, Iodine, Iron, Manganese, Molybdenum, Nickel, Silicon, Vanadium and Zinc*. Washington, DC: National Academies Press; 2001:290.

35. Omenn GS, Goodman GE, Thornquist MD, et al. Effects of a combination of beta carotene and vitamin A on lung cancer and cardiovascular disease. *N Engl J Med*. 1996; 334:1150-1155.

36. Feskanich D, Singh V, Willett WC, et al. Vitamin A intake and hip fractures among postmenopausal women. *JAMA*. 2002;287:47-54.

37. Vollset SE, Clarke R, Lewington S, et al.; B-Vitamin Treatment Trialists' Collaboration. Effects of folic acid supplementation on overall and site-specific cancer incidence during the randomised trials: meta-analyses of data on 50,000 individuals. *Lancet*. 2013;381:1029-1036.

38. Tian T, Yang KQ, Cui JG, et al. Folic acid supplementation for stroke prevention in patients with cardiovascular disease. *Am J Med Sci*. 2017;354(4):379-387.

39. Galasko DR, Peskind E, Clark CM, et al; Alzheimer's Disease Cooperative Study. Antioxidants for Alzheimer disease: a randomized clinical trial with cerebrospinal fluid biomarker measures. *Arch Neurol*. 2012;69:836-841.

40. Bjelakovic G, Nikolova D, Gluud LL, et al. Antioxidant supplements for prevention of mortality in healthy participants and patients with various diseases. *Cochrane Database Syst Rev*. 2012;3: CD007176.

41. Institute of Medicine, Food and Nutrition Board. *Dietary Reference Intakes for Vitamin C, Vitamin E, Selenium, and Carotenoids*. Washington, DC: National Academies Press; 2000.

42. Stranges S, Marshall JR, Natarajan R, et al. Effects of long-term selenium supplementation on the incidence of type 2 diabetes. *Ann Intern Med*. 2007;147:217-223.

43. Bleys J, Navas-Acien A, Guallar E. Serum selenium and diabetes in U.S. adults. *Diabetes Care*. 2007;30:829-834.

44. Bleys J, Navas-Acien A, Guallar E. Serum selenium levels and all-cause, cancer, and cardiovascular mortality among US adults. *Arch Intern Med*. 2008;168:404-410.

45. Rees K, Hartley L, Day C, et al. Selenium supplementation for the primary prevention of cardiovascular disease. *Cochrane Database Syst Rev*. 2013;1:CD009671.

46. Zhang X, Liu C, Guo J, et al. Selenium status and cardiovascular diseases: meta-analysis of prospective observational studies and randomized controlled trials. *Eur J Clin Nutr*. 2016;70:162-169.

47. U.S. Food and Drug Administration. Letter Regarding Dietary Supplement Health Claim for Selenium and Certain Cancers (Docket No. 02P-0457). 2003.

48. Vinceti M, Filippini T, Del Giovane C, et al. Selenium for preventing cancer. *Cochrane Database Syst Rev*. 2018;1:CD005195.

49. Ross AC, Taylor CL, Yaktine AL, et al, eds.; Institute of Medicine (US) Committee to Review Dietary Reference Intakes for Vitamin D and Calcium. *Dietary Reference Intakes for Calcium and Vitamin D*. Washington, DC: National Academies Press; 2011.

50. Cosman F, De beur SJ, Leboff MS, et al. Clinician's guide to prevention and treatment of osteoporosis. *Osteoporos Int*. 2014;25:2359-2381.

51. Bolland MJ, Barber PA, Doughty RN, et al. Vascular events in healthy older women receiving calcium supplementation: randomised controlled trial. *BMJ*. 2008;336:262-266.

52. Bolland MJ, Grey A, Avenell A, Gamble GD, Reid IR. Calcium supplements with or without vitamin D and risk of cardiovascular events: reanalysis of the Women's Health Initiative limited access dataset and meta-analysis. *BMJ*. 2011;342:d2040.

53. Mao PJ, Zhang C, Tang L, et al. Effect of calcium or vitamin D supplementation on vascular outcomes: a meta-analysis of randomized controlled trials. *Int J Cardiol*. 2013;169:106-111.

54. Bolland MJ, Avenell A, Baron JA, et al. Effect of calcium supplements on risk of myocardial infarction and cardiovascular events: meta-analysis. *BMJ*. 2010;341:c3691.

55. Michaëlsson K, Melhus H, Warensjö Lemming E, Wolk, A, Byberg, L. Long term calcium intake and rates of all cause and cardiovascular mortality: community based prospective longitudinal cohort study. *BMJ*. 2013;346:f228.

56. Xiao Q, Murphy RA, Houston DK, Harris TB, Chow WH, Park Y. Dietary and supplemental calcium intake and cardiovascular disease mortality: the National Institutes of Health-AARP diet and health study. *JAMA Intern Med*. 2013;173:639-646.

57. Chung M, Tang AM, Fu Z, et al. Calcium intake and cardiovascular disease risk: an updated systematic review and meta-analysis. *Ann Intern Med*. 2016;165: 856-866.

58. Kopecky SL, Bauer DC, Gulati M, et al. Lack of evidence linking calcium with or without vitamin D supplementation to cardiovascular disease in generally healthy adults: a clinical guideline from the

National Osteoporosis Foundation and the American Society for Preventive Cardiology. *Ann Intern Med.* 2016;165:867-868.

59. Bikle DD. Vitamin D metabolism, mechanism of action, and clinical applications. *Chem Biol.* 2014;21:319-329.

60. Holick MF, Binkley NC, Bischoff-Ferrari HA, et al. Evaluation, treatment, and prevention of vitamin D deficiency: an Endocrine Society clinical practice guideline. *J Clin Endocrinol Metab.* 2011;96:1911-1930.

61. American Geriatrics Society Workgroup on Vitamin D Supplementation for Older Adults. Recommendations abstracted from the American Geriatrics Society consensus statement on vitamin D for prevention of falls and their consequences. *J Am Geriatr Soc.* 2014;62:147-152.

62. Rooney MR, Harnack L, Michos ED, et al. Trends in use of high-dose vitamin D supplements exceeding 1000 or 4000 International Units daily, 1999-2014. *JAMA.* 2017;317(23):2448-2450.

63. Bjelakovic G, Gluud LL, Nikolova D, et al. Vitamin D supplementation for prevention of mortality in adults. *Cochrane Database Syst Rev.* 2014;1:CD007470.

64. Avenell A, Mak JC, O'Connell D. Vitamin D and vitamin D analogues for preventing fractures in post-menopausal women and older men. *Cochrane Database Syst Rev.* 2014;4:CD000227.

65. Chowdhury R, Kunutsor S, Vitezova A, et al. Vitamin D and risk of cause specific death: systematic review and meta-analysis of observational cohort and randomized intervention studies. *BMJ.* 2014;348:g1903.

66. Schöttker B, Jorde R, Peasey A, et al. Vitamin D and mortality: meta-analysis of individual participant data from a large consortium of cohort studies from Europe and the United States. *BMJ.* 2014;348:g3656.

67. Bjelakovic G, Gluud LL, Nikolova D, et al. Vitamin D supplementation for prevention of cancer in adults. *Cochrane Database Syst Rev.* 2014;6:CD007469.

68. Elamin MB, Abu Elnour NO, Elamin KB, et al. Vitamin D and cardiovascular outcomes: a systematic review and meta-analysis. *J Clin Endocrinol Metab.* 2011;96:1931-1942.

69. Ford JA, Maclennan GS, Avenell A, et al. Cardiovascular disease and vitamin D supplementation: trial analysis, systematic review, and meta-analysis. *Am J Clin Nutr.* 2014;100:746-755.

70. Chung M, Lee J, Terasawa T, et al. Vitamin D with or without calcium supplementation for prevention of cancer and fractures: an updated meta-analysis for the U.S. Preventive Services Task Force. *Ann Intern Med.* 2011;155:827-838.

71. Chung M, Lee J, Terasawa T, Lau J, Trikalinos TA. Correction: vitamin D with or without calcium supplementation for prevention of cancer and fractures. *Ann Intern Med.* 2014;161:615.

72. Michael YL, Whitlock EP, Lin JS, et al. Primary care relevant interventions to prevent falling in older adults: a systematic evidence review for the U.S. Preventive Services Task Force. *Ann Intern Med.* 2010;153:815-825.

73. Wu H, Pang Q. The effect of vitamin D and calcium supplementation on falls in older adults: a systematic review and meta-analysis. *Der Orthopade.* 2017;46(9):729-736.

74. Zhao JG, Zeng XT, Wang J, Liu L. Association between calcium or vitamin D supplementation and fracture incidence in community-dwelling older adults: a systematic review and meta-analysis. *JAMA.* 2017;318(24):2466-2482.

75. Moyer VA. Vitamin D and calcium supplementation to prevent fractures in adults: U.S. Preventive Services Task Force recommendation statement. *Ann Intern Med.* 2013; 158:691-696.

76. Institute of Medicine, Food and Nutrition Board. *Dietary Reference Intakes for Energy, Carbohydrate, Fiber, Fat, Fatty Acids, Cholesterol, Protein, and Amino Acids (Macronutrients).* Washington, DC: National Academies Press; 2005.

77. He K, Daviglus ML. A few more thoughts about fish and fish oil. *J Am Diet Assoc.* 2005;105:350-351.

78. Wilson JF. Balancing the risks and benefits of fish consumption. *Ann Intern Med.* 2004;141:977-980.

79. Foran JA, Carpenter DO, Hamilton MC, et al. Risk-based consumption advice for farmed Atlantic and wild Pacific salmon contaminated with dioxins and dioxin-like compounds. *Environ Health Perspect.* 2005;113:552-556.

80. American Heart Association. Fish 101. 2015. www.heart.org/HEARTORG/GettingHealthy/NutritionCenter/Fish-101_UCM_305986_Article.jsp. Accessed April 7, 2017.

81. U.S. Food and Drug Administration. Summary of qualified health claims subject to enforcement discretion. 2014.

82. Bang HO, Dyerberg J, Sinclair HM. The composition of the Eskimo food in north western Greenland. *Am J Clin Nutr*. 1980;33:2657-2661.

83. Roncaglioni MC, Tombesi M, Silletta MG. n-3 fatty acids in patients with cardiac risk factors. *N Engl J Med*. 2013; 369:781-782.

84. Bosch J, Gerstein HC, Dagenais GR, et al. n-3 fatty acids and cardiovascular outcomes in patients with dysglycemia. *N Engl J Med*. 2012;367:309-318.

85. Kromhout D, Giltay EJ, Geleijnse JM; Alpha Omega Trial Group. n-3 fatty acids and cardiovascular events after myocardial infarction. *N Engl J Med*. 2010;363:2015-2026.

86. Bonds DE, Harrington M, Worrall BB, et al. Effect of long-chain omega-3 fatty acids and lutein + zeaxanthin supplements on cardiovascular outcomes: results of the age-related eye disease Study 2 (AREDS2) randomized clinical trial. *JAMA Intern Med*. 2014;174:763-771.

87. Kwak SM, Myung SK, Lee YJ, et al. Efficacy of omega-3 fatty acid supplements (eicosapentaenoic acid and docosahexaenoic acid) in the secondary prevention of cardiovascular disease: a meta-analysis of randomized, double-blind, placebo-controlled trials. *Arch Intern Med*. 2012;172:686-694.

88. Rizos EC, Ntzani EE, Bika E, et al. Association between omega-3 fatty acid supplementation and risk of major cardiovascular disease events: a systematic review and meta-analysis. *JAMA*. 2012;308:1024-1033.

89. Chowdhury R, Stevens S, Gorman D, et al. Association between fish consumption, long chain omega 3 fatty acids, and risk of cerebrovascular disease: systematic review and meta-analysis. *BMJ*. 2012;345:e6698.

90. Chowdhury R, Warnakula S, Kunutsor S, et al. Association of dietary, circulating, and supplement fatty acids with coronary risk: a systematic review and meta-analysis. *Ann Intern Med*. 2014;160:398-406.

91. Balk EM, Adam GP, Langberg V, et al. Omega-3 fatty acids and cardiovascular disease: an updated systematic review. Evidence Report/Technology Assessment No. 223. (Prepared by the Brown Evidence-based Practice Center under Contract No. 290-2012-00012-I.) AHRQ Publication No. 16-e002-ef. Rockville, MD: Agency for Healthcare Research and Quality; 2016. www.effectivehealthcare.ahrq.gov/reports/final.cfm. Accessed April 7, 2017.

92. Siscovick DS, Barringer TA, Fretts AM, et al. Omega-3 polyunsaturated fatty acid (fish oil) supplementation and the prevention of clinical cardiovascular disease: a science advisory from the American heart association. *Circulation*. 2017;135:e867-e884.

93. Aung T, Halsey J, Kromhout D, et al. Associations of omega-3 fatty acid supplement use with cardiovascular disease risks: meta-analysis of 10 trials involving 77 917 individuals. *JAMA Cardiol*. 2018;3(3):225-234.

94. Pradhan AD, Manson JE. Update on the vitamin D and OmegA-3 trial (VITAL). *J Steroid Biochem Mol Biol*. 2016; 155:252-256.

95. Bassuk SS, Manson JE, Lee IM, et al. Baseline characteristics of participants in the VITamin D and OmegA-3 TriaL (VITAL). *Contemp Clin Trials*. 2016;47:235-243.

# Therapeutic Advances in Common Geriatric Hospital Presentations

# Therapeutic Advances in Hyponatremia: Fluids, Diuretics, Vaptans, and More

Shu Yang, MD and Mark Goldin, MD

**CHAPTER 5**

## BACKGROUND

**Hyponatremia** is defined as serum sodium concentration <135 mEq/L and is particularly common in older adults because of reduced ability to excrete free water.[1] It can be found in up to 7% of ambulatory and 53% of institutionalized **geriatric** patients.[2-5] Associated morbidity is significant and can range from subtle encephalopathy or gait disturbance in mild cases to lethargy and seizure in severe cases. Severe **hyponatremia** (sodium <125 mmol/L) has an estimated mortality of 27% to 40%.[6,7]

Chronic **hyponatremia** has been associated with bone loss.[2,8] In particular, cross-sectional human data have shown that **hyponatremia** is associated with significantly increased odds of osteoporosis at the hip (odds ratio = 2.85; 95% confidence interval [CI], 1.03-7.86; $P < 0.01$).[9,10] This, plus the neurocognitive effects of chronic **hyponatremia**, increases fall risk in older adults. Moreover, even mild asymptomatic **hyponatremia** is associated with increased fracture incidence in ambulatory elderly patients.[11]

**Hyponatremia** is primarily a disorder of water, not of sodium. The first step in evaluation is to determine whether low serum sodium represents true hyposmotic **hyponatremia**, defined by serum osmolality <280 mOsm/kg (Figure 5.1). This contrasts with isosmotic (eg, caused by hypertriglyceridemia or hyperproteinemia) or hyperosmotic (eg, caused by hyperglycemia or mannitol) **hyponatremia**. Subsequent assessment of volume, urine sodium, and urine osmolality guides diagnosis (Figure 5.2). Treatment of **hyponatremia** depends on its acuity, symptoms, and underlying etiology (Table 5.1).

Elderly patients are at increased risk of dehydration. In acute hypovolemic **hyponatremia** with urine sodium < 20 mEq/L, treatment is volume repletion with isotonic saline ([Na] = 154 mEq/L), which restores intravascular volume and suppresses

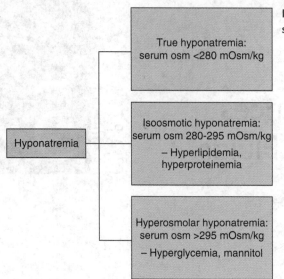

**FIGURE 5.1** Approach to hyponatremia based on serum osmolality. Osm, osmolality.

arginine vasopressin peptide (AVP), allowing diuresis.[12] Isotonic saline should be avoided in patients with hypervolemic **hyponatremia** because it can worsen fluid overload, and in those with severe syndrome of inappropriate antidiuretic hormone (SIADH) because sodium will be excreted and free water retained, potentially worsening **hyponatremia**. This is particularly important because approximately 50% of true **hyponatremia** in the elderly is caused by SIADH. This is characterized by euvolemia, urine osmolality $> 100$ mOsm/L, and urine sodium $> 20$ mEq/L. Causes of SIADH are summarized in Table 5.2. Treatment consists of fluid restriction; generally,

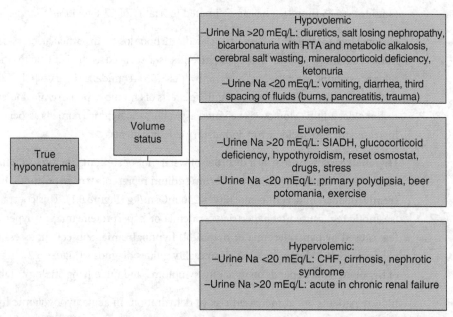

**FIGURE 5.2** Approach to hyponatremia based on volume status. CHF, congestive heart failure; RTA, renal tubular acidosis; SIADH, syndrome of inappropriate antidiuretic hormone; UNa, urine sodium.

**TABLE 5.1 • Management of Hyponatremia**

| | |
|---|---|
| Hypovolemic hyponatremia | Volume repletion with normal saline |
| Hypervolemic hyponatremia (CHF, cirrhosis, nephrotic syndrome) | Fluid restriction, loop diuretics, vaptans |
| Euvolemic hyponatremia (SIADH) | Fluid restriction, vaptans, salt tablets, urea |

CHF, congestive heart failure; SIADH, syndrome of inappropriate antidiuretic hormone.

recommended total fluid intake by oral (especially fruits and soups), intravenous (IV), or any route is <800 mL/d. However, patients often have difficulty with compliance in the long term because of increased thirst with fluid restriction.

In addition to fluid restriction, salt tablets can be used to treat mild SIADH.[13] Nine grams of oral salt provides a quantify of sodium similar to 1 L of isotonic saline but without any water. Other adjunctive treatments for SIADH include

**TABLE 5.2 • Causes of SIADH**

| |
|---|
| **CNS disease** |
| Trauma |
| Stroke |
| Infection |
| Tumor |
| Intracranial hemorrhage |
| Neoplastic disease |
| **Lung disease** |
| Malignancy |
| In particular small cell lung cancer |
| Lymphoma |
| Throat (squamous cell carcinoma) |
| Prostate adenocarcinoma |
| Pancreatic adenocarcinoma |
| **Medications** |
| Thiazide diuretics |
| Nonsteroidal anti-inflammatory drugs |
| Antipsychotics |
| Antidepressants (especially selective serotonin reuptake inhibitors) |
| Vasopressin |
| Antiepileptics |
| Chemotherapies (eg, cyclophosphamide, vincristine) |

CNS, central nervous system; SIADH, syndrome of inappropriate antidiuretic hormone.

demeclocycline and lithium, which act on collecting tubule cells and interfere with the renal action of vasopressin, promoting diuresis by inducing nephrogenic diabetes insipidus within days to a week.[14,15] Demeclocycline, a tetracycline antibiotic, works by inhibiting adenylyl cyclase activation after AVP binds to its V2 receptor in the kidney, thus allowing water diuresis. However, demeclocycline is not approved by the U.S. Food and Drug Administration (FDA) to treat **hyponatremia** and can be nephrotoxic in patients with cirrhosis and heart failure. Likewise, the use of lithium is limited by its nephrotoxicity and central nervous system effects. Demeclocycline can also be nephrotoxic in patients with cirrhosis and heart failure, has poor gastrointestinal tolerability, and can also exert hepatotoxic effects. An additional treatment for SIADH is urea, which acts as an osmotic diuretic and induces osmotic diuresis and augments free water excretion. Typical effective doses of urea are 30 to 90 g daily in divided doses. However, urea is not available in the United States and is not approved by the FDA for treatment of **hyponatremia**. Despite effects such as poor palatability leading to poor patient compliance, and diarrhea at high doses, urea may be effective in treating patients in critical care with SIADH and brain edema, especially in patients with feeding tubes in whom palatability is not a concern and those with high fluid intake as part of their nutritional or medication requirement.[16-17] Lastly, furosemide (20-40 mg/d) with sodium chloride (NaCl, or high salt intake 200 mEq/d) has been used in the treatment of chronic euvolemic **hyponatremia** in some patients.

Hypervolemic **hyponatremia** in congestive heart failure (CHF), cirrhosis, or nephrotic syndrome is treated with loop diuretics. These agents block the sodium/potassium/2 chloride cotransporter in the thick ascending limb of the loop of Henle, diminishing medullary hypertonicity required to reabsorb water. There are important pharmacokinetic differences between the loop diuretics. Bumetanide is more extensively metabolized than furosemide and therefore has a shorter half-life. Torsemide is less metabolized, has greater and more predictable bioavailability, and has a longer half-life than furosemide. Given oral bioavailability of approximately 50%, oral furosemide dose should be approximately double that of an equivalent IV dose.

It should be noted that diuretics, in fact, frequently cause **hyponatremia**. This is particularly true of thiazides, which inhibit the sodium/chloride cotransporter in the distal convoluted tubule, impairing the nephron's diluting capacity. Loop diuretics cause **hyponatremia** less commonly. Diuretic-induced **hyponatremia** frequently co-occurs with hypokalemia. Because potassium is as osmotically active as sodium, and intracellular and extracellular osmolality maintain equilibrium, supplementing potassium is crucial to raise serum sodium.[18-20]

In cases of acute severe **hyponatremia**, standard treatment is hypertonic 3% saline. When **hyponatremia** is chronic or of unknown duration, the recommended rate of sodium correction is <0.5 mEq/L/h or <6 to 8 mEq/L/d to avoid central pontine myelinolysis (CPM) or osmotic demyelination syndrome (ODS). Osmotic demyelination is caused by brain dehydration and osmotic brain shrinkage following rapid correction of chronic **hyponatremia**. It is also related to the disruption of the blood–brain barrier, which can lead to an influx of complements into the brain, resulting in brain myelinolysis from the neurotoxic effects of complements on the oligodendrocytes that produce and maintain myelin sheaths of neurons.[21-23] ODS is a devastating complication of rapid **hyponatremia** correction characterized by paraplegia, dysarthria, and dysphagia. Overly rapid correction should be reversed with deamino-delta-D-arginine vasopressin (dDAVP) and 5% dextrose in water (D5W) infusion.

# AREAS OF UNCERTAINTY

The broad range of etiologies and treatments of **hyponatremia** make this a challenging condition to evaluate. Despite long-established physiology and familiarity with treatments, there remain areas of uncertainty. The foregoing discussion of hypertonic saline use in severe symptomatic **hyponatremia** illustrates this well; in fact, several strategies have been suggested for achieving a target rate of sodium correction while minimizing complications. A rough estimate of initial 3% hypertonic saline infusion rate is weight (kilogram) $\times$ desired correction rate (mEq/L/h) to treat patients with severe symptomatic **hyponatremia**, manifested by seizures, respiratory distress due to pulmonary edema, obtundation, or coma. For example, for a 75-kg individual with a desired correction rate of 8 mEq/L/24 h = 1/3 mEq/L/h, the infusion rate is about 75/3 = 25 mL/h. An even simpler alternative regimen is to administer an initial 100-mL bolus of 3% hypertonic saline and repeat once in 30 minutes if necessary, especially in the setting of severe exercise-induced **hyponatremia**.[24] This is expected to increase serum sodium by 2 to 3 mEq/L and reduce the degree of cerebral edema.

A further strategy posits that concurrent administration of hypertonic saline with DDAVP may avoid overcorrection in severe chronic **hyponatremia** with mild/moderate symptoms. It has been shown that 1- to 2-mg dDAVP (either IV or subcutaneous) every 4 to 8 hours for 24 to 48 hours, during an infusion of hypertonic saline at 15 to 30 mL/h can correct **hyponatremia** slowly and safely.[25] Treatment of hypervolemic **hyponatremia** also continues to stir debate. Given the pharmacokinetic variation among loop diuretics, it has been suggested that torsemide may be preferable to furosemide in treating CHF. A subgroup analysis of the Acute Study of Clinical Effectiveness of Nesiritide in Decompensated Heart Failure (ASCEND-HF) compared the efficacy of torsemide versus furosemide in 1741 patients. Although there was a trend toward fewer events (defined as 30-day mortality plus CHF hospitalization) (odds ratio, 0.85; 95% CI, 0.62-1.29; $P < 0.05$) and lower 180-day mortality (hazard ratio, 0.86; 95% CI, 0.63-1.19) in the torsemide group, results did not achieve statistical significance.[26]

This question of optimal agent is particularly relevant in light of research showing a mortality risk in hypervolemic **hyponatremia** related to CHF. A post hoc analysis of 949 patients from the Outcomes of a Prospective Trial of Intravenous Milrinone for

Exacerbations of Chronic Heart Failure (OPTIME-CHF) revealed that patients with serum sodium of 132 to 135 mEq/L had significant increases in mortality both in hospital (5.9% vs 1%-2.3%) and at 30 days (15.9% vs 6.4%-7.8%).[27] These data highlight the need for randomized controlled trials.

At the same time, the benefits of adjunctive fluid restriction in hypervolemic **hyponatremia** have been questioned, notably for patients with highly concentrated urine ($>$500 mOsm/kg $H_2O$) and in those with daily urine output $<$1.5 L/d. One method of determining the effectiveness of fluid restriction is to calculate the electrolyte-free water clearance. Electrolyte-free water clearance = urine volume X (1-(UNa + UK)/SNa). Therefore, if the ratio of (UNa + UK)/SNa = 1, the electrolyte-free water clearance will be positive. If this ratio is low enough (eg, $<$0.5), serum sodium will likely rise with fluid restriction. Conversely, a ratio of (UNa + UK)/SNa $>$ 1 predicts negative electrolyte-free water clearance and net water retention. In this scenario, serum sodium will not rise with fluid restriction alone.[28]

In recent years, the uncertainty around even established treatments has driven the advent of newer agents. The best studied class of therapeutics is the arginine vasopressin receptor antagonists (AVPR antagonists) or **vaptans**, to which the discussion now turns.

# THERAPEUTIC ADVANCES

**Vaptans** (conivaptan and tolvaptan) are competitive receptor antagonists of AVP V2 receptors and are approved by the FDA for the treatment of euvolemic and hypervolemic **hyponatremia**. They induce water diuresis by competing with AVP for its receptor and thus blocking the action of AVP in the distal convoluted tubule and collecting duct. The effect is a decrease in water reabsorption in the distal nephron and therefore an increase in electrolyte-free water excretion. The net effect is a reduction in total body water without natriuresis, leading to an increase in serum [Na]. The starting dose of tolvaptan is 15 mg on the first day, and the dose can be titrated to 30 mg and 60 mg at 24-hour intervals if serum [Na] remains $<$135 mEq/L or increase in serum [Na] $<$5 mEq/L in 24 hours. The efficacy of tolvaptan, a selective vasopressin receptor (V2) antagonist, was established in two prospective, randomized, double-blind, placebo-controlled multicenter trials (SALT-1 and SALT-2), which studied 448 patients with **hyponatremia** (mean sodium 129 mEq/L) caused by SIADH, CHF, or liver cirrhosis. Tolvaptan significantly increased the serum sodium at day 4 (increase = 3.5 $\pm$ 2.4 mEq/L vs 0.3 $\pm$ 2.3, $P$ $<$0.001; total 134-135 vs 130 mEq/L) and day 30 (increase = 4.2 $\pm$ 3.4 mEq/L vs 1.2 $\pm$ 3.5, $P$ $<$0.001; total 136 vs 131 mEq/L).[29] The proportion of patients with serum sodium $>$135 mEq/L by day 4 was 41% in the tolvaptan group compared with 11% in the placebo group ($P$ = 0.002), and the proportions were 33% versus 19%, respectively, at day 30. Seven days after tolvaptan withdrawal in the study group, serum declined nearly to values in the placebo group. Among patients with a serum sodium, 130 mEq/L, tolvaptan was also associated with a statistically significant improvement in mental status scores as measured using the 12-item Short-Form General Health Survey from baseline to day 30.[29] These results show that tolvaptan can rapidly increase serum sodium and that this increase can be largely sustained. Furthermore, the clear, measurable improvements in cognitive well-being are of particular benefit in the **geriatric** population.

Conivaptan, a V1a/V2 receptor blocker, is the only IV vasopressin receptor antagonist approved in the United States. As with tolvaptan, conivaptan is metabolized by the liver cytochrome P450 isozyme, CYP3A4. Conivaptan increases serum [Na] by an average of 4 to 8 mEq/L within 24 to 48 hours, which is significantly more efficacious than fluid restriction.[30] Conivaptan is given as an IV 20-mg loading dose over 30 minutes, followed by a continuous infusion of 20 to 40 mg/d for a maximum of 4 days because of drug interactions with other agents metabolized by the CYP3A4 hepatic isoenzyme (Table 5.3).

In using **vaptans** it is crucial to monitor the serum [Na] closely, at least every 6 to 8 hours and more frequently in patients at risk for developing osmotic demyelination, such as severe **hyponatremia**, alcoholism, malnutrition, liver disease, and hypokalemia. Free water restriction should be lifted so as to allow patient to drink free water to counteract the vigorous free water excretion. The goal of serum [Na] correction should be ≦8 mEq/L/d. Rapid overcorrection can potentially lead to devastating osmotic demyelination and should be reversed by stopping vaptan and giving water (either oral or IV D5W) and dDAVP if needed.

Several studies have evaluated the benefit of **vaptans** in patients with CHF. In a large, multicenter, randomized, double-blind, placebo-controlled trial in patients with symptomatic heart failure, conivaptan reduced pulmonary capillary wedge pressure and right atrial pressure compared with placebo, although it did not show a mortality benefit.[31] Another randomized, placebo-controlled, multicenter trial administered IV conivaptan for 48 hours along with loop diuretics to 170 hospitalized patients with acute decompensated heart failure and found an average 1 to 1.5 L/d increase in urine output.[31]

| TABLE 5.3 • Comparison of Vaptans | Tolvaptan | Conivaptan |
|---|---|---|
| Receptor antagonism | V1a/V2 | V2 |
| Administration route | Intravenous (IV) | Oral |
| Effect on urine osmolality | ↓ | ↓ |
| Half-life, h | 3.1-7.8 | 6-8 |
| Metabolism | Liver metabolism (CYP3A4) | Liver metabolism (CYP3A4) |
| Dosing | Loading dose of 20 mg IV (infused over 30 min), followed by continuous infusion of 20-40 mg/d for a maximum of 4 d | Start with 15 mg. Dose can be titrated upward to 30-60 mg depending on efficacy. |

Two recent studies focus on the use of conivaptan in neurologic or neurosurgical patients with **hyponatremia**. One study retrospectively evaluated the effect of a single 20-mg dose of conivaptan in 32 patients in critical care with baseline mean sodium of 129.8 mEq/L. Conivaptan increased serum sodium to 133.1 ± 3.2 mEq/L at 6 hours, 134.2 ± 3.2 mEq/L by 24 hours, and 134.7 ± 3.6 in 48 hours. Serum sodium increased by ≥4 mEq/L in 18 patients (56%).[32] However, in the EVEREST Outcome trial that included over 4100 patients hospitalized for worsening heart failure who were randomly assigned to tolvaptan or placebo, although tolvaptan increased the serum sodium within the first 7 days (5.5 vs 1.9 mEq/L) with placebo, there was no survival benefit and no improvement in long-term outcomes in patients who received tolvaptan. Therefore, despite encouraging and promising data from short-term studies, long-term trials of **vaptans** have failed to show a mortality benefit.[33]

The main side effects of **vaptans** are frequent urination, thirst, dry mouth, fatigue, polyuria and polydipsia, nausea, orthostatic hypotension, and a small but important risk of liver injury as reported in a study of tolvaptan in the treatment of autosomal dominant polycystic kidney disease.[34,35] In general, tolvaptan should not be used in any patient with liver disease because of potential hepatotoxicity, gastrointestinal bleeding, and drug-drug interactions relating to cytochrome P450 metabolism. These risks, as well as a lack of mortality benefit, led the FDA to caution against the use of **vaptans** in patients with underlying liver disease. A further clinical consideration, particularly in the elderly, is the risk of rapid diuresis and sodium overcorrection that can occur if patients are fluid restricted while treated with **vaptans**.

In addition to these adverse effects, the high cost of **vaptans** limits their use. For example, the cost of tolvaptan can be as high as $300 per tablet (~$11 000 for 30 tablets). However, **vaptans** may shorten length of hospital stay; and cost analyses in the United States and South Korea have shown a small but significant savings for patients admitted for treatment of chronic **hyponatremia**. In the US study, using data from the SIADH subgroup in the SALT trials and two studies, investigators found that the cost of tolvaptan for 4 days was offset by the reduction in length of stay by 1.11 days, with a net savings of $694.[36]

# SUMMARY

**Hyponatremia** is frequently encountered in **geriatric** patients and is associated with significant morbidity and mortality. Of special interest is an increased risk of confusion and ataxia due to metabolic encephalopathy and increased incidence of falls and fractures in the elderly population. Randomized controlled studies are needed to assess whether treatment of **hyponatremia** can mitigate this risk. Traditional management approaches have targeted underlying causes, such as volume repletion with normal saline in dehydrated patients, loop diuretics and fluid restriction in hypervolemic patients, and fluid restriction and salt tablets in euvolemic patients. Elderly patients are at particular risk for hypovolemic **hyponatremia** because of dehydration, as well as the SIADH. In addition to fluid restriction, SIADH may be treated with salt tablets and demeclocycline; however, its use is limited by nephrotoxicity especially in patients with heart failure and cirrhosis. In severe symptomatic **hyponatremia**, standard therapy is the infusion of hypertonic (3%) saline. Judicious monitoring is paramount because rapid overcorrection is associated with central pontine myelinolysis. Newer agents such as arginine vasopressin receptor antagonists (tolvaptan, conivaptan) have been shown to be effective in the treatment of euvolemic and hypervolemic chronic **hyponatremia**. In two randomized, double-blind, placebo-controlled multicenter trials (SALT-1 and SALT-2), tolvaptan significantly increased serum sodium at days 4 and 30 in 448 patients with mean baseline serum sodium 129 mEq/L. However, **vaptans** can cause liver damage, and the FDA has cautioned against their use in patients with underlying liver disease. The cost of **vaptans** has been a major barrier, but this may be offset by decreases in length of stay in hospitalized patients. A potential role for **vaptans** in the treatment of congestive heart failure (EVEREST) showed short-term improvement in dyspnea, but no long-term survival benefit or improvement in mortality. Thus, although **vaptans** have shown promise in the treatment of euvolemic and hypervolemic chronic **hyponatremia,** they have not shown long-term mortality benefits. More randomized studies are needed.

## References

1. Adrogue HJ, Madias NE. Hyponatremia. *N Engl J Med.* 2000;342:1581-1589.
2. Verbalis JG, Barsony J, Sugimura Y, et al. Hyponatremia induced osteoporosis. *J Bone Miner Res.* 2010;25:554-563.
3. Kleinfeld M, Casimir M, Borra S. Hyponatremia as observed in a chronic disease facility. *J Am Geriatr Soc.* 1979;27:156-161.
4. Hawkins RC. Age and gender as risk factors for hyponatremia and hypernatremia. *Clin Chim Acta.* 2003;337:169-172.
5. Chen LK, Lin MH, Hwang SJ, et al. Hyponatremia among the institutionalized elderly in two long-term care facilities in Taipei. *J Chin Med Assoc.* 2006;69:115-119.
6. Miller M, Morley JE, Rubenstein LZ. Hyponatremia in a nursing home population. *J Am Geriatr Soc.* 1995;43:1410-1413.
7. Lindner G, Funk GC, Schwarz C, et al. Hypernatremia in the critically ill is an independent risk factor for mortality. *Am J Kidney Dis.* 2007;50:952-957.
8. Verbalis JG, Drutarosky MD. Adaptation to chronic hypoosmolality in rats. *Kidney Int.* 1988;34:351-360.
9. Looker AC, Orwoll ES, Johnston CC Jr, et al. Prevalence of low femoral bone density in older US adults from NHANES III. *J Bone Miner Res.* 1997;12:1761-1768.
10. Looker AC, Johnston CC Jr, Wahner HW, et al. Prevalence of low femoral bone density in older US women from NHANES III. *J Bone Miner Res.* 1995;10:796-802.
11. Gankam KF, Andres C, Sattar L, et al. Mild hyponatremia and risk of fracture in the ambulatory elderly. *Q J Med.* 2008;101:583-588.
12. Verbalis JG, Goldsmith SR, Greenberg A, et al. Diagnosis, evaluation, and treatment of hyponatremia: expert panel recommendations. *Am J Med.* 2013;126(suppl 1):S1-S42.
13. Kerns E, Patel S, Cohen DM. Hourly oral sodium chloride for the rapid and predictable treatment of hyponatremia. *Clin Nephrol.* 2014;82:397.
14. Forrest JN Jr, Cox M, Hong C, et al. Superiority of demeclocycline over lithium in the treatment of chronic syndrome of inappropriate secretion of antidiuretic hormone. *N Engl J Med.* 1978;298:173.

15. Cox M, Guzzo J, Morrison G, et al. Demeclocycline and therapy of hyponatremia. *Ann Intern Med.* 1977;86:113.

16. Decaux G, Genette F. Urea for long term treatment of syndrome of inappropriate secretion of antidiuresis of antidiuretic hormone. *BMJ Clin Res.* 1981;283:1081-1083.

17. Rocque BG. Manucher Javid, urea, and the rise of osmotic therapy for intracranial pressure. *Neurosurgery.* 2012;70:1049-1054.

18. Laragh JH. The effect of potassium chloride on hyponatremia. *J Clin Invest.* 1954;33:807.

19. Kamel KS, Bear RA. Treatment of hyponatremia: a quantitative analysis. *Am J Kidney Dis.* 1993;21:439.

20. Edelman IS, Leibman J, O'Meara MP, et al. Interrelations between serum sodium concentration, serum osmolarity and total exchangeable sodium, total exchangeable potassium and total body water. *J Clin Invest.* 1958;37:1236-1256.

21. Adler S, Verbalis JG, Williams D. Effect of rapid correction of hyponatremia on the blood–brain barrier of rats. *Brain Res.* 1995;679:135-143.

22. Adler S, Martinez J, Williams DS, et al. Positive association between blood–brain barrier disruption and osmotically induced demyelination. *Mult Scler.* 2000;6(1):24-31.

23. Baker EA, Tian Y, Adler S, et al. Blood–brain barrier disruption and complement activation in the brain following rapid correction of chronic hyponatremia. *Exp Neurol.* 2000;165(2):221-230.

24. Hew-Butler T, Rosner MH, Fowkes-Godek S, et al. Statement of the third international exercise-associated hyponatremia consensus development conference, Carisbad, California, 2015. *Clin J Sport Med.* 2015;25:303.

25. Sood L, Sterns RH, Hix JK, et al. Hypertonic saline and desmopressin: a simple strategy for safe correction of severe hyponatremia. *Am J Kidney Dis.* 2013;61:571.

26. Mentz RJ, Hasselblad V, DeVore AD, et al. Torsemide versus furosemide in patients with acute heart failure (from the ASCEND-HF Trial). *Am J Cardiol.* 2016;117:404-411.

27. Gheorghiade M, Abraham WT, Albert NM, et al. Relationship between admission serum sodium concentration and clinical outcomes in patients hospitalized for heart failure: an analysis from the OPTIMIZE-HF registry. *Eur Heart J.* 2007;28:980-988.

28. Furst H, Hallows KR, Post J, et al. The urine/plasma electrolyte ratio: a predictive guide to water restriction. *Am J Med Sci.* 2000;319:240-244.

29. Schrier RW, Gross P, Gheorghiade M, et al. Tolvaptan, a selective oral vasopressin V2-receptor antagonist, for hyponatremia. *N Engl J Med.* 2006;355:2099-2112.

30. Zeltser D, Rosansky S, van Rensburg H, et al. Assessment of the efficacy and safety of intravenous conivaptan in euvolemic and hypervolemic hyponatremia. *Am J Nephrol.* 2007;27(5):447-457.

31. Goldsmith SR, Elkayam U, Haught WH, et al. Efficacy and safety of the vasopressin V1A/V2-receptor antagonist conivaptan in acute decompensated heart failure: a dose-ranging pilot study. *J Card Fail.* 2008;14:641-647.

32. Marik PE, Rivera R. Therapeutic effect of conivaptan bolus dosing in hyponatremic neurosurgical patients. *Pharmacotherapy.* 2013;33:51-55.

33. Konstam MA, Gheorghiade M, Burnett JC Jr, et al. Efficacy of vasopressin antagonism in heart failure outcome study with tolvaptan (EVEREST) investigators. Effects of oral tolvaptan in patients hospitalized for worsening heart failure: the EVEREST outcome trial. *JAMA.* 2007;297:1319-1331.

34. Higashihara E, Torres VE, Chapman AB, et al. Tolvaptan in autosomal dominant polycystic kidney disease: three years' experience. *Clin J Am Soc Nephrol.* 2011;6:2499.

35. Torres VE, Chapman AB, Devuyst O, et al. Tolvaptan in patients with autosomal domain polycystic kidney disease. *N Engl J Med.* 2012;367:2407.

36. Dasta JF, Chiong JR, Christian R, Lin J. Evaluation of costs associated with tolvaptan-mediated hospital length of stay reduction among US patients with the syndrome of inappropriate antidiuretic hormone secretion, based on SALT-1 and SALT-2 trials. *Hosp Pract. (1995).* 2012;40:7-14.

# Updates in Management of Complicated Urinary Tract Infections: A Focus on Multidrug-Resistant Organisms

CHAPTER 6

Adrienne H. Ma, PharmD and Gregory J. Hughes, PharmD, BCPS, BCGP

## BACKGROUND

Urinary tract infections (UTIs) are some of the most common infections in both younger and older populations. In 2010, it was one of the foremost reasons for hospital admission in older patients, only behind heart failure, pneumonia, and septicemia.[1] As patients age, the management of UTIs becomes more difficult due to accumulating comorbidities, impairment of organ function, decreased physiologic reserve, increased frequency of reinfection, and higher prevalence of drug-drug interactions.[2] Optimal treatment of UTIs requires knowledge of the pathophysiology, awareness of likely causative organisms, and appropriate use of pharmacologic options.[3]

Types of UTIs vary in terms of severity and symptomatology, described with different sets of nomenclature. Uncomplicated UTIs are those that occur in healthy premenopausal females who lack functional or anatomic abnormalities of the genitourinary systems, whereas all other scenarios are considered complicated. UTIs are also described by anatomic sites. Cystitis refers to infection of the bladder (lower urinary tract) and pyelonephritis refers to infection of the kidney (upper urinary tract). Presentations of UTIs include asymptomatic, local urinary symptoms and can include systemic findings such as sepsis.[3] Asymptomatic bacteriuria has been found in up to 19% of older patients and is generally not associated with adverse outcomes, even without treatment.[4] Older adults in the community and institutional settings do not have a reduction in the development of symptomatic UTIs after treatment of asymptomatic bacteriuria and screening and treatment are therefore not recommended in these patients.[5] Treatment of asymptomatic bacteriuria unnecessarily exposes patients to antibiotics, which can lead to microbial resistance and, in one study, higher recurrence of symptomatic **UTIs**.[6] Catheter-associated **urinary tract infections** (CA-UTIs) are of particular concern because many patients are catheterized inappropriately or chronically, and there is a paucity of available literature on their management.

Risk factors for **UTIs** can be medical, behavioral, and genetic. Increasing age and structural or functional urinary tract impairments that prevent the normal flow of urine are the primary risk factors of **UTIs**. Although premenopausal women experience more **UTIs** than do equivalent aged men, in the older population the incidence of both genders increases and equalizes.[3] Medical conditions such as a history of previous **UTIs**, diabetes, and vaginitis are known risk factors for a new **UTI**.[7] Behaviors such as sexual activity, use of a diaphragm with spermicide, and not voiding before/after intercourse are also associated with **UTIs**.[8] Other etiologies that cause impairment to the flow of urine can include genetic structural abnormalities, trauma from instrumentation, urinary stones, or an enlarged prostate.

In uncomplicated **UTIs**, gram-negative organisms such as *Escherichia coli*, *Proteus mirabilis*, and *Klebsiella pneumoniae* are the common pathogens, with *E. coli* accounting for 75% to 95% of events. For complicated **UTI** and CA-UTI, the most common pathogens include the same gram-negative organisms mentioned, but with *E. coli* being less frequent and a more diverse group of bacteria and fungi such as Serratia, Citrobacter, Enterobacter, *Pseudomonas aeruginosa*, and gram-positives such as Staphylococci and Enterococci. Prolonged duration of catheterization increases reinfection rates and the likelihood that each subsequent infection may be due to new or more resistant organisms. Polymicrobial **UTIs**, increasing resistance rates, and bacteria that produce biofilm make selecting an ideal antimicrobial regimen a difficult task.[9]

# AREAS OF UNCERTAINTY

The difficulties in management of **UTIs** lie with the more complicated patient scenarios. Although management of an uncomplicated **UTI** is relatively straightforward with clear empiric treatment options available, more ambiguity exists in patients with numerous reinfections, infections by resistant organisms, or the sustained need for catheterization. In these scenarios, the clinician is often uncertain whether the patient should even receive antibiotics. Distinguishing asymptomatic bacteriuria from a **UTI**, or sterile pyuria from a **UTI**, can be a difficult task clinically and it is a limitation of the available literature study methodology. In patients who are catheterized for prolonged periods of time, colonization is an important part of **UTI** pathogenesis and decisions on whether or how to reduce colonization are unclear at this time. In the older population, these tasks are even more difficult because of the frequent difficulty in symptom ascertainment.[10]

Interest has been taken in prevention strategies for certain high-risk populations to prevent **UTIs** from recurring. The main pharmacologic options are antibiotics, but cranberry juice, topical estrogens, and probiotics have also been studied.[11]

The role of prophylactic antibiotics is well established in nonpregnant adult patients experiencing multiple **UTIs** per year. A Cochrane Review included 10 trials of various low-dose, continuous antibiotic regimens compared to placebo. The authors concluded that daily antibiotic use had a 0.15 relative risk of clinical recurrence compared to placebo with a number needed-to-treat of 2.2.[12] Alternative antibiotic dosing strategies that have proved effective other than continuous daily dosing include postcoital antibiotic use, in addition to self-start antibiotics because select patients have a very high accuracy in self-diagnosis.[13] Prophylactic antibiotics are not recommended in catheterized patients because of the paucity of evidence and the risks of adverse drug reaction (ADR) and the development of resistance.[10]

One alternative option with a less-established role in prevention of recurrent **UTIs** is cranberry juice. The extract proanthocyanidin in cranberry juice has been shown to reduce the adhesion of *E. coli* to the uroepithelial lining, potentially reducing the risk of **UTIs**.[14] Studies have used cranberry juice in capsule and tablet form containing proanthocyanidin and compared them with placebo, water, antibiotics, and probiotics with contradicting results.[15] A Cochrane Review of 24 studies concluded that there was no benefit to cranberry product supplementation for reduction of symptomatic UTI and the Infectious Diseases Society of America (IDSA) CA-UTI guidelines recommend against the routine use of cranberry products in catheterized or intermittently catheterized patients.[10,15] Probiotics are another appealing strategy that has been studied in many populations for reducing infections, including the development of **UTI**. Probiotics are of interest because they may potentially protect the urinary tract from ascension of pathogenic organisms or their adherence and colonization. There is only a sparse amount of literature available on this topic and it was compiled in a recent Cochrane Review. The authors concluded that there was no significant reduction in the development of recurrent symptomatic bacterial **UTIs** in those who received probiotics compared to placebo.[16]

Antimicrobial resistance is an encroaching global threat affecting not just **UTIs** but across the entire spectrum of infectious diseases. Within the past 5 years, <10 antibacterial agents have been approved by the U.S. Food and Drug Administration (FDA), an approval rating greatly outpaced by other classes of medications.[17] Many of these antibiotics have unique features, making them effective for organisms with specific resistance profiles. The specific nuances of these newer medications and their place in therapy will be reviewed.

# APPROACH TO TREATMENT OF URINARY TRACT INFECTIONS

The challenge of treating the proliferation of extended-spectrum β-lactamase (ESBL) and fluoroquinolone (FQ)-resistant pathogens has burgeoned into an international crisis. In an effort to combat the rise of resistance, uncomplicated **UTI** guidelines further emphasized first-line therapies such as nitrofurantoin (NTF), sulfamethoxazole/trimethoprim (SMZ/TMP), and oral fosfomycin and relegated FQs to last-line therapy (Table 6.1). NTF has shown efficacy against multidrug-resistant (MDR)

**TABLE 6.1** Overview of Empiric First-Line Antimicrobials for Uncomplicated and Complicated UTI[91-114]

| Type | Drug | Dosing | Renal Dose Adjustment | Adverse Side Effects | Commentary (DDIs, etc) |
|---|---|---|---|---|---|
| Uncomplicated UTIs | Sulfamethoxazole/trimethoprim | One 160/800 mg tablet bid for 3 d | 50% decrease if CrCl 15-30 | Nausea, vomiting, rash, and pruritus (usually 7-14 d after start), pseudoelevation of SrCr, hyperkalemia, bone marrow suppression, hepatitis, photosensitivity, acute kidney injury, neurologic toxicity, SJS/TENs | Contraindicated in patients with sulfa allergy |
| | Nitrofurantoin monohydrate/macrocrystal | 100 mg bid for 5 d | FDA – CrCl < 60 – Contraindicated | Brown urine, rash, hypersensitivity (acute pulmonary sx and pneumonitis), pulmonary fibrosis, peripheral neuropathy, hepatitis | Preferred form of NTF is extended release Macrobid, not immediate release Macrodantin |
| | Fosfomycin | 3 g × 1 dose | None | Diarrhea, nausea, dyspepsia, headache, dizziness | Males may be dosed 3 g q72h for 3 doses Antacids and food decrease fosfomycin absorption. |
| Second Line for Uncomplicated UTIs | Levofloxacin | 250 mg po daily for 3 d | CrCl < 20: 250 mg q48h Hemodialysis (HD): 500 mg × 1 dose, then 250 mg q48h after HD | BBW: Tendon rupture, tendinitis, peripheral neuropathy, myalgia, worsening of myasthenia gravis, CNS effects (hallucinations, anxiety, depression, insomnia, severe headaches, confusion) ADRs: Qtc prolongation | Reserve for use in complicated UTIs. FDA warning AGAINST use in uncomplicated UTI, acute bacterial sinusitis, acute bacterial exacerbation of chronic bronchitis. |
| | Ciprofloxacin | 250 mg po bid for 3 days | CrCl 5-29: 250 mg q18h HD: 250 mg q12h or 250 q24h post dialysis | | |

| Complicated UTIs | Ceftriaxone | 1-2 g IV q24h | None | Pseudocholelithiasis/sludging in gallbladder, rash, diarrhea, bone marrow suppression, hemolytic anemia | Do not coadminister with calcium-containing solution. In adults, may flush infusion line thoroughly for sequential use |
|---|---|---|---|---|---|
| | Ampicillin + gentamicin/tobramycin | Ampicillin: 1 to 2 g q4-6h (Adjust for CrCl) Gentamicin/tobramycin: 5 mg/kg IV q24h (extended interval) Or 1.7-2 mg/kg q8h (traditional) (adjust for CrCl) | | Ampicillin: Aminoglycosides: nephrotoxicity, ototoxicity, neurotoxicity | Extended interval dosing for aminoglycosides preferred. Refer to Hartford nomogram for monitoring. |
| | Fluoroquinolones | Levofloxacin 750 mg po for 5 d | CrCl 20-49: 750 mg q48h CrCl < 20: 750 mg × 1, then 500 mg q48h | Refer to second line therapy | Refer to second line therapy |

Allergan. Positive phase III results demonstrate efficacy of antibiotic medicine AVYCAZ™ (Ceftazidime-Avibactam) in complicated urinary tract infections. http://www. allergan.com/news/news/thomson-reuters/positive-phaseiii-results-demonstrate-efficacy-of. Accessed January 14, 2017; Avycaz (R) [package insert]. Verona, Italy: GlaxoSmithKline; 2017; Carmeli Y, Armstrong J, Laud PJ, et al. Ceftazidime-avibactam or best available therapy in patient with ceftazidime-resistant Enterobacteriaceae and Pseudomonas aeruginosa complicated urinary tract infections or complicated intra-abdominal infections: a randomised, pathogen-directed, phase 3 study. Lancet. 2016;16:661-673; Mazuski JE, Gasink LB, Armstrong J, et al. Efficacy and safety of ceftazidime-avibactam plus metronidazole versus meropenem in the treatment of complicated intraabdominal infection. Clin Infect Dis. 2016;62:1380-1389; The Medicines Company. The Medicines Company announces positive top- line results for Phase 3 TANGO 1 clinical trial of Carbavance (Meropenem-Vaborbactam). http://www.themedicinescompany. com/investors/news/medicines-company-announcespositive-top-line-results-phase-3-tango-1-clinical-trial. Accessed January 17, 2017; ClinicalTrials.gov. Safety and efficacy of ZTI-01 (IV Fosfomycin) Vs piperacillin/tazobactam for treatment cUTI/AP infections (ZEUS). https://clinicaltrials.gov/ct2/show/NCT02753946. Accessed February 4, 2017; Garau J. Other antimicrobials of interest in the era of extended-spectrum b-lactamases: fosfomycin, nitrofurantoin and tigecycline. Clin Microbiol Infect. 2008;14:198-202.

Abbreviations: ADRs, adverse drug reactions; BBW, black box warning; bid, twice a day; CNS, central nervous system; CrCl, creatinine clearance; DDIs, drug-drug interactions; FDA, U.S. Food and Drug Administration; NTF, nitrofurantoin; po, orally; SrCr, serum creatinine; SJS/TENs, Stevens-Johnson Syndrome/Toxic Epidermal Necrolysis; UTI, urinary tract infection.

*E. coli* in the outpatient setting.[18] Oral pivmecillinam is also a first-line agent used often in Nordic countries, but unavailable in the United States. The judicious use of antimicrobials starts with outreach and education of providers in the emergency department. In a 439-bed teaching hospital, as a result of an education intervention, appropriate empiric antibiotic selection rates increased from 44.8% to 83% ($n = 350$) (difference, 38.2%, 95% CI, 33-43; $P < 0.001$), although this patient population was young (average 29.5-31.8 years).[19]

The FDA had issued a nationwide safety alert on July 26, 2016, to curtail the overuse of FQs. FQs should be restricted as a last-line option in acute bacterial sinusitis, acute bacterial exacerbation of chronic bronchitis, and uncomplicated UTIs.[20] FQs are far from benign and have a black box warning on disabling and/or permanently debilitating ADRs, including tendon rupture, tendinitis, peripheral neuropathy, myalgia, and worsening of myasthenia gravis.

Healthcare providers, in particular, may now reconsider NTF in elderly women with creatinine clearance (CrCl) > 30 mL/min in light of the 2015 revision of the Beers Criteria. A retrospective chart review of 356 patients in Canada showed that an estimated cure rate of 76% (95% CI, 69-83) versus 75% (95% CI, 69-81) between normal renal function (mean age 67 years, estimated glomerular filtration rate [eGFR], > 50 mL/min) and renal impairment (mean age 86 years, eGFR, ≤ 50 mL/min).[21] No serious side effects due to low renal CrCl were observed. Another retrospective review analyzed the inefficacy and ADR occurrence leading to hospitalization of NTF in comparison with SMZ/TMP in two cohorts ($n = 21\,317$ NTF group, $n = 7926$ SMZ/TMP group). The study found that NTF treatment was not associated with ineffectiveness or in a subgroup of women with moderate renal impairment (30-50 mL/min/1.73 m$^2$ calculated with the Modification of Diet in Renal Disease [MDRD] equation).[22] The only serious ADRs found were pulmonary reactions in 0.16% of the cohort. A third Canadian retrospective chart review ($n = 9223$) analyzed the likelihood of receiving a prescription for a second antibiotic or a hospitalization after being prescribed NTF between women with high eGFR (median 69 mL/min/1.73 m$^2$) or low eGFR (median 38 mL/min/1.73 m$^2$).[23] Similar rates of both outcomes were observed across both groups, although an overall lower efficacy rate in comparison with other FQs and SMZ/TMP was noted. This efficacy rate may be accounted for by lower Canadian rates of resistance against FQs or SMZ/TMP.

UTIs in men should be treated with caution given the complex nature of the infection. In older men, hypertrophy of the prostate may cause urinary retention and turbulent urine flow, predisposing them to chronic prostatitis. The chronically inflamed prostate predisposes men to recurrent UTIs, because of the formation of calculi that entrap bacteria. A retrospective chart review of outpatient male veterans between 2004 and 2013 ($n = 1551$, mean age 73) evaluated the rate of clinical cure and the degree of renal impairment in patients receiving NTF. Although the rates of ADRs did not differ, a minimum CrCl of 60 mL/min was associated with an 80% cure rate.[24] A post hoc modified intention to treat (mITT) and microbiologically evaluable analysis of specifically male and female patients, with complicated UTIs (cUTIs) and without acute pyelonephrosis, showed that a 5-day oral course of levofloxacin 750 mg daily may be considered. They suggest it specifically for outpatient treatment of men with proven susceptible organisms and in an area where resistance to levofloxacin is low.[25]

Complicated lower or upper UTIs (specifically acute pyelonephritis) that necessitate hospitalization will require an induction period of intravenous therapy for at least 48 hours before transitioning to oral agents.[26-29] Initial empiric treatment options include a third-generation cephalosporin, aminoglycoside with ampicillin, or carbapenem and should be chosen in accordance with the local hospital's antibiogram. For patients with penicillin allergies, an aminoglycoside or an FQ may be an appropriate option. Tigecycline is not recommended to treat UTI with sepsis because of the difficulty in maintaining appropriate systemic and urinary levels and a black box warning on increased mortality risk.[26,27] Patients with a history of UTIs or ESBL infections should start with a carbapenem. Ertapenem should not be used for *P. aeruginosa* because of ineffectiveness. In patients with vancomycin-resistant enterococcus UTIs, ampicillin or amoxicillin has been shown to be as effective and represents a less expensive option over linezolid and daptomycin. Patients with vancomycin-resistant enterococcus cystitis may receive treatment with NTF, fosfomycin, or doxycycline depending on sensitivities.[28]

Duration of therapy for complicated cystitis is typically 7 to 10 days and 10 to 14 days for complicated pyelonephritis.[29,30] The optimal duration of therapy is unknown, with a lack of rigorous data assessing when to convert from intravenous to oral therapy. A 2008 double-blind trial did show noninferiority of levofloxacin 750 mg daily for 5 days to ciprofloxacin 400/500 mg twice daily for 10 days for cUTI, although with increasing FQ resistance, the results may no longer be applicable for certain populations.[31]

In light of antibiotic resistance, multidisciplinary antibiotic stewardship programs are recommended nationwide to help guide de-escalation, appropriate oral conversions, and selection of antibiotics. Appropriate selection should consider side effects, drug-drug interactions, dosing regimen, and cost (Table 6.2). Antibiotic therapy should be narrowed when susceptibilities and minimum inhibitory concentrations (MICs) are known. ESBL-producing *E. coli* and ESBL-producing *K. pneumoniae* may be resistant to conventional cephalosporin, FQ, and aminoglycoside therapy. In these cases, NTF and fosfomycin are useful alternatives for acute cystitis.[28] Oral fosfomycin 3 g every other day for three doses has been shown to be noninferior and effective in vitro and also in several retrospective cohort and observational studies for ESBL-Enterobactericiae.[32,33] New antibiotics ceftolozane/tazobactam (CTZ/TZB) and ceftazidime/avibactam (CFT/AVI) should be restricted to third or last line with an identified pathogen and not be used empirically. CFT/AVI should be targeted toward cases of MDR/ESLB-producing *P. aeruginosa*, whereas CTZ/TZB should be aimed at treating ceftazidime-resistant or *K. pneumoniae* carbapenemase (KPCs) strains. Other alter-

**TABLE 6.2 • Overview of Specific Agents and Other Second-line MDR-Resistant Antimicrobial Agents [91-114]**

| Tier | Drug | Dosing | Renal Dose Adjustment | Adverse Side Effects | Comments |
|---|---|---|---|---|---|
| Second Line - Empiric | Piperacillin/Tazobactam | 4.5 g-3.375 g IV q8h | CrCl < 20: 2.25 g IV q8h extended infusion | Rash, diarrhea, bone marrow suppression, acute tubular necrosis | For additional pseudomonas and anaerobic coverage |
| | Aztreonam | 500 mg to 1 g every 8 to 12 h | CrCl 10-30: 50% reduction at usual interval<br><10 and HD: 75% reduction at usual interval | Bone marrow suppression, infusion site reactions, diarrhea, rash, LFT elevations, seizures | For penicillin-allergic patients. Covers pseudomonas and ONLY gram negatives |
| ESBL Pathogens and Other MDR Organisms | Imipenem/Cilastatin | 500 mg IV q6h or 1000 mg q8h (max 4 g/d) | CrCl 30-70: 50% reduction q6-8h<br>CrCl 20-30: 63% reduction q8-12h<br>CrCl 6-20: 75% reduction q12h<br>CrCl <6: Not recommended unless HD within 48 h<br>HD: 75% reduction q12h after dialysis | Seizures, confusion, cross hypersensitivity reaction with penicillin allergy, local phlebitis/thrombophlebitis | Drug of choice for ESBL. Covers pseudomonas and anaerobes. If MIC of meropenem > 16 µg/mL, consider another agent or dual carbapenem-based regimen |
| | Meropenem | 1 g IV q8h. High dose – 2000 mg q8h over 4 h for CRE | CrCl 26-50: 1g q12h<br>CrCl 10-25: 50% reduction q12h<br>CrCl <10: 50% reduction q24h<br>HD: Give additional 1 g after dialysis or dose 1 g q12h post dialysis | | |
| | Aminoglycosides | May consider Amikacin 15-20 mg/kg IV q24h if Gent/Tobra resistant. Refer to extended interval nomogram for monitoring. | | Nephrotoxicity, neurotoxicity, and ototoxicity | Appropriate for combination therapy for CRE infections |
| | Colistin | *Pharmacokinetic dosing*<br>LD: 3.5–4[a] (2.5 µg/mL*) × 2 × ideal body weight<br>[a]Appropriate for organism with MIC ≤ 1 µg/mL<br>Maintenance: 3.5–4[a] (2.5 µg/mL) × 1.5 × CrCl + 30<br>MAX daily dose = 475 mg (divided q12h) | | Nephrotoxicity, neurotoxicity. Avoid coadministering with aminoglycosides | Prodrug colistimethate converted to active colistin, meaning delay with achieving adequate plasma colistin conc. Recommended in combination with tigecycline, carbapenem |

| | Dose | Renal Adjustment | Adverse Effects | Comments |
|---|---|---|---|---|
| **Vancomycin-Resistant Enterococcus** | | | | |
| Tigecycline | 100 mg IV Loading dose, followed by 50 mg IV bid | None | BBW: Increase in all-cause mortality shown in meta-analysis; Vomiting, nausea, hyperbilirubinemia, rash, pancreatitis, hepatitis | Avoid in diabetic foot infections, VAP, and severe infections + bacteremia; Reserve for VRE infections; Only 22% excreted in urine as active drug |
| Ampicillin | 1-2 g IV q4-6h | CrCl 10-50: 1-2 g q6-12h; CrCl < 10: 1-2 g q12-24h; HD: 1-2 g q12-24h post dialysis | Hypersensitivity, rash, diarrhea | Drug of choice for enterococcus; May be switched to oral amoxicillin 500 mg bid |
| Daptomycin | Use ideal body weight 6 mg/kg IV q24h | CrCl < 30: 6 mg/kg q48h; HD: 6 mg/kg q48h after hemodialysis | Rhabdomyolysis | Monitor creatine kinase levels at baseline and weekly and DDIs |
| Linezolid | 600 mg IV or po bid | No empiric adjustment; Give dose after hemodialysis | Long-term bone marrow suppression and peripheral neuropathy; Serotonin syndrome | DDI with SSRIs/SNRIs/TCAs |

New agents ceftazidime/avibactam and ceftolozane/tazobactam are suitable for CRE/KPC-type infections—Refer to Table 6.4

[a] Appropriate for organism with MIC < 1 µg/mL

Cho YH, Jung SI, Chung HS, et al. Antimicrobial susceptibilities of extended-spectrum beta-lactamase-producing Escherichia coli and Klebsiella pneumoniae in health care-associated urinary tract infection: focus on susceptibility to fosfomycin. Int Urol Nephrol. 2015;47:1059-1066; Falagas ME, Kastoris AC, Kapaskelis AM, Karageorgopoulos DE. Fosfomycin for the treatment of multidrug-resistant, including extended-spectrum β-lactamase producing, Enterobacteriaceae infections: a systematic review. Lancet Infect Dis. 2010;10:43-50; ClinicalTrials. gov. Imipenem/relebactam/cilastatin versus piperacillin/tazobactam for treatment of participants with bacterial pneumonia (MK-7655A-014) (RESTORE-IMI 2). https://www.clinicaltrials. gov/ct2/show/NCT02493764?term5relebactam&rank52. Accessed January 17, 2017; ClinicalTrials.gov. Efficacy and safety of imipenem + cilastatin/relebactam (MK-7655A) versus colisti-methate sodium + imipenem + cilastatin in imipenem-resistant bacterial infection (MK-7655A-013) (RESTORE-IMI 1). https://www.clinicaltrials.gov/ct2/show/NCT02452047?term5rele-bactam&rank51. Accessed January 17, 2017; Toussaint KA, Gallagher JC. β-lactam/β-lactamase inhibitor combinations: from then to now. Ann Pharmacother. 2015;49:86-98; Tetraphase Pharmaceuticals, Inc.. Tetraphase announces top line results from IGNITE2 phase 3 clinical trial of eravacycline in cUTI. http://ir.tphase.com/releasedetail.cfm?releaseid5930613. Accessed January 17, 2017; Solomkin J, Evans D, Slepavicius A, et al. Assessing the efficacy and safety of eravacycline vs ertapenem in complicated intra-abdominal infections in the investigating gram-negative infections treated with eravacycline (IGNITE 1) trial: a randomized clinical trial. JAMA Surg. 2017;152:224-232; Aggen JB, Armstrong ES, Goldblum AA, et al. Synthesis and spectrum of the neoglycoside ACHN-490. Antimicrob Agents Chemother. 2010;54:4636-4642.

Abbreviations: BBW, bid, twice a day; CrCl, creatinine clearance; CRE, carbapenem-resistant Enterobacteriaceae; DDIs, ESBL, extended-spectrum beta lactamase; HD, hemodialysis; IV, intravenous; KPC, Klebsiella pneumoniae carbapenemase; LD, loading dose; LFT, liver function test; MDR, multidrug-resistant; po, orally; SNRIs, serotonin–norepinephrine reuptake inhibitors; SSRI, selective serotonin reuptake inhibitors; TCAs, tricyclic antidepressants ; VAP, ventilator-associated pneumonia; VRE, Vancomycin-resistant enterococcus.

native ways of treating KPCs also include dual gentamicin/carbapenem and colistin/polymixin B with a carbapenem on the basis of limited cohort and case review data (Table 6.3).[34-37] Patients with a penicillin allergy may need to resort to tigecycline ± colistin–based therapy for treatment of KPCs.[37]

## Special Patient Populations: Catheter-Associated Urinary Tract Infections and Fungal Urinary Infections

### Catheter-Associated Urinary Tract Infections

The FDA has placed new emphasis on infection control to prevent the incidence of inappropriate catheter use. The Comprehensive Unit-Based Safety Program was tested in 603 hospitals nationwide and was found to reduce catheter use and rates of catheter-associated **urinary tract infections** (CA-UTIs) in all non-ICU units.[10] This result coupled with a 2016 Cochrane Review on policies for replacing long-term indwelling urinary catheters implies that ICU and long-term nursing home CA-UTI management requires further research or individual institution fine tuning.[38] The 2014 Update on CA-UTI prevention recommends against antimicrobial-impregnated catheters. In the UK Catheter Trial, there was no statistically significant clinical difference between a standard latex catheter, a latex silver alloy–coated catheter, and a silicone nitrofurazone–impregnated catheter.[39] The small difference found with the nitrofurazone silicone catheter used may be due to either the silicone or nitrofurazone component (odds ratio [OR], 0.68; 97.5% CI, 0.48-0.99; $P = 0.017$). Condom catheters may be a safer option than indwelling options except in the case of men with a smaller penile size, skin ulceration, or neurogenic bladders due to spinal cord injury. Further, perioperative indwelling catheters should be removed as soon as possible.

Given the significantly higher rates of MDR organisms in this population, treatment of CA-UTI should only proceed after ruling out other causes, because pyuria in this population may not be indicative of infection. Indeed, treatment of asymptomatic bacteriuria is only appropriate in patients at a high risk of complications (ie, acute pyelonephritis, bloodstream infections).[40,41] Catheters should also not be regularly irrigated with antimicrobials or changed. Empiric treatment should assume to cover multiple MDR organisms, because data support two or more organisms causing infection. Of note, the likelihood of Proteus infection increases with the duration of indwelling catheter and in obstructed catheters. Proteus species are known for producing greater amounts and more persistent biofilms because of their ability to produce urease at rates greater than those of other species.[41] The 2009 guidance on CA-UTIs suggests a 7-day treatment duration if symptoms resolve quickly or 10 to 14 days if the patient seems to heal slowly. A 3-day duration of treatment is generally not appropriate for women 65 years or older. Candida has also been attributed to 28% of CA-UTIs reported in ICUs, but has not been known to cause complications.[40] Should candidemia truly be suspected, the 2016 IDSA guidelines have been updated to support the use of either an echinocandin (ie, micafungin 100 mg daily, caspofungin loading dose (LD) 70 mg, then 50 mg daily, anidulafungin LD 200 mg, then 100 mg daily or fluconazole intravenous or oral LD 800 mg (12 mg/kg) then 400 mg (6 mg/kg) daily, as first-line agents in nonneutropenic patients.[42] In neutropenic patients, an echinocandin is considered as efficacious as liposomal amphotericin B, but safer, and treatment duration should be approximately 14 days.

# NEW THERAPIES

As we consider the treatment of complicated UTIs and MDR pathogens, additional antibiotics have arrived in our arsenal for the treatment of UTI with sepsis. Two recent cephalosporin/β-lactamase inhibitors in the US market are CTZ/TZB and CFT/AVI.[43,44] Both of these drugs were fast-tracked and approved on the basis of phase II data and without the completion of all phase III trials. Pipeline drugs pending approval are the following: fosfomycin sodium (intravenous formulation), aztreonam-AVI, imipenem/cilastatin/relebactam, eravacycline, and plazomicin.

CTZ/TZB is a novel parenteral antibiotic comprising a cephalosporin/β-lactamase inhibitor. An aminothiadiazole ring at the 7-position side chain of CTZ confers enhanced gram-negative activity against *P. aeruginosa*, whereas a pyrazolium ring at the 3-position protects against hydrolysis of the β-lactam ring by AmpC β-lactamase via steric hindrance.[45-47] Tazobactam provides irreversible inhibition of certain ESBL-producing Enterobacteriaceae. CTZ/TZB is bactericidal and works by inhibiting bacterial cell wall synthesis through binding penicillin-binding proteins (PBPs). In particular, it binds PBP1b, PBP1c, and PBP3 exhibited by *P. aeruginosa* and PBP3 exhibited by *E. coli*. However, the lack of PBP4 exhibited by *P. aeruginosa* renders CTZ/TZB a weak inducer of AmpC expression.[45,48] CTZ/TZB remains susceptible to metallo-β-lactamase and KPCs.[45,49]

CTZ/TZB's pivotal evidence comes from aggregated data from the Assessment of the Safety Profile and Efficacy of ceftolozane/tazobactam-complicated UTI (ASPECT-cUTI) and ASPECT-complicated intra-abdominal infections (cIAI) trials.[50,51] In the ASPECT-cUTI phase III double-blind, double-dummy, noninferiority randomized controlled trial (RCT), evaluated hospitalized patients ($n = 1083$) diagnosed with pyelonephritis or complicated UTI (cUTI) received either CTZ/TZB 1.5 g intravenously every 8 hours or high-dose levofloxacin 750 mg intravenously every day for 7 days. Of this, 25.1% and 24.6% of the CTZ/TZB and levofloxacin arms, respectively, included patients over the age of 65 years. The composite cure of CTZ/TZB was found to be noninferior to levofloxacin (306/398 [76.9%] CTZ/TZB arm versus 275/402 [68.4%], 95% CI, 2.3-14.6). Notably, the protocol did not include attempts to convert to oral antibiotics. CTZ/TZB is also approved for treatment of cIAI in combination with metronidazole 500 mg intravenously every 8 hours and another ongoing phase III ASPECT-NP (nosocomial pneumonia) with CTZ/TZB 3 g intravenously every 8 hours is due to be completed in 2018.[52] Overall, CTZ/TZB is well tolerated, with nausea, diarrhea, headache, infusion-related reactions, and pyrexia as the most common side effects. Incidences of adverse events were similar between 185/533 (34.7%) of

**TABLE 6.3 • Overview of New Agents**[42-71,91-114]

| Drug | Dosing | Renal Dose Adjustment | Adverse Side Effects | Commentary |
|---|---|---|---|---|
| Ceftolozane/tazo-bactam (Zerbaxa) | 2.5 g q8h | CrCl 30-50: 750 mg q8h<br>CrCl 15-29: 375 mg q8h<br>HD: LD 750 mg following by 150 mg q8h post dialysis | Nausea, diarrhea, headache, fever, renal impairment | Covers ESBLs |
| Ceftazidime/avi-bactam (Avycaz) | 1.5g q8h | CrCl 31-50: 1.25 g q8h<br>CrCl 16-30: 0.94 g q12h<br>CrCl 6-15: 0.94 g q24h<br>CrCl < 5 or HD: 0.95 g q48h post dialysis | Seizures, consti-pation, diarrhea, nausea, vomiting, anxiety | Covers KPCs Approved for cIAI with metronida-zole and cUTIs |
| IV Fosfomycin | Optimal dosing not determined IV 1-16 daily div-ided q6-12h | Not determined. Cap of 16 g suggested for patients on renal replacement therapy | IV: Hypokale-mia(26%), local pain, heart failure | Pending FDA approval |
| Meropenem/vaborbactam (Vabomere) | 4 g q8h over 3 h infusion | Yes<br>eGFR 30-49: 2 g q8h<br>eGFR 15-29: 2 g q12h<br>eGFR < 15: 1 g q12h | Seizures, head-ache, phlebitis, diarrhea | Approved for cUTIs |
| Imipenem/Cilas-tatin/Relebactam | 200/100 mg to 500/250 mg q6h over 30 min | Yes—exact adjust-ment pending | Thrombocytosis, nausea, headache, decreased creati-nine clearance | Undergoing phase III trials |
| Cefiderocol | 2 g q8h over 1 h infusion | Yes—exact adjust-ment pending | Diarrhea, *Clostridi-um. difficile* colitis | Pending FDA approval |
| Plazomicin | 15 mg/kg q24h | Yes—exact adjust-ment pending | Nephrotoxicity, neurotoxicity, ototoxicity | Aminoglyco-side-pending FDA approval |

Abbreviations: cIAI = complicated intra-abdominal infection; CrCl, creatinine clearance; cUTIs, complicated urinary tract infection; eGFR, estimated glomerular filtration rate; ESBLs, extended-spectrum β-lactamase; FDA, U.S. Food and Drug Admin-istration; HD, hemodialysis; IV, intravenous; KPCs, *Klebsiella pneumoniae* carbapenemases; LD, loading dose.

CTZ/TZB arm and 184/535 (34.4%) of levofloxacin arm. However, serious episodes of *Clostridium difficile* infection were reported in both clinical trials (rate <1%).

The second newcomer is AVI, available in combination with CFT and currently under phase II trials in combination with aztreonam.[53,54] Trial data intriguingly show efficacy against previously resistant ceftazidime infections. AVI represents a unique, new, non–β-lactam-based approach, where a diazabicyclooctane moiety forms an important carbamate linkage after binding the active β-lactamase (β-L) inhibitor and initiates additional strong hydrogen bonds. The inhibition of the β-L enzyme is further strengthened by the displacement of water molecules, meaning that unlike other conventional β-L inhibitors, the inhibited β-L complex cannot be broken by hydrolysis, only reversed by deacylation.[55,56] In fact, upon deacylation of this intermediate structure, AVI reverts to the original active compound and is ready to defend its cephalosporin component again.[56] With this mechanism of action, AVI exhibits potent inhibition against Ambler class A carbapenemases (includes KPCs) and Class C and Class D OXA-48 carbapenemase. CFT/AVI has little or no activity against anaerobic, gram-positive organisms, Stenotrophomonas, and Ambler class B metallo-β-lactamases.[55,57,58] P. aeruginosa has varying susceptibility to CFT/AVI, and Acinetobacter is resistant against CFT/AVI.

CFT/AVI is now approved for treatment of cUTIs and in combination with metronidazole for cIAI. The efficacy and safety of CFT/AVI has been shown in three phase III trials: REPROVE, REPRISE, RECAPTURE.[50,59,60] REPRISE ($n = 333$) was a phase III open-label RCT that randomized patients with either ceftazidime-resistant cIAI ($n = 21$) or cUTI ($n = 281$) to either CFT/AVI 2.5 g intravenously every 8 hours or best available therapy (97% carbapenem) for 5 to 21 days. The average age of REPRISE cUTI arms was 64.3 (SD: 14.6) and 61.3 (SD: 15.3), respectively, with 26% of the CFT/AVI and 20% of best available therapy between 75 and 90 years. According to microbial mITT analysis, 140/154 (90.9%) (95% CI, 85.6-94.7) of the CFT/AVI group and 135/148 (91.2%) (95% CI, 85.9-95) of the best available group achieved clinical cure 21 to 35 days after initiation of therapy. RECAPTURE primarily assessed CFT/AVI 2.5 g intravenously every 8 hours ($n = 393$) against doripenem 500 mg intravenously every 8 hours ($n = 417$) in patients with cUTI to measure the proportion with symptomatic resolution at visit day 5 without or with pathogen eradication at test-of-cure visit (21-25 days post initiation), respectively. Patients could be switched to oral antibiotics after 5 days of treatment. The trial analyzed a younger population with average age 51.4 (SD: 20.2) and 53.3 (18.6), respectively, in the treatment and comparator groups. Noninferiority was achieved with total cure rate at 280/293 (71.2%) in the CFT/AVI group and 269/417 (64.5%) in the doripenem group (difference, 6.7%, 95% CI, 0.3-13.2). Trial data show that the most common ADRs are nausea, vomiting, and diarrhea (rates $< 3\%$), with cases of C. difficile infection reported in the CFT/AVI arm. However, ceftazidime must be dose-adjusted for renal clearance due to neurotoxicity (eg, seizures, encephalopathy). It may also interact with probenecid.[58]

Specifically, in patients with carbapenem-resistant Enterobacteriaceae (CRE) bloodstream infections, CFT/AVI has been shown to be clinically and statistically advantageous in comparison with the best available treatment options. In rates of 30-day clinical successes, CFT/AVI treatment was associated with an 11/13 (85%) success rate in comparison with 12/25 (48%) ($P = 0.04$) with carbapenems, 12/30 (40%) ($P = 0.009$) with aminoglycosides, and 15/41 (37%) ($P = 0.004$) with carbapenem[61] and colistin.

The CFT/AVI group contained 5/13 patients who received short-term gentamicin (median duration 4 days, range 3-7 days). Rates of success with monotherapy and combination CFT/AVI therapy were 6/8 (75%) and 5/5 (100%), respectively.

Both CTZ/TZB and CFT/AVI have had published[61-63] reports of resistance in *Klebsiella pneumoniae* and MDR *P. aeruginosa*, implying that these agents should be used judiciously and placed on restricted formulary as last-line agents. Alarmingly, a retrospective case analysis at the University of Pittsburg Medical Center showed that resistance to CFT/AVI (MIC > 8 mcg/mL) developed within 10 to 19 days in 3/10 (30%) of microbiologic failure subgroup patients infected with CRE[64] out of an overall failure rate of 27% (10/37). This cohort consisted of patients with median age 64 years (range 26-78) and 30% of transplant recipients.

Meropenem/vaborbactam (M-V) has recently become the first antibiotic marketed specifically for CRE. Vaborbactam is the first novel cyclic boronic inhibitor designed specifically against serine carbapenemases, also known as KPCs. The addition of vaborbactam 4 µg/mL in vitro has been effective in suppressing class A and class B carbapenemases, but failed to restore potency against class B metallo-β-lactamases and class D OXA-48 carbapenemases. Vaborbactam remains vulnerable to mutations in the OmpK35/36 porins, which normally allows vaborbactam into the cell.[58]

The Targeting Antibiotic Nonsusceptible Gram-negative Organisms (TANGO-I) phase III trial specifically for cUTIs has been published. By mITT analysis, meropenem 2 g/vaborbactam 2 g intravenously every 8 hours overall success rates (189/192 (98.4%)) is noninferior to piperacillin/tazobactam 4.5 g intravenously every 8 hours (171/182 (94%)) (difference 4.5% [95% CI, 0.7% to 9.1%], $P < 0.001$). Pip/TZB was not given as an extended infusion. Overall success is defined as a composite of clinical cure and improvement and microbial eradication. Of note, TANGO-I only had 19.5% (30/154) patients who were nonsusceptible to piperacillin/tazobactam[65-67] and five CRE patients. The targeted TANGO-II trial, which tested M-V ($n = 28$) against the best available therapy against CRE ($n = 15$), was stopped early for superior efficacy results. Best available therapy included myriad options such as carbapenem, aminoglycoside, polymyxin B, colistin, tigecycline alone or in combination,[68] or CFT/AVI alone. A staggering difference was noted in all-cause mortality at day 28 in patients with cUTI/acute pyelonephritis of 4/15 (25%) in the M-V group and 4/9 (44.4%) in the best available therapy group. Overall success at end of therapy was 8/11 (72%) in the M-V group and 2/4 (50%) in the best available therapy group.[69]

Parenteral fosfomycin disodium is also making its way from the European markets to the FDA, with the phase III trial ZEUS.[70] The drug has been available as generic in the United Kingdom since 2013 and brand name 2 g since May 8, 1980, and 8 g since December 28, 2006.[71] Fosfomycin works in a unique pathway by which it exerts a bactericidal action by inhibiting phosphoenolpyruvate transferase, an earlier step in peptidoglycan synthesis, and thereby bacterial cell wall inhibition.[32,72] Its spectrum of activity is the most extensive out of the new agents, including the following: methicillin-resistant Staphylococcus, vancomycin-resistant Enterococcus, *P. aeruginosa*,

*E. coli*, and against ESBL-producing *K. Pneumoniae* and *E. coli*, and *Proteus mirabilis*, metallo-β-lactamase-producing pathogens, and KPCs. Listeria monocytogenes and Bacteroides fragilis are resistant against fosfomycin. The efficacy of fosfomycin against ESBL and KPCs has been shown in multiple case studies, and several observational/prospective or retrospective inpatient studies of parenteral fosfomycin in ESBL and KPCs have shown good outcomes in combination with colistin or other antibiotics.[32,33,60,71-73] Dose of fosfomycin used ranged from 2 to 8 g intravenously three to four times a day with a cap of 16 g for patients on renal replacement therapy. It has been used at least once in the United States through successful New Drug Application (NDA) to the FDA.

Finally, imipenem-cilastatin-relebactam (I-C-R), plazomicin, and cefiderocol are future antimicrobials under consideration. Currently tested in phase III RESTORE trials, relebactam falls under the same mechanism of action as does AVI[73,60] and is effective against class A and class C β-lactamases.[74,75] However, in vitro data show that relebactam has a narrower spectrum of activity and is not effective against class D enzymes (eg, OXA-48 enzymes) or imipenem-resistant *Acinetobacter baumannii*, *Stenotrophomonas*, and most anaerobes. I-C-R has passed two phase II trials in cUTI and cIAIs and established noninferiority to imipenem/cilastatin alone.[76-78] Significant ADRs leading to discontinuation of therapy include decreased CrCl, thrombocytosis, nausea, and increased alanine transaminase (ALT). Two phase III trials (RESTORE-IMI 1) for bacterial pneumonia compared to piperacillin/tazobactam with linezolid and RESTORE-IMI 2 for imipenem-nonsusceptible cIAI compared to colistimethate sodium plus imipenem/cilastatin are ongoing.[79,80]

Eravacycline, a fluorocycline relative of tetracycline,[81] has fallen out of favor because of both the inferior results of the Investigating Gram-Negative Infections Treated with Eravacycline (IGNITE 2) phase III trial and IGNITE-3 trial that specifically tested the intravenous-only formulation.[82] The parenteral to oral regimen where patients could convert to oral antibiotics after 3 days of eravacycline 1 g intravenously daily was inferior to levofloxacin 750 mg daily; whereas in IGNITE-3, it failed to show noninferiority to ertapenem for treatment of cUTI.[83]

The next-generation aminoglycoside, plazomicin, has been modified to resist inactivation by O-adenylylation, O-phosphorylation, or N-acetylation, but it should also be viewed with caution.[84] In a multicenter, randomized, double-blind phase 2 study, patients ($n = 145$) were randomized to either plazomicin 10 mg/kg, 15 mg/kg or levofloxacin 750 mg daily. By mITT analysis, at 5 to 12 days after the last day, 66.7%, 70.6%, and 65.5% of patients met[85] criteria for clinical cure, respectively. In the Evaluating Plazomicin in cUTI (EPIC trial), preliminary results showed an 89.5% (171/191) versus 74.6% (147/197) microbiological eradication rate (95% CI 7.0-22.7) in comparison with meropenem 15 to 19 days after initiation of therapy. At follow up, 24 to 32 days later, 1.8% (3/170) versus 7.9% (14/178)[86] of the meropenem group experienced clinical relapse. Specifically, in aminoglycoside-resistant to amikacin, gentamicin, and tobramycin enterobacteriaceae, plazomicin achieved a

78.8% (41/52) eradication at test of cure (15 to 19 days after start of therapy).[88,89] Two cases of reversible ototoxicity were noted in both study groups, with 3.7% (11/300) of plazomicin-treated patients developing a >0.5 mg/dL increase in serum creatinine. In the Combating Antibiotic-Resistant Enterobacteriaceae (CARE) phase 3 trial, plazomicin 15 mg/kg daily over 30 minutes ($n = 18$) was evaluated against colistin alone ($n = 21$) for patients with known or suspected CRE bloodstream infections in two cohorts—one randomized ($n = 39$) and one observational.[83,87] In the randomized cohort, all-cause mortality at day 28 or significant complications was 23.5% (4/17) in the plazomicin group versus 50.0% (10/20) in the colistin-only treated group. Results should be treated with caution because colistin is typically used in combination with either carbapenem or tigecycline in CRE bloodstream infections. Patients with coinfections of non-Enterobacteriaceae gram-negative pathogens (ie, *P. aeruginosa*, *Acinetobacter* spp) were excluded.[88]

Finally, a new class of cephalosporins known as the siderophore cephalosporins may emerge and provide[89-91] the broadest spectrum of action with activity against all classes of β-lactamases and carbapenem-resistant *A. baumannii*, *P. aeruginosa*, and *Stenotrophomonas maltophilia*. Cefiderocol (S-649266) is a unique cephalosporin with an attached catechol moiety on the 3-position side chain. The catechol group facilitates the formation of a cefiderocol-iron complex. This complex takes advantage of the bacterial ferric iron active transporter system and delivers cefiderocol into the bacterium for subsequent cell way synthesis inhibition. Cefiderocol has completed both a targeted carbapenem-resistant phase II trial (CREDIBLE-CR) and phase III trial (APEKS-cUTI) successfully. APEKS-cUTI evaluated cefiderocol 2 g parenterally against imipenem/ cilastatin 1 g every 8 hours for 7 to 14 days in a multicenter, double-blind randomized phase III trial without any oral step-down antibiotics. Cefiderocol achieved a 183/252 (72.6%) composite of clinical and microbiological response rates over 65/119 (54.6%) that of the imipenem group. The clinical response rate between two agents was similar at 226/252 (89.7%) and 104/119 (87.4%), respectively. *C. difficile colitis* cases were reported in both groups. However, data for specifically in vivo efficacy rates in comparison with current standards of therapy for CRE pathogens have not been published.

**UTIs** with specific class B metalloproteases remain a challenge, but developing drugs to address this challenge include zidebactam and aztreonam with avibactam.[92,93] Other drugs that may come to fruition also include BAL30072, a siderophore monosulfactam (no ongoing trials) and finafloxacin.[94-96]

# CONCLUSIONS

From physicians to pharmacists to nurses, all healthcare providers play a pivotal role in managing the appropriate empiric use and de-escalation of antibiotic treatment of uncomplicated and complicated **UTIs**. Antibiotic stewardship committees are essential for inpatient management on all emergency department, internal medicine, and surgical and specialty floors to ensure that inappropriate use of antimicrobials does not increase the prevalence of MDR pathogens. SMZ/TMP, NTF, and fosfomycin are effective first-line agents for uncomplicated **UTIs**, particularly in the emergency department setting. For ESBLs or MDR acute cystitis, NTF and fosfomycin are still effective agents because of high urine concentrations and unique mechanisms of action. For **UTIs** with sepsis due to ESBLs or carbapenem-resistant Enterobacteriaceae-producing pathogens, carbapenems are the first line while ampicillin still remains a strong alternative for VRE infections. Older antibiotics like colistin/polymixin or newer antibiotics such as CTZ/TZB for MDR pseudomonas or CFT/AVI for carbapenem-resistant Enterobacteriaceae may be necessary for highly resistant cases and dependent on the basis of the type of β-lactamase involved.

# SUMMARY

UTI treatment can be difficult in the geriatric population. These patients often require a more nuanced approach because of recurrent, resistant, and catheter-associated infections. Although some attempts have been made to prevent **UTIs** using cranberry products, probiotics, and nonpharmacologic means, current interest lies largely with the development of new antibiotics to treat increasingly resistant organisms.

Efforts to reduce the development of resistance start with judicious and appropriate empiric use of antibiotics. FQs are no longer recommended as first-line therapy because of adverse reactions and the development of resistance. Complicated and upper **UTIs** require broader empiric coverage, and measures should be taken to de-escalate treatment as early as possible. **Antimicrobial stewardship** programs are recommended to aid in these efforts in addition to antibiotic selection in the presence of **multidrug-resistant organisms** such as those producing extended-spectrum β-lactamase or carbapenemase. **Multidrug-resistant organisms** are often present in catheter-associated **UTIs**, so broad empiric coverage should be initially started. Catheter-associated **UTIs** should generally be treated for 7 to 14 days depending on the rate of clinical improvement, and fungal coverage is often also necessary. Ceftolozane/tazobactam, ceftazidime/avibactam, and meropenem/vaborbactam were recently approved in the United States for treating **multidrug-resistant organisms**; and several more agents are in development, such as parenteral fosfomycin. Ceftolozane/tazobactam is effective in treating *P. aeruginosa* and other gram-negative organisms, even those that produce extended-spectrum beta-lactamases. Ceftazidime/avibactam is effective solely for gram-negative organisms, including those that produce various carbapenemases, but efficacy for *P. aeruginosa* is variable. Both combinations are approved for complicated **UTIs** in addition to cIAIs. Several medications are currently in the pipeline to treat **multidrug-resistant organisms**. Meropenem/vaborbactam was approved for complicated **UTIs** and its coverage includes carbapenem-resistant Enterobacteriaceae. Fosfomycin, currently available orally and first line for uncomplicated **UTIs**, is being evaluated for intravenous use for methicillin-resistant Staphylococcus, vancomycin-resistant Enterococcus, and gram-negative bacilli that produce both extended-spectrum β-lactamase and carbapenemase.

UTIs are a common cause of hospitalization in older adults. Antibiotic selection and **antimicrobial stewardship** programs are important given the increasing prevalence of **multidrug-resistant organisms**.

## References

1. Pfuntner A, Wier LM, Stocks C. *Most Frequent Conditions in U.S. Hospitals, 2010*. HCUP Statistical Brief #148. January 2013. Rockville, MD: Agency for Healthcare Research and Quality; 2010. https://www.hcup-us.ahrq.gov/reports/statbriefs/sb148.pdf. Accessed January 28, 2017.

2. Hughes GJ, Beizer JL. Appropriate prescribing. In: Ham RJ, Sloane PG, Warshaw GA, et al, eds. *Ham's Primary Care Geriatrics: A Case-Based Approach*. 6th ed. Philadelphia, PA: Elsevier; 2014:67-76.

3. Coyle EA, Prince RA. Chapter 94. Urinary tract infections and prostatitis. In: DiPiro JT, Talbert RL, Yee GC, et al, eds. *Pharmacotherapy: A Pathophysiologic Approach*. 9th ed. New York, NY: McGraw-Hill; 2014.

4. Nicolle LE. Asymptomatic bacteriuria: when to screen and when to treat. *Infect Dis Clin North Am*. 2003;17:367-394.

5. Nicolle LE, Bradley S, Colgan R, Rice JC, Schaeffer A, Hooton TM. Infectious Diseases Society of America guidelines for the diagnosis and treatment of asymptomatic bacteriuria in adults. *Clin Infect Dis*. 2005;40:643-654.

6. Cai T, Nesi G, Mazzoli S, et al. Asymptomatic bacteriuria treatment is associated with a higher prevalence of antibiotic resistant strains in women with urinary tract infections. *Clin Infect Dis*. 2016;61:1655-1661.

7. Marques LP, Flores JT, Barros O, et al. Epidemiological and clinical aspects of urinary tract infection in community-dwelling elderly women. *Braz J Infect Dis*. 2012;16:436-441.

8. Foxman B, Chi JW. Health behavior and urinary tract infection in college-aged women. *J Clin Epidemiol*. 1990;43:329-337.

9. Nicolle LE. Catheter-related urinary tract infection. *Drugs Aging*. 2005;22:627-639.

10. Hooton TM, Bradley SF, Cardenas DD, et al. Diagnosis, prevention, and treatment of catheter-associated urinary tract infections in adults: 2009 International clinical practice guidelines from the Infectious Diseases Society of America. *Clin Infect Dis*. 2010;50:625-663.

11. Nicolle LE. Urinary tract infections in the older adult. *Clin Geriatr Med*. 2016;32:523-538.

12. Albert X, Huertas I, Pereiró II, et al. Antibiotics for preventing recurrent urinary tract infection in non-pregnant women. *Cochrane Database Syst Rev*. 2004:CD001209.

13. Gupta K, Hooton TM, Roberts PL, et al. Patient-initiated treatment of uncomplicated recurrent urinary tract infections in young women. *Ann Intern Med*. 2001;135:9-16.

14. Lavigne JP, Bourg G, Combescure C, et al. In-vitro and in-vivo evidence of dose-dependent decrease of uropathogenic Escherichia coli virulence after consumption of commercial Vaccinium macrocarpon (cranberry) capsules. *Clin Microbiol Infect*. 2008;14:350-355.

15. Jepson RG, Williams G, Craig JC. Cranberries for preventing urinary tract infections. *Cochrane Database Syst Rev*. 2012;17:10.

16. Schwenger EM, Tejani AM, Loewen PS. Probiotics for preventing urinary tract infections in adults and children. *Cochrane Database Syst Rev*. 2015:CD008772.

17. U.S. Food and Drug Administration. Novel Drug Approvals for 2017. http://www.fda.gov/Drugs/DevelopmentApprovalProcess/DrugInnovation/ ucm537040.htm Accessed January 31, 2017.

18. Sanchez GV, Baird AM, Karlowsky JA, et al. Nitrofurantoin retains antimicrobial activity against multidrug-resistant urinary Escherichia coli from US outpatients. *J Antimicrob Chemother*. 2014;69:3259-3262.

19. Percival KM, Valenti KM, Schmittling SE, et al. Impact of an antimicrobial stewardship intervention on urinary tract infection treatment in the ED. *Am J Emerg Med*. 2015;33:1129-1133.

20. U.S. Food & Drug Administration. FDA Drug Safety Communication: FDA updates warnings for oral and injectable fluoroquinolone antibiotics due to disabling side effects. http://www.fda.gov/Drugs/DrugSafety/ucm511530.htm. Accessed January 10, 2017.

21. Bains A, Buna D, Hoag NA. A retrospective review assessing the efficacy and safety of nitrofurantoin in renal impairment. *Can Pharm J.* 2009;142:248-252.

22. Geerts FJ, Eppenga WL, Heerdink R, et al. Ineffectiveness and adverse events of nitrofurantoin in women with urinary tract infection and renal impairment in primary care. *Eur J Clin Pharmacol.* 2013;69:1701-1707.

23. Singh N, Gandhi S, McArthur E, et al. Kidney function and the use of nitrofurantoin to treat urinary tract infections in older women. *CMAJ.* 2015;187:648-656.

24. Ingalsbe ML, Wojciechowski AL, Smith KA, et al. Effectiveness and safety of nitrofurantoin in outpatient male veterans. *Ther Adv Urol.* 2015;7:186-193.

25. Mospan GA, Wargo KA. 5-Day versus 10-day course of fluoroquinolones in outpatient males with a urinary tract infection (UTI). *J Am Board Fam Med.* 2016;29:654-662.

26. Thaden JT, Pogue JM, Kaye KS. Role of newer and reemerging older agents in the treatment of infections caused by carbapenem-resistant Enterobacteriaceae. *Virulence.* 2016;6:1-14.

27. Pallett A, Hand K. Complicated urinary tract infections: practical solutions for the treatment of multiresistant Gram-negative bacteria. *J Antimicrob Chemother.* 2010;65(suppl 3):iii25-iii33.

28. Heintz BH, Halilovic J, Christensen CL. Vancomycin-resistant enterococcal urinary tract infections. *Pharmacotherapy.* 2010;30:1136-1149.

29. Gupta K, Hooton TM, Naber KG. International clinical practice guidelines for the treatment of acute uncomplicated cystitis and pyelonephritis in women. Clin Infect Dis. 2011;52:e103-e120.

30. Badalato G, Kaufmann M: Adult UTI. American Urological Association Website. https://www .auanet.org/education/auauniversity/education-and-career-resources/for-medical-students/ medical-student-curriculum/adult-uti. Accessed January 15, 2017.

31. Peterson J, Kaul S, Khashab M, Fisher AC, Kahn JB. A double-blind, randomized comparison of levofloxacin 750 mg once-daily for five days with ciprofloxacin 400/500 mg twice-daily for 10 days for the treatment of complicated urinary tract infections and acute pyelonephritis. *Urology.* 2008;71:17-22.

32. Reffert JL, Smith WJ. Fosfomycin for the treatment of resistant gram-negative bacterial infections. *Pharmacotherapy.* 2014;34:845-857.

33. Veve MP, Wagner JL, Kenney RM, et al. Comparison of fosfomycin to ertapenem for outpatient or step-down therapy of extended-spectrum β-lactamase urinary tract infections. *Int J Antimicrob Agents.* 2016;48:56-60.

34. Nation Rl, Velkov TY, Li J, et al. Peas in a pod, or chalk and cheese? *Clin Infect Dis.* 2014;59:88-94.

35. Morrill H, Pogue JM, Kaye KS, et al. Treatment options for carbapenem-resistant Enterobacteriaceae infections. *Open Forum Infect Dis.* 2015;2:ofv050.

36. Lee GC, Burgess DS. Treatment of Klebsiella pneumonia carbapenemase (KPC) infections: a review of published case series and case reports. *Ann Clin Microbiol Antimicrob.* 2012;11:32.

37. Hirsch EB, Tam VH. Detection and treatment options for Klebsiella pneumoniae carbapenemases (KPCse): an emerging cause of multidrug-resistant infection. *J Antimicrob Chemother.* 2010;65:1119-1125.

38. Saint S, Greene T, Krein S, et al. A program to prevent catheter-associated urinary tract infection in acute care. *N Engl J Med.* 2016;374:2111-2119.

39. Pickard R, Lam T, MacLennan G, et al. Antimicrobial catheters for reduction of symptomatic urinary tract infection in adults requiring short-term catheterization in hospital: a multicentre randomised controlled trial. *Lancet.* 2012;380:1927-1935.

40. Chenoweth CE, Gould CV, Saint S. Diagnosis, management, and prevention of catheter associated urinary tract infections. *Infec Dis Clin N Am.* 2014;28:105-119.

41. Nicolle LE. Catheter associated urinary tract infections. *Antimicrob Resist Infect Control.* 2014;3:23.

42. Pappas PG, Kauffman CA, Andes DR, et al. Clinical practice guideline for the management of candidiasis: 2016 update by the infectious diseases society of America. *Clin Infect Dis.* 2016;62:e1-e50.

43. U.S. Food and Drug Administration: FDA Approves New Antibacterial Drug Zerbaxa. Available at: http:// www.fda.gov/NewsEvents/Newsroom/PressAnnouncements/ucm427534.htm. Accessed February 2, 2017.

44. IDSA website. FDA approves new antibacterial drug Zerbaxa. https://www.idsociety.org/ FDA_20141222/. Accessed February 2, 2017.

45. Cluck D, Lewis P, Stayer B, et al. Ceftolozane–tazobactam: a new-generation cephalosporin. *Am J Health Syst Pharm.* 2015;72:2135-2146.

46. Zerbaxa (R) [package insert]. Whitehouse station, NJ: Merck & Co, Inc; 2015.

47. Murano K, Ymanaka T, Toda A, et al. Structural requirements for the stability of novel cephalosporins to AmpC beta-lactamase based on 3D-structure. *Bioorg Med Chem*. 2008;18:2261-2275.

48. Moya B, Zamorano L, Juan C, et al. Activity of a new cephalosporin, CXA-101 (FR264205) against β-lactam-resistant Pseudomonas aeruginosa mutants selected in vitro and after antipseudomonal treatment of intensive care unit patients. *Antimicr Agents Chemother*. 2010;54:1213-1217.

49. Golan Y. Empiric therapy for hospital-acquired, Gram-negative complicated intra-abdominal infection and complicated urinary tract infections: a systematic literature review of current and emerging treatment options. *BMC Infect Dis*. 2015;15:313.

50. Wagenlehner FM, Umeh O, Steenbergen J, et al. Ceftolozane-tazobactam compared with levofloxacin in the treatment of complicated urinary-tract infections, including pyelonephritis: a randomised, double-blind, phase 3 trial. *Lancet*. 2015;385:1949-1956.

51. Solomkin J, Hershberger E, Miller B, et al. Ceftolozane/tazobactam plus metronidazole for complicated intraabdominal infections in an era of multidrug resistance: results from a randomized, double-blind, phase 3 trial. *Clin Infect Dis*. 2015;60:1462-1471.

52. ClinicalTrials.gov. Safety and efficacy study of ceftolozane/tazobactam to treat ventilated nosocomial pneumonia (MK-7625A-008) (ASPECT-NP). https://clinicaltrials.gov/ct2/show/NCT02070757. Accessed January 14, 2017.

53. ClinicalTrials.gov. Determine the PK and Safety and Tolerability of ATM-AVI for the Treatment of cIAIs in Hospitalized Adults (REJUVENATE). https://clinicaltrials.gov/ct2/show/NCT02655419?term5Aztreonam+Avibactam&rank52. Accessed January14, 2017.

54. Singh R, Kim A, Tanudra MA, et al. Pharmacokinetics/pharmacodynamics of a b-lactam and b-lactamase inhibitor combination: a novel approach for aztreonam/avibactam. *J Antimicrob Chemother*. 2015;70:2618-2626.

55. Zasowski EJ, Rybak JM, Rybak MJ. The β-lactams strike back: ceftazidime-avibactam. *Pharmacotherapy*. 2015;35:755-770.

56. Lahiri SD, Johnstone MR, Ross PL, et al. Avibactam and class C β-lactamases: mechanism of inhibition, conservation of the binding pocket, and implications for resistance. *Antimicrob Agents Chemother*. 2014;58:5704-5713.

57. Allergan. Positive Phase III results demonstrate efficacy of antibiotic medicine AVYCAZ™ (Ceftazidime-Avibactam) in complicated urinary tract infections. http://www. allergan.com/news/news/thomson-reuters/positive-phaseiii-results-demonstrate-efficacy-of. Accessed January 14, 2017.

58. Avycaz (R) [package insert]. Verona, Italy: GlaxoSmithKline; 2017.

59. Carmeli Y, Armstrong J, Laud PJ, et al. Ceftazidime-avibactam or best available therapy in patient with ceftazidime-resistant Enterobacteriaceae and Pseudomonas aeruginosa complicated urinary tract infections or complicated intra-abdominal infections: a randomised, pathogen-directed, phase 3 study. *Lancet*. 2016;16:661-673.

60. Mazuski JE, Gasink LB, Armstrong J, et al. Efficacy and safety of ceftazidime-avibactam plus metronidazole versus meropenem in the treatment of complicated intraabdominal infection. *Clin Infect Dis*. 2016;62:1380-1389.

61. Shields RK, Hong Nyugyen M, Chen L, et al. Ceftazidime-avibactam is superior to other treatment regimens against carbapenem-resistant Klebsiella pneumoniae bacteremia. *Antimicrob Agents Chemother*. 2017;61(8):e00883-17.

62. Shields RK, Chen L, Cheng S, et al. Emergency of ceftazidime-avibactam resistance due to plasmid-borne blaKPC-3 mutations during treatment of carbapenem-resistant Klebsiella pneumoniae infections. *Antimicrob Agents Chemother*. 2017;61:e02097-16.

63. Giddins MG, Macesic N, Annavajhala MK, et al. Successive emergence of ceftazidime-avibactam resistance through distinct genomic adaptations in blaKPC-2-harboring Klebsiella pneumoniae Sequence Type 307 Isolates. *Antimicrob Agents Chemother*. 2018;62(3):e02101-17. doi:10.1128/AAC.02101-17.

64. Fraile-Ribot PA, Cabot G, Mulet X, et al. Mechanisms leading to in vivo ceftolozane/tazobactam resistance development during the treatment of infections caused by MDR Pseudomonas aeruginosa. *J Antimicrob Chemother*. 2018;63:658-663. doi:10.1093/jac/dkx424

65. Shields RK, Potoski BA, Haidar G, et al. Clinical outcomes, drug toxicity, and emergence of ceftazi-dime-avibactam resistance among patients treated for carbapenem-resistant Enterobacteriaceae infections. *Clin Infect Dis.* 2016;63(12);1615-1618.

66. Lomovskaya O, Sun D, Rubio-Aparicio D, et al. Vaborbactam: spectrum of beta-lactamase inhibition and impact of resistance mechanisms on activity in Enterobacteriaceae. *Antimicrob Agents Chemother.* 2017;61(11):e01443-17.

67. Kaye KS, Bhowmick T, Metallidis S, et al. Effect of meropenem-vaborbactam vs piperacillin-tazobactam on clinical cure or improvement and microbial eradication in complicated urinary tract infection. *JAMA.* 2018;319(8):788-799.

68. Walsh TJ, Bhowmick T, Darouiche R, et al. Meropenem-vaborbactam vs. piperacillin-tazobactam in TANGO I (a phase 3 randomized, double-blind trial): outcomes by baseline MIC in adults with complicated urinary tract infections or acute pyelonephritis [poster abstract]. *OFID.* 2017;4(suppl 1):S536.

69. Tan JL, Jorgenson SCJ, Rybak MG. Carbapenem-resistant Enterobacteriaceae (CRE): new treatment options against *Klebsiella pneumoniae* carbapenemase (KPC). *MAD-ID Newsletter.* Fall 2017;7(3):6-23.

70. Wunderink R, Bourboulis EG, Rahav G, et al. Meropenem-vaborbactam vs. best available therapy for carbapenem-resistant Enterobacteriaceae infections in TANGO II: primary outcomes by site of infection [poster abstract]. *OFID.* 2017;4(suppl 1):S536.

71. The Medicines Company. The Medicines Company announces positive top- line results for Phase 3 TANGO 1 clinical trial of Carbavance (Meropenem-Vaborbactam). http://www.themedicinescompany.com/investors/news/medicines-company-announcespositive-top-line-results-phase-3-tango-1-clinical-trial. Accessed January 17, 2017.

72. ClinicalTrials.gov. Safety and efficacy of ZTI-01 (IV Fosfomycin) Vs piperacillin/tazobactam for treatment cUTI/AP infections (ZEUS). https://clinicaltrials.gov/ct2/show/NCT02753946. Accessed January 14, 2017.

73. Nordic Pharma Limited. Fomicyt 40 mg/ml powder for solution for infusion. Available at: https://www.medicines.org.uk/emc/medicine/28971/. Accessed February 4, 2017.

74. Garau J. Other antimicrobials of interest in the era of extended-spectrum b-lactamases: fosfomycin, nitrofurantoin and tigecycline. *Clin Microbiol Infect.* 2008;14:198-202.

75. Cho YH, Jung SI, Chung HS, et al. Antimicrobial susceptibilities of extended-spectrum beta-lactamase-producing Escherichia coli and Klebsiella pneumoniae in health care-associated urinary tract infection: focus on susceptibility to fosfomycin. *Int Urol Nephrol.* 2015;47:1059-1066.

76. Falagas ME, Kastoris AC, Kapaskelis AM, Karageorgopoulos DE. Fosfomycin for the treatment of multidrug-resistant, including extended-spectrum β-lactamase producing, Enterobacteriaceae infections: a systematic review. *Lancet Infect Dis.* 2010;10:43-50.

77. ClinicalTrials.gov. Imipenem/relebactam/cilastatin versus piperacillin/tazobactam for treatment of participants with bacterial pneumonia (MK-7655A-014) (RESTORE-IMI 2). https://www.clinicaltrials.gov/ct2/show/NCT02493764?term5relebactam&rank52. Accessed January 17, 2017.

78. ClinicalTrials.gov. Efficacy and safety of imipenem + cilastatin/relebactam (MK-7655A) versus colistimethate sodium + imipenem + cilastatin in imipenem-resistant bacterial infection (MK-7655A-013) (RESTORE-IMI 1). https://www.clinicaltrials.gov/ct2/show/NCT02452047?term5relebactam&rank51. Accessed January 17, 2017.

79. Wright H, Bonomo RA, Paterson DL. New agents for the treatment of infections with Gram-negative bacteria: restoring the miracle or false dawn? *Clin Microbiol Infect.* 2017;23(10):704-712. doi:10.1016/j.cmi.2017.09.001

80. Zhanel GG, Lawrence CK, Adam H, et al. Imipenem-relebactam and meropenem-vaborbactam: two novel carbapenem-β-lactamase inhibitor combinations. *Drugs.* 2018;78(1):65-98. doi:10.1007/s40265-017-0851-9

81. Sims M, Mariyanovski V, McLeroth P, et al. Prospective, randomized, double-blind, Phase 2 dose-ranging study comparing efficacy and safety of imipenem/cilastatin plus relebactam with imipenem/cilastatin alone in patients with complicated urinary tract infections. *J Antimicrob Chemother.* 2017;72(9):2616-2626. doi:10.1093/jac/dkx139

82. Lucasti C, Vasile L, Sandesc D, et al. Phase 2, dose-ranging study of relebactam with imipenem-cilastatin in subjects with complicated intra-abdominal infection. *Antimicrob Agents Chemother*. 2016;60(10): 6234-6243.

83. ClinicalTrials.gov. A phase III, randomized, double-blind, active comparator-controlled clinical trial to estimate the efficacy and safety of imipenem/cilastatin/relebactam (MK-7655a) versus colistimethate sodium + imipenem/cilastatin in subjects with imipenem-resistant bacterial infection. (RESTORE-IMI 1). https://www.clinicaltrials.gov/ct2/show/NCT02452047. Accessed February 18, 2018.

84. Tetraphase Pharmaceuticals, Inc. Tetraphase announces top-line results from ignite3 phase 3 clinical trial of eravacycline in complicated urinary tract infections (cUTI). https://globenewswire.com/news-release/2018/02/13/1340188/0/en/Tetraphase-Announces-Top-Line-Results-from-IGNITE3-Phase-3-Clinical-Trial-of-Eravacycline-in-Complicated-Urinary-Tract-Infections-cUTI.html. Accessed February 18, 2018.

85. Toussaint KA, Gallagher JC. β-lactam/β-lactamase inhibitor combinations: from then to now. *Ann Pharmacother*. 2015;49:86-98.

86. Tetraphase Pharmaceuticals, Inc.. Tetraphase announces top line results from IGNITE2 phase 3 clinical trial of eravacycline in cUTI. https://ir.tphase.com/news-releases/news-release-details/tetraphase-announces-top-line-results-ignite2-phase-3-clinical. Accessed January 17, 2017.

87. Solomkin J, Evans D, Slepavicius A, et al. Assessing the efficacy and safety of eravacycline vs ertapenem in complicated intra-abdominal infections in the investigating gram-negative infections treated with eravacycline (IGNITE 1) trial: a randomized clinical trial. *JAMA Surg*. 2017;152:224-232.

88. Connolly LE, Riddle V, Cebrik D, Armstrong ES, Miller LG. Efficacy and safety of plazomicin compared with levofloxacin in the treatment of complicated urinary tract infection and acute pyelonephritis: a multicenter, randomized, double-blind, phase 2 study. *Antimicrob Agents Chemother*. 2018;62(4):e01989-17. doi:10.1128/AAC.01989-17

89. Cloutier DJ, Miller LG, Komirenko AS, et al. Evaluating once-daily plazomicin versus meropenem for the treatment of complicated urinary tract infection and acute pyelonephritis: results from a phase 3 study (EPIC). Presented at the American Society of Microbiology Microbe; June 1-5, 2017; New Orleans, LA.

90. Aggen JB, Armstrong ES, Goldblum AA, et al. Synthesis and spectrum of the neoglycoside ACHN-490 . *Antimicrob Agents Chemother*. 2010;54:4636-4642.

91. Connolly LE, Jubb AM, O'Keeffe B, et al. Plazomicin is associated with improved survival and safety compared with colistin in the treatment of serious infections due to carbapenem-resistant Enterobacteriaceae: results of the CARE study. Presented at 27th European Congress of Clinical Microbiology and Infectious Diseases (ECCMID); April 22-25, 2017; Vienna, Austria.

92. Portsmouth S, Van Veenhuyzen D, Echols R, et al. Clinical response of cefiderocol compared with imipenem/cilastatin in the treatment of adults with complicated urinary tract infections with or without pyelonephritis or acute uncomplicated pyelonephritis: results from a multicenter, double-blind, randomized study (APEKS-cUTI). *OFID*. 2017:4(suppl 1):S537-S538.

93. ClinicalTrials.gov Identifier: NCT03329092. A study to determine the efficacy, safety and tolerability of aztreonam-avibactam (atm-avi) ± metronidazole (mtz) versus meropenem (mer) ± colistin (col) for the treatment of serious infections due to gram negative bacteria (REVISIT). https://clinicaltrials.gov/ct2/show/NCT03329092. Accessed February 18, 2018.

94. Achaogen, Inc. Achaogen completes patient enrollment in phase 3 EPIC clinical trial of plazomicin. September 1, 2016. http://investors.achaogen.com/news-releases/news-release-details/achaogen-completes-patient-enrollment-phase-3-epic-clinical. Accessed January 17, 2017.

95. ClinicalTrials.Gov. Study of S-649266 or best available therapy for the treatment of severe infections caused by carbapenem-resistant gram-negative pathogens (CREDIBLE-CR). https://clinicaltrials.gov/ct2/show/NCT02714595. Accessed January 17, 2017.

96. Bartoletti R, Cai T, Perletti G, et al. Finafloxacin for the treatment of urinary tract infections. *Expert Opin Investig Drugs*. 2015;24:957-963.

97. Shionogi. Shionogi announces positive top-line results for cefiderocol pivotal cUTI clinical trial. January 12, 2017. http://www.prnewswire.com/news-releases/shionogi-announces-positive-top-line-results-for-cefiderocol-pivotal-cuti-clinical-trial-300389912.html. Accessed May 30, 2017.

98. Micromedex Healthcare Series. *Ceftriaxone.* Greenwood Village, CO: Thomson Micromedex. https://www.micromedexsolutions.com/home/dispatch/ssl/true. Accessed May 30, 2017.

99. Micromedex Healthcare Series. *Nitrofurantoin.* Greenwood Village, CO: Thomson Micromedex. Available at: https://www.micromedexsolutions.com/home/dispatch/ssl/true. Accessed May 30, 2017.

100. Micromedex Healthcare Series. *Sulfamethoxazole/Trimethoprim.* Greenwood Village, CO: Thomson Micromedex. Available at: https://www.micromedexsolutions.com/home/dispatch/ssl/true. Accessed May 30, 2017.

101. Micromedex Healthcare Series. *Fosfomycin.* Greenwood Village, CO: Thomson Micromedex. Available at: https://www.micromedexsolutions.com/home/dispatch/ssl/true. Accessed May 30, 2017.

102. Micromedex Healthcare Series. *Ampicillin.* Greenwood Village, CO: Thomson Micromedex. Available at: https://www.micromedexsolutions.com/home/dispatch/ssl/true. Accessed May 30, 2017.

103. Micromedex Healthcare Series. *Gentamicin/Tobramycin.* Greenwood Village, CO: Thomson Micromedex. Available at: https://www.micromedexsolutions.com/home/dispatch/ssl/true. Accessed May 30, 2017.

104. Micromedex Healthcare Series. *Levofloxacin.* Greenwood Village, CO: Thomson Micromedex. Available at: https://www.micromedexsolutions.com/home/dispatch/ssl/true. Accessed May 30, 2017.

105. Micromedex Healthcare Series. *Ciprofloxacin.* Greenwood Village, CO: Thomson Micromedex. Available at: https://www.micromedexsolutions.com/home/dispatch/ssl/true. Accessed May 30, 2017.

106. Micromedex Healthcare Series. *Piperacillin/Tazobactam.* Greenwood Village, CO: Thomson Micromedex. Available at: https://www.micromedexsolutions.com/home/dispatch/ssl/true. Accessed May 30, 2017.

107. Micromedex Healthcare Series. *Aztreonam.* Greenwood Village, CO: Thomson Micromedex. Available at: https://www.micromedexsolutions.com/home/dispatch/ssl/true. Accessed May 30, 2017.

108. Micromedex Healthcare Series. *Imipenem/Cilastin.* Greenwood Village, CO: Thomson Micromedex. Available at: https://www.micromedexsolutions.com/home/dispatch/ssl/true. Accessed May 30, 2017.

109. Micromedex Healthcare Series. *Meropenem.* Greenwood Village, CO: Thomson Micromedex. Available at: https://www.micromedexsolutions.com/home/dispatch/ssl/true. Accessed May 30, 2017.

110. Micromedex Healthcare Series. *Daptomycin.* Greenwood Village, CO: Thomson Micromedex. Available at: https://www.micromedexsolutions.com/home/dispatch/ssl/true. Accessed May 30, 2017.

111. Micromedex Healthcare Series. *Linezolid.* Greenwood Village, CO: Thomson Micromedex. Available at: https://www.micromedexsolutions.com/home/dispatch/ssl/true. Accessed May 30, 2017.

112. Pham PA, Auwaerter PG. Tigecycline. https://www.micromedexsolutions.com/home/dispatch/ssl/true. Accessed May 30, 2017.

113. Dzintars K, Pham PA. Gentamicin. https://www.micromedexsolutions.com/home/dispatch/ssl/true. Accessed May 30, 2017.

114. Pham PA, Bartlett JG. Colistimethate (Colistin). https://www.micromedexsolutions.com/home/dispatch/ssl/true. Accessed May 30, 2017.

# CHAPTER 7

# Therapeutic Advances in the Management of Orthostatic Hypotension

Karishma Patel, MD, Kinga Kiszko, DO, and Ali Torbati, MD

## BACKGROUND

### Introduction and Epidemiology

The time course of postural blood pressure (BP) responses changes as we age.[1] **Orthostatic hypotension (OH)**, also known as postural hypotension, is characterized by a significant fall in BP on standing. This phenomenon has the greatest impact on the elderly population, affecting an estimated 20% of individuals over the age of 65 years and 30% of individuals over the age of 75 in the general community. The prevalence is as high as 50% in frail elderly nursing home residents.[2] Most available studies have been performed in extended care facilities because the prevalence of **OH** in hospitalized patients is unclear; yet, as many as 60% of hospitalized adults have been observed to experience **OH**.[2] This is especially important in the setting of acute illness, decreased mobility, and the use of polypharmacy during hospitalization all of which make elderly patients particularly vulnerable to consequences of **OH**, especially falls. A study of 210 hospitalized elderly patients over 4 years showed that patients with **orthostatic hypotension** have higher mortality, morbidity, and cardiovascular disease compared to patients without **orthostatic hypotension**.[3]

### Symptoms

Symptomatic individuals may experience dizziness, lightheadedness, nausea, weakness, angina, syncope, and strokes. In addition, elderly individuals with **OH** often experience alterations in cognition, slurring of speech, visual impairments, and falls. However, it is important to note that individuals who do not display symptoms are still at risk of syncope and falls. A trial of 1094 patients (AASK trial) showed that patients with **OH** are more likely to present with symptoms of **orthostatic hypotension**, because the lack of consensus regarding the definition of **orthostatic hypotension** does not exclude the clinical symptoms. It is important to consider that the symptoms associated with **OH** may also be the result of dehydration, medication side effects, or symptoms of existing medical conditions.[4,5]

## Diagnosis

**OH** is diagnosed when there is a sustained drop of at least 20 mm Hg in systolic blood pressure (SBP) and/or at least 10 mm Hg drops in diastolic BP when changing from supine to upright positioning. Sound measuring technique such as proper cuff size and ensuring that the arm is at heart level are important for accuracy. There is no clear consensus as to how long the individual must assume a supine position, although 5 minutes is generally recommended followed by 2 to 5 minutes of quiet standing before measuring vital signs.[2] One small study of elderly hospitalized patients, which included normotensive and hypertensive patients 60 to 90 years old, demonstrated a greater SBP fall after 7 to 9 minutes as compared with the first 3 minutes, suggesting that some patients may require a longer than normal monitoring time.[6] The American Heart Association guidelines for BP measurement do not specify whether the individual should be supine or sitting, before standing when evaluating for **OH**.[7] The European Federation of Neurological Societies guidelines for BP measurement recommend measuring supine BP followed by standing BP.[8] If the patient complains of any symptoms of **OH** on changing to upright position, such as dizziness or weakness, the examination should be terminated so as to ensure patient safety.[2] There is no clear consensus on methods of diagnosing **OH** in the hospital setting; thus, both head-up tilt-table testing and active standing approaches can be used.[2] A positive head-up table result demonstrates the above-described BP changes, within 3 minutes in the head-up and tilt position, at an angle of at least 60 degrees.[9] The American Academy of Neurology and American Autonomic Society do not include changes in heart rate (HR) within their definition of **OH**. HR monitoring may be of use in patients who do not fully meet criteria depending on their BP readings because an increased HR may represent a compensatory mechanism for rapid BP drop.[9,10]

## Pathophysiology

It is estimated that assuming an upright posture results in pooling of 500 to 1000 mL of blood in the lower extremities, and the pulmonary and splanchnic circulation.[2,11] There is also a fluid shift in the lower extremities secondary to increased hydrostatic pressure on standing, resulting in extravasation of intravascular fluid into the interstitial space. Subsequently, there is a rapid drop in cardiac output and BP because of a decrease in venous return to the heart. This sets off a cascade of regulatory mechanisms involving both the central and peripheral nervous systems. Baroreceptors in the carotid sinus, aortic arch, heart, and lungs become activated and sympathetic outflow increases, elevating peripheral vascular resistance and HR. The renin-angiotensin-aldosterone system also becomes activated contributing to peripheral vasoconstriction. If properly functioning, the abovementioned compensatory mechanisms allow for only a small drop in SBP (5-10 mm Hg), an increase in diastolic BP (5-10 mm Hg), and an increase in HR of 10 to 25 beats/min.

OH can be categorized into two groups: acute OH and chronic OH. Acute OH occurs when there is a sudden change in circulating blood volume. This can be due to volume depletion or as a result of sepsis, myocardial infarction, cardiac arrhythmias, and adrenal crisis. Elderly patients have less baseline cardiovascular reserve as compared to younger patients; thus, they are more likely to present with OH in the setting of volume depletion or diuretic use.[12] Commonly administered medications can also lead to OH, including antipsychotics, diuretics, α- and β- blockers, tricyclic antidepressants, narcotics and sedatives, vasodilators, anti-parkinsonian medications, and illicit drugs such as marijuana (Figures 7.1-7.3).

Chronic OH results from autonomic dysfunction, which is commonly attributed to the aging process. The decrease in stroke volume that is seen in congestive heart failure, more often in diastolic dysfunction in which ventricular filling is impaired, can also be a risk factor for OH development, especially in conjunction with diuretic use.[13] Supine hypertension also contributes to OH. Sustained uncontrolled BP negatively affects the ability to respond to positional changes and increases the risk of falls.

**FIGURE 7.1** Causes of acute orthostatic hypotension (OH).

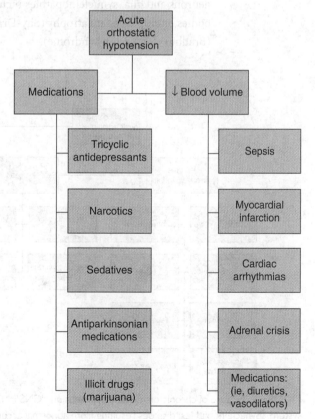

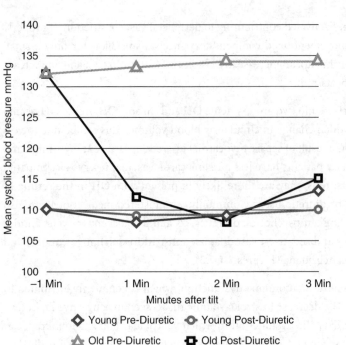

**FIGURE 7.2** Mean SBP response to 60-degree upright tilt before and after diuretic-induced volume depletion in six old and six young subjects. SBP, systolic blood pressure. Adapted from Bradley JG, Davis KA. Orthostatic hypotension. *Am Fam Physician*. 2003;68:2393-2399.

Autonomic dysfunction and **OH** are part of the clinical presentation of certain diseases. Named after the abnormal accumulation of alpha synuclein (Lewy body) in neurons and glia, synucleinopathies include Parkinson disease, dementia with Lewy bodies, multiple system atrophy (Shy-Drager syndrome), and pure autonomic failure (Bradbury-Eggleston syndrome).

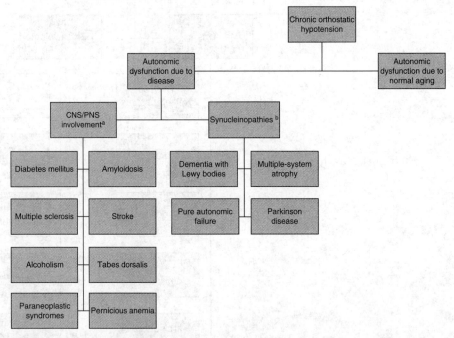

**FIGURE 7.3** Cause of chronic orthostatic hypotension. [a]CNS/PNS: central nervous system/peripheral nervous system. [b]Synucleinopathies: diseases resulting from abnormal accumulation of alpha synuclein in neurons and glia.

In addition, autonomic failure leading to **OH** has also been observed in diseases affecting the peripheral and central nervous system, including diabetes, amyloidosis, multiple sclerosis, stroke, alcoholism, paraneoplastic syndromes, pernicious anemia, and tabes dorsalis.[4,11] Other age-related risk factors for development of **OH** (especially late **OH**) have to do with impairment of the renin-angiotensin-aldosterone system, which compromises the body's ability to adequately respond to dehydration or periods of fluid restriction.[4] It has been shown that acutely ill elderly inpatients experience **OH** and/or its symptoms more often on first morning standing after bed rest.[6] Bed rest affects postural BP through several mechanisms, including an increased compliance of dependent veins and decreased baroreceptor function after periods of supine rest.[14,15] If initial assessment after first mobilization is inconsistent with **OH**, likelihood of subsequent development is likely to be low; however, some studies suggest at least once-daily **OH** monitoring may be of benefit in patients after periods of prolonged bed rest.[2]

## Long-Term Morbidity and Mortality

Data analysis from multiple studies has demonstrated a positive association between **OH** and increased morbidity and mortality. **OH** is recognized as an independent risk factor for recurrent falls in geriatric nursing home residents.[16] It has been shown that individuals with baseline **OH** had more cardiovascular events (ie, myocardial infarction and strokes) and increased all-cause mortality.

Data analysis from a Swedish study found an **OH** prevalence of 6.2% in their population. There was a positive association between **OH** and the presence of other factors including hypertension, diabetes, anti-hypertensive treatment, and increased HR. **OH** was found to be an independent risk factor for all-cause mortality and coronary events (particularly in individuals, 42 years and younger). The risk of poor outcomes was even higher with SBP drops of 30 mm Hg and diastolic BP drops of 15 mm Hg. The highest risk was observed in individuals with **OH** both at baseline and at follow-up.[17,18] Furthermore, data from subjects who were hospitalized for nonischemic heart failure demonstrated a positive association between **OH** and long-term incidence of heart failure–related hospitalizations (especially among middle-aged adults).[18]

A large study in the Netherlands observed individuals 55 years or older, with **OH** but without previous cardiovascular disease or history of stroke. After adjusting for cardiovascular risk factors including diabetes mellitus and hypertension, there was an increase in all-cause mortality and incidence of coronary heart disease (at mean follow-up period 6.0 ± 3.5 years) and stroke (at mean follow-up period 6.7 ± 3.6 years), suggesting that **OH** is an independent risk factor for these events.[19] Another study of elderly American Japanese men in Honolulu found an increase in the risk of 4-year all-cause mortality in subjects with **OH**, even after the data were adjusted for confounders such as diabetes, coronary artery disease, stroke, and cancer.

In fact, there was an 18% increase in all-cause mortality for every 10 mm Hg drop in SPB when rising to standing from a supine position.[20] A large study of middle-aged subjects who were previously free of heart disease or stroke found a significant association between the presence of **OH** and increased risk for ischemic stroke.[21] Last, examination of home-dwelling individuals in northern Finland found that individuals with **OH** have a significant increase in vascular deaths.[21]

The above-described evidence is compelling and should alert the healthcare provider to pay closer attention to postural hypotension during hospitalization and on discharge. A routine measurement of orthostatic BP on admission and before discharge can help identify those individuals most at risk of persistence of **OH**, and associated complications, especially in relation to falls, cardiovascular events, and mortality.

# AREAS OF UNCERTAINTY IN TREATMENT

**OH** is a common finding in elderly adults who are oftentimes asymptomatic. There is clear evidence that **OH** is a risk factor for cardiovascular disease, ischemic stroke, and mortality.[3,16,20,21] Although certain treatments have demonstrated some success in improving **OH**, it is unclear whether these interventions have any effect on clinical outcomes such as falls, syncope, and mortality.[4,22,23] A recent trial of individuals aged $69 \pm 10.3$ years found that low BP (systolic $< 120$ mm Hg and diastolic $< 70$ mm Hg) and **OH** ($P > 0.10$) were not associated with increased concern about falling (The Falls Efficacy Scale-International).[24] Given the possible side effects of available pharmaceutical interventions for elderly adults and the limited evidence regarding supporting improvement in clinical outcomes, treatment should center around reversible causes of **OH** and symptom relief with nonpharmaceutical interventions, especially lifestyle modification.[25,26] In addition, and commonly seen in practice, not treating baseline supine hypertension because of the concern for inappropriate postural BP changes, can have major clinical outcomes in **geriatric** patients.[27,28]

Treatment for **OH** in the acute setting starts with addressing the reversible causes of **OH**. The next step is non pharmacologic interventions, with an emphasis on patient education regarding associated symptoms (presyncope, syncope, and falls) and lifestyle modifications.[26] An important step in geriatric patients with polypharmacy and multiple medical problems is avoidance or minimization of medications, which can induce the development of **OH**. Patients should be educated on the importance of hydration, dietary changes, daily physical activity, and the use of physical countermaneuvers that can help manage their symptoms of **OH**.[29] If these measures are ineffective and the patient remains persistently symptomatic, one may try a variety of pharmacotherapeutic agents, such as fludrocortisone, nonsteroidal anti-inflammatory drugs (NSAIDs), and midodrine. Given the uncertainty about the benefits of current treatment options and limited studies in elderly adults with multiple medical problems, we provide the following recommendations to implement in your clinical practice.

# THERAPEUTIC ADVANCES

## Nonpharmacologic Treatment

Management of **OH** in an acute setting begins with addressing acute medical conditions (pain, sepsis, volume depletion, acute heart failure, stroke, cardiac arrhythmia, or anemia), educating patients on the nature of **OH** and possible clinical outcomes such as falls, syncope and presyncope, and discussing implementation of lifestyle modifications.[26] For patients with **OH** secondary to volume depletion, fluid replacement should be initiated and diuretic use should be decreased or avoided. Other medications that could cause **OH**, such as nitrates, tricyclic antidepressants, diuretics, neuroleptics, and α-blockers, should also be minimized or discontinued, if allowable. In certain situations, using compression stockings, ace bandages, or abdominal binders can be helpful in increasing venous return, decreasing drops in orthostatic SBP, and reducing symptoms in elderly patients with progressive hypotension.[30-32] One study that looked at patients with progressive **OH** demonstrated a decrease in BP drop with the use of compression bandages ($P = 0.002$) and symptom relief continued after 1 month of use ($P = 0.001$).[30]

Early mobilization and avoidance of physical deconditioning in the acute care setting has a cardinal role in treating and preventing **OH** in hospitalized older patients.[6,14]

For patients who have been restricted to the bed, physical countermaneuvers, such as changing body position, squatting or leaning forward as opposed to sitting, and encouraging activity can be helpful in preventing and treating **OH**. Of these maneuvers, the isometric handgrip, in which the patient tenses the arms for 2 minutes or until the first sign of impending syncope, has shown to improve BP and **OH** symptoms, especially in patients with neurocardiogenic syncope.[33] Meanwhile, lower body muscle tensing for approximately 40 seconds after standing from squatting position has also showed to improve BP and its symptoms.[31] Simple positional changes can be an easy way to improve **OH** without using medications in the elderly. Clinicians should consider educating their patients on lower extremity exercises with or without leg crossing, putting their head between their knees, or squatting exercises to improve their symptoms.[32]

In a study of patients with severe **OH** because of autonomic failure, rapid ingestion of room temperature 480 mL of tap water 5 minutes before standing improved orthostatic drop in BP ($P = 0.001$).[34] Older patients who drink water with their meals have less episodes of postprandial hypotension than do patients who do not drink water. The effect of water is more apparent within 1 hour of drinking fluids. Some clinicians believe that drinking water early in the morning after getting out of bed and liberal intake of salt and water to achieve a 24-hour urine volume of 1.5 to 2 L may attenuate fluid loss commonly seen in autonomic insufficiency.[35]

Small observational studies have suggested that raising the head of the bed by 5 to 10 degrees (15 cm) at night in patients with autonomic failure can reduce supine hypertension; however, the benefit of this intervention in the acute setting is unclear.[36]

## Pharmacologic Interventions

Numerous pharmacologic agents are available to treat **OH** if the patient remains symptomatic despite nonpharmacologic interventions. The two main approaches to treating hypotension are using pharmaceutical agents that aid in increasing blood volume and peripheral vascular resistance.

Increasing blood volume is a long-term strategy that works by increasing the baseline BP throughout the day.[26] One of the most potent agents is fludrocortisone, a synthetic mineralocorticoid, with a primary mode of action being reduction of salt loss and expansion of blood volume. In a small study of diabetic patients with symptomatic **OH**, use of 0.1 mg of fludrocortisone twice daily showed improvement in symptoms, and an increase in SBP, total plasma volume, and body weight. Patients with lower albumin showed less clinical improvement and lower extremities edema.[37] The recommended starting dose is 0.1 mg daily early in the morning with potential weekly increase up to 0.3 mg/d. There are a few key items to monitor such as supine BP, fluid overload, lower extremities edema, hypokalemia, heart failure, and headache.[4] Fludrocortisone should not be viewed as an isolated therapy, but a next step after dietary salt and water expansion with the goal of increasing blood volume.

Recombinant erythropoietin (EPO) is commonly used as a volume expansion agent in patients with severe symptomatic autonomic failure and concomitant anemia. In a small study of patients with chronic **OH**, use of 50 U/kg of subcutaneous EPO three times a week for 6 to 10 weeks showed improvement in symptoms and **OH**, with no effect on plasma volume and supine BP.[38] Common barriers to using EPO are cost and the need for injections rather than oral administration.[39] Major side effects include hypertension, stroke, deep vein thrombosis, and myocardial infarction. A close monitoring of hemoglobin levels is required.[38]

In patients with chronic **OH** who continue to be symptomatic despite volume expansion, the next treatment approach is to use direct and indirect sympathomimetic agents to increase peripheral vascular resistance. Short-acting peripheral selective alpha-1 adrenergic agonist medications are commonly used. At this time, the only medication in this group that has been approved by the U.S. Food and Drug Administration for the treatment of **OH** is midodrine. In a review of clinical trials involving patients with symptomatic **OH** and recurrent reflex syncope, use of midodrine showed low/moderate improvement in clinically important outcomes.[23,24] The starting dose of midodrine is 2.5 mg three times/d, which can be slowly titrated to a maximum of 10 mg three times/d. Because of the short half-life of midodrine, the morning dose should be given early and the evening dose no later than 6 PM.[26,40] Midodrine works within 20 to 30 minutes of administration and can last up to 4 hours. Because of possible side effects, midodrine should not be used in patients with heart disease, cardiac arrhythmias, urinary retention, and uncontrolled supine hypertension. Given the increased potential for underlying cardiovascular diseases in geriatric patients, Midodrine should be used cautiously in acute illness. Clinicians should monitor BP, HR, and urinary retention when treating elderly patients with midodrine, especially when taking medications for supine hypertension, HR control, and benign prostatic hyperplasia. A systematic review of several clinical trials revealed insufficient and low quality of evidence supporting midodrine for **OH** especially in supine to standing SBP, and, in fact, its use caused more harm than good.[40]

Some patients may benefit from the use of prostaglandin inhibitors, such as NSAIDs, which block the vasodilating effects of prostaglandins, thereby increasing BP. Owing to an increased risk of gastrointestinal bleeding, renal failure, and electrolytes abnormalities in elderly adults, use of NSAIDs, especially high potent NSAIDs such as indomethacin, should be limited.[41]

Another class of medications that can be used for **OH** especially in Parkinson disease includes the alpha-2 adrenergic agonists, namely, clonidine and yohimbine. Both of these agents work on alpha-2 adrenergic receptors in the central and peripheral nervous system. Clonidine may improve **OH** in patients with central nervous system autonomic failure by promoting peripheral venoconstriction, thereby increasing venous return to the heart.[4,42] Yohimbine is a central α-2 adrenergic antagonist that can increase central sympathetic outflow in some patients with residual sympathetic nervous system efferent output.[43] Yohimbine was originally on the market for erectile dysfunction. At this time, yohimbine is no longer manufactured, although it is still available through compounding pharmacies. Pyridostigmine, a peripheral acetylcholinesterase inhibitor, is another potential medication for the management of **OH**. Pyridostigmine acts to increase synaptic acetylcholine concentrations in the autonomic ganglia. Because pyridostigmine does not directly activate the receptor, but rather it increases the neurotransmitter concentration, it may have more pressor action when a patient is upright than while supine. It has been shown that pyridostigmine significantly reduces falls in standing diastolic BP, with no significant difference in supine BP. This finding was seen both with pyridostigmine alone and with concurrent midodrine.[44]

A different intervention that can be used to improve **OH** includes methylxanthine caffeine administered in a dose of 200 mg every morning in the form of two cups of brewed coffee or by tablet. Methylxanthine caffeine may attenuate symptoms of **OH** in some patients. Caffeine is an adenosine-receptor blocker that inhibits adenosine-induced vasodilatation. To avoid tolerance and insomnia, caffeine should not be given more than once in the morning.[4] A combination of caffeine and dihydroergotamine also has been found to be effective in treatment of **OH**.[45] Last, there are alternative medications such as Cafergot, octreotide, or droxidopa that are used in patients who are refractory to the abovementioned treatment options. Cafergot is often used with midodrine, which causes vasoconstriction through a nonsympathomimetic mechanism.[4]

## Treatment of Supine Hypertension in the Setting of Orthostatic Hypotension

The presence of supine hypertension in patients with **OH** is a common clinical finding. Managing these two conditions simultaneously can be extremely challenging.[46] Although there is clear evidence that not treating supine hypertension leads to end-organ damage, there is no accepted protocol regarding how to manage hypertension in patients with **OH**.[28] Previous studies have demonstrated that patients without previous **OH** are at low risk of having **OH** after antihypertensive treatment.[47] Indeed, better BP control decreases the incidence of **OH**; however, antihypertensive medications may also exacerbate underlying **OH**.[48-50] It is not clear which group of antihypertensive medications should be used in this patient population, but some studies favor the use of β-blockers and angiotensin-converting enzyme inhibitors/angiotensin receptor blockers, over alpha-receptor antagonists and diuretics.[50-52] Overall, blunted sympathetic nerve activity and high baseline BP has an important role in the development of **OH** in hypertensive elderly patients.[50]

# SUMMARY

**Orthostatic hypotension** (**OH**) is a common condition in hospitalized geriatric patients. These patients have a worse outcome compared to patients without **OH**. In addition, they are more susceptible to **OH** during acute sickness, dehydration, and volume depletion.

**OH** can be asymptomatic. There is clear evidence that **OH** is a risk factor for cardiovascular disease, ischemic stroke, and mortality. Although certain treatments have demonstrated some success in improving **OH**, it is unclear whether these interventions have any effect on clinical outcomes such as falls, syncope, and mortality.

Initial approaches to treatment should focus on nonpharmaceutical interventions, such as education about symptom recognition, lifestyle modifications, promotion of early mobilization, and avoidance of unnecessary bed rest orders. Pharmaceutical treatments are only indicated if the patient continues to be symptomatic in spite of nonpharmacologic interventions. The two main approaches to treating hypotension with pharmaceuticals include increasing blood volume and peripheral vascular resistance. Fludrocortisone should not be used as an isolated therapy, but a next step after dietary salt and water expansion. The recommended starting dose of fludrocortisone is 0.1 mg daily early in the morning with potential weekly increase up to 0.3 mg/d.

If fludrocortisone is unsuccessful, midodrine may be used to increase peripheral vascular resistance. Given the increased potential for underlying cardiovascular diseases in geriatric patients, midodrine should be used cautiously in acute illness. The use of prostaglandin inhibitors that is nonsteroidal anti-inflammatory drugs to raise blood pressure should be limited because of the increased risk of gastrointestinal bleeding, renal failure, and electrolyte abnormalities in elderly adults. Other agents that may be of benefit include clonidine, yohimbine, pyridostigmine, methylxanthine, dihydroergotamine, Cafergot, octreotide, and droxidopa; however, their use is conditional to certain etiologies behind **OH**, and the supporting evidence is low.

Although there is clear evidence that not treating supine hypertension leads to end-organ damage, there is no accepted protocol regarding how to manage hypertension in patients with **orthostatic hypotension**. Some studies favor the use of beta-blockers and angiotensin-converting enzyme inhibitors/angiotensin receptor blockers, over alpha-receptor antagonists and diuretics.

## References

1. Finucane C, O'Connell MDL, Fan CW, et al. Age-related normative changes in phasic orthostatic blood pressure in large population study (TILDA). *Circulation*. 2014;130: 1780-1789.

2. Feldstein C, Weder AB. Orthostatic hypotension: a common, serious, and under-recognized problem in hospitalized patients. *J Am Soc Hypertens*. 2012;6:27-39.

3. Lindstedt I, Edvinsson L, Lindberg A, Olsson M, Dahlgren C, Edvinsson ML. Increased all-cause mortality, total cardiovascular disease and morbidity in hospitalized elderly patients with orthostatic hypotension. *Arch Gen Intern Med*. 2018;2(1):8-15.

4. Gupta V, Lipsitz L. Orthostatic hypotension in the elderly: diagnosis and treatment. *Am J Med*. 2007;120:841-847.

5. Rutan GH, Hermanson B, Bild DE, et al. Orthostatic hypotension in older adults: the cardiovascular health study. *Hypertension*. 1992;19:508-519.

6. Fotherby M, Iqbal P, Potter J. Orthostatic blood pressure changes on prolonged standing in elderly hospital patients. *Blood Press*. 1997;6:343-348.

7. Pickering TG, Hall JE, Appel LJ, et al. Recommendations for blood pressure measurement in humans and experimental animals: part 1: blood pressure measurement in humans: a statement for professionals from the Subcommittee of Professional and Public Education of the American Heart Association Council on High Blood Pressure Research. *Circulation*. 2005;111:697-716.

8. Lahrmann H, Cortelli P, Hilz M, et al. EFNS guidelines on the diagnosis and management of orthostatic hypotension. *Eur J Neurol*. 2006;13:930-936.

9. Schatz IJ, Bannister R, Freeman RL, et al. Consensus statement on the definition of orthostatic hypotension, pure autonomic failure and multiple system atrophy. *Clin Auton Res*. 1996;6:125-126.

10. Bradley JG, Davis KA. Orthostatic hypotension. *Am Fam Physician*. 2003;68:2393-2399.

11. Iwanczyk L, Weintraub NT, Rubenstein LZ. Orthostatic hypotension in nursing hone setting. *J Am Med Dir Assoc*. 2006;7:163-167.

12. Shannon R, Wei J, Rosa R, et al. The effect of age and sodium depletion on cardiovascular response to ortho-static. *Hypertension*. 1986;8:438-443.

13. van Kraaij DJ, Jansen RW, Bouwels LH, Hoefnagels WHL. Furosemide withdrawal improves postprandial hypotension in elderly patients with heart failure and preserved left ventricular systolic function. *Arch Intern Med*. 1999;159:1599-1605.

14. Kolegard R, Mejkavic IB, Eiken O. Increased distensibility in dependent veins following prolonged periods of bed rest. *Eur J Appl Physiol*. 2009;106:547-554.

15. Xiao X, Mukkamama R, Sheynberg N, et al. Effects of prolonged bed rest on the total peripheral resistance baroreflex. *Comput Cardiol*. 2002;39:53-56.

16. Ooi W, Hossain M, Lipstiz L. The association between Orthostatic hypotension and recurrent falls in nursing home residents. *Am J Med*. 2000;108:106-111.

17. Federowski A, Stavenow L, Hedblad B, et al. Orthostatic hypotension predicts all-cause mortality and coronary events in middle aged individuals (The Malmo Preventive Project). *Eur Heart J*. 2010;31:85-91.

18. Federowski A, Stavenow L, Hedblad B, Melander O. Consequences of orthostatic hypotension predicts incidence of heart failure: the Malmo Preventive Project. *Am J Hypertens*. 2010;23:1209-1215.

19. Verwoert GC, Mattace-Raso FU, Hofman A, et al. Ortho-static hypotension and risk of cardiovascular disease in elderly people: the Rotterdam study. *J Am Geriatric Soc*. 2008;56:1816-1820.

20. Masaki KH, Schatz IJ, Burchfiel CM, et al. Orthostatic hypotension predicts mortality in elderly men: the Honolulu Heart Program. *Circulation*. 1998;98:2290-2295.

21. Eigenbrodt ML, Rose KM, Couper DJ, et al. Orthostatic hypotension is a risk factor for stroke: the atherosclerosis risk in communities (ARIC) study, 1987–1996. *Stroke*. 2000;31:2037-2313.

22. Miller E, Appel L. High prevalence but uncertain clinical significance of orthostatic hypotension without symptoms. *Circulation*. 2014;130:1722-1774.

23. Izcovich A, Malla CG, Manzotti M, et al. Midodrine for orthostatic hypotension and recurrent reflex syncope. *Neurology*. 2014;83:1170-1177.

24. Berlowitz DR, Breaux-Shropshire T, Foy CG, et al. Hypertension treatment and concern about falling: base-line data from the systolic blood pressure intervention trial. *J Am Geriatr Soc*. 2016;64:2302-2306.

25. Ward CR, Gray JC, Gilroy JJ, et al. Midodrine: a role in the management of neurocardiogenic syncope. *Heart*. 1998;79:45-49.

26. Raj SR, Coffin ST. Medical therapy and physical maneuvers in the treatment of the vasovagal syncope and ortho-static hypotension. *Prog Cardiovas Dis*. 2013;55:425-433.

27. The SPRINT Research Group. A randomized trial of intensive standard blood pressure control. *N Engl J Med*. 2015;373:2103-2116.

28. Sandroni P, Benarroch EE, Wijdicks EF. Caudate hemorrhage as a possible complication of midodrine induced supine hypertension. *Mayo Clin Proc*. 2001;76:1275.

29. Mills P, Fund C, Travlos A, et al. Non-pharmacological management of orthostatic hypotension. *Arch Phys Med Rehabil*. 2015;96:366-375.

30. Podoleanau C, Maggi R, Brignole M, et al. Lower limb and abdominal compression bandages prevent progressive orthostatic hypotension in elderly persons. *J Am Coll Cardiol*. 2006;48:1425-1432.

31. Krediet CT, Go-Schon IK, Kim YS, et al. Management of initial orthostatic hypotension: lower body muscle tensing attenuates the transient arterial blood pressure decrease upon standing from squatting. *Clin Sci*. 2007;113:401-407.

32. Krediet CT, van Dijk N, Linzer M, et al. Management of vasovagal syncope: controlling or aborting faints by leg crossing and muscle tensing. *Circulation*. 2002;106:1684-1689.

33. Brignole M, Croci F, Menozzi C, et al. Isometric arm counter-pressure maneuvers to abort impending vasovagal syncope. *J Am Coll Cardiol*. 2002;40:2053-2059.

34. Shannon JR, Diedrich A, Biaggioni I, et al. Water drinking as a treatment of orthostatic syndromes. *Am J Med*. 2002;112:355-360.

35. Fedorowski A, Melander O. Syndromes of orthostatic intolerance: a hidden danger. *J Intern Med.*. 2013;273:322-335.

36. Wieling W, Raj SR, Thijs RD. Are small observational studies sufficient for a recommendation of head-up sleeping in all patients with debilitating orthostatic hypotension? *Clin Auton Res*. 2009;19:8-12.

37. Campbell W, Ewing DJ, Clarke BF. 9-Alpha-fluorohydrocortisone in the treatment of postural hypotension in diabetic autonomic neuropathy. *Diabetes*. 1975;24:381-384.

38. Hoeldtke RD, Streetan DHP. Treatment of orthostatic hypotension with erythropoietin. *N Engl J Med*. 1993; 329:611–615.

39. Singh AK, Szczech L, Tang KL, et al; CHOIR Investigators. Correction of anemia with erythropoietin alfa in chronic kidney disease. *N Engl J Med*. 2006;355:2085-2098.

40. Parsaik A, Singh B, Altayar O, et al. Midodrine for orthostatic hypotension: a systematic review and meta-analysis of clinical trials. *J Gen Intern Med*. 2013;38:1496-1503.

41. Wright RA, Kaufmann HC, Perera R, et al. A double-blind, dose-response study of Midodrine in neurogenic orthostatic hypotension. *Neurology*. 1998;51:120-124.

42. Logan I, Withman MD. Efficacy of treatment for ortho-static hypotension. *Age and Aging*. 2012;41:587-594.

43. Jordan J, Shannon JR, Biaggioni I, et al. Contrasting actions of pressor agents in severe autonomic failure. *Am J Med*. 1998;105:116-124.

44. Singer W, Sandroni P, Opfer-Gehrking TL, et al. Pyridostigmine treatment trial in neurogenic orthostatic hypotension. *Arch Neurol.* 2006;63:513-518.

45. Hoeldtke R, Cavanaugh S, Hughs J, et al. Treatment of orthostatic hypotension with Dihydroergotamine and caffeine. *Ann Intern Med.* 1986;105:168-173.

46. Dhruva SS, Redberg RF. Accelerated approval and possible withdrawal of Midodrine. *JAMA.* 2010;304:2172-2173.

47. Vagaonescu TD, Saadia D, Tuhrim S, et al. Hypertensive cardiovascular damage in patients with primary autonomic failure. *Lancet.* 2000;355:725-726.

48. Saez T, Suarez C, Sierra MJ, et al. Orthostatic hypotension in the aged and its association with antihypertensive treatment. *Med Clin (Barc).* 2000;114:525-529.

49. Fotherby MD, Iqbal P. Antihypertensive therapy and orthostatic responses in elderly hospital in-patients. *J Hum Hypertens.* 1997;11:291-294.

50. Masuo K, Mikami H, Ogihara T, Tuck ML. Changes in frequency of orthostatic hypotension in elderly hypertensive patients under medications. *Am J Hypertens.* 1996;9:263.

51. Brignole M, Alboni P, Benditt D, et al; Task Force Report. Guidelines on management (diagnosis and treatment) of syncope. *Eur Heart J.* 2001;22:1256-1306.

52. Mader SL. Orthostatic hypotension. *Med Clin North Am.* 1989;73:1337-1349.

53. Juraschek S, Miller E, Appel L. Orthostatic hypotension and symptoms in the AASK trial. *Am J Hypertens.* 2018;31(6):665-671.

# CHAPTER 8

# Therapeutic Advances in the Perioperative Period for Older Adults

Philip Solomon, MD, Brooke Calabrese, MD, and Sean LaVine, MD

## BACKGROUND

The unique needs of segments of the surgical population have helped drive the field of **perioperative** medicine in the inpatient setting. Consultative medicine and medical comanagement of surgical patients by hospitalists have become the norm in many inpatient facilities. As the population of the United States continues to increase, with an exponential increase expected in individuals older than 65 years,[1] the number of adults older than 65 years undergoing surgeries should increase as well. The inpatient **perioperative** care of this segment of the population has unique challenges that are not currently well studied or outlined.

The American College of Cardiology/American Heart Association (ACC/AHA) 2014 Guidelines have become the standard of care for preoperative cardiac evaluation, with many implications on the **perioperative** management of geriatric patients. They have helped standardize medication management and provide algorithms for **perioperative** testing.

According to these guidelines, emergency procedures should not be delayed for testing unless there is active cardiac disease. Patients with acute coronary syndrome should be treated and then reevaluated before **surgery**. Other patients should be risk stratified for **perioperative** cardiac events using a risk calculator. The Revised Cardiac Risk Index (RCRI) and National Surgical Quality Improvement Program calculator are two widely used tools to estimate risk based on patient and **surgery** characteristics. There is no clear benefit of one risk calculator over the other. Patients with less than 1% risk of a major adverse cardiac event (MACE) do not need further testing. Those with greater than 1% risk of MACE may need further cardiac testing, but only if this testing will affect decision making in the **perioperative** period.[2] In preoperative evaluation, special consideration must be made for geriatric patients, including discussion about advanced directives, management of polypharmacy, and potentially shortening the fluid fast preoperatively.[3]

# AREAS OF UNCERTAINTY

**Perioperative** management of geriatric patients remains a moving target, with much of the data extrapolated from studies that did not necessarily focus on patients older than 65 years. Which patients need to be screened and have a full cardiac workup remains unclear. In a study from the American University of Beirut Medical Center, only 1% of 522 patients had preoperative cardiac evaluation that changed the surgical or anesthetic plan (cancelled **surgery**, change in the type of anesthesia given, or referral to cardiac **surgery**), although the patients in this study were relatively low risk. This study, however, did find that age older than 65 years was predictive of a need for further preoperative testing.[4] This is important to remember when evaluating older adults because they are more likely to need advanced cardiac testing before surgical procedures.

A 2013 study analyzing Medicare data found that between 1996 and 2008, approximately 56 000 Medicare recipients had unnecessary preoperative stress testing.[5] Although this study reflected that overtesting was occurring, it did not look at their resultant effects on patients. A 2012 retrospective study also found that overscreening was more common than underscreening (95% vs 5% of incorrectly screened cases). It also found that overscreening in preoperative cardiac evaluation before hip fracture **surgery** often led to a delay in **surgery**. Patients with a delay of 48 hours or more had a statistically significant increase in postoperative complications, including death, up to 1 month postoperatively.

Overscreening was found to be most common in patients who fell under the "intermediate risk" category.[6] A 2015 retrospective study in the *Journal of Orthopaedic Trauma* replicated the results that unnecessary preoperative cardiac consultation increased delay to **surgery**. This study did not find a difference in complication rates postoperatively. It did, however, find that none of the patients who had unnecessary stress testing or echocardiograms required cardiac **surgery** or catheterization, indicating that the increased testing did not alter outcomes or management.[7] A 2012 study in the *Journal of Nuclear Medicine* found that myocardial perfusion imaging was predictive of MACE when patients were tested appropriately on the basis of ACC/AHA **perioperative** guidelines, but the results were nonpredictive in patients who were inappropriately tested.[8]

There is building evidence that evaluation of frailty may become an important tool in the preoperative assessment of older adults. Frailty can be defined as a decline in multiple physiologic systems that occur with advanced age and may be a better predictor of morbidity and mortality than advanced age. A systematic review found that there is a correlation between increased frailty score and postoperative mortality and complications, increased length of stay, decreased postoperative functional status, and decreased quality of life.[9] A 2013 study found that older patients with high frailty scores undergoing both cardiac and colorectal surgery had increased postoperative complications, length of stay, and readmissions compared with their nonfrail counterparts.[10] Gait speed was found to be an independent predictor of postoperative morbidity and mortality in a 2010 study.[11] On the basis of these trials, frailty evaluation should become a routine part of the screening of older adults before surgery because it will help to further risk stratify patients.

# THERAPEUTIC ADVANCES

## β-Blockers

The pendulum for perioperative β-blocker use has swung in favor and against over the past two decades, but recent retrospective studies and a 2014 meta-analysis have helped consolidate recommendations from the ACC/AHA. However, specific data on geriatric cohorts remain sparse.

For patients who are on chronic β-blocker therapy (ie, medication started >30 days before surgery), it is a class I, level B recommendation to continue the medication, as per the updated ACC/AHA guidelines from 2014 (Tables 8.1 and 8.2).[2] Despite the consensus opinion, this recommendation is based on numerous robust retrospective studies. A large retrospective cohort study from 2005 reviewed over 700 000 patients undergoing noncardiac surgery from 329 hospitals in the United States, 18% of whom received β-blockers perioperatively. There was no benefit in mortality for patients with an RCRI of 0 to 1, but adjusted odds ratios for in-hospital mortality were 0.88 (95% confidence interval [CI], 0.80-0.98), 0.71 (95% CI, 0.63-0.80), and 0.58 (95% CI, 0.50-0.67) for patients with an RCRI of 2, 3, or 4, respectively.[12] A 2014 Danish cohort study identified more than 28 000 patients with ischemic heart disease undergoing noncardiac surgery and further divided them on the basis of a history of heart failure (28% of participants) and perioperative β-blocker use (53% of patients with heart failure and 37% of patients with no history of heart failure).[13] The study's primary endpoints were MACE and all-cause mortality at 30-day follow-up. Among patients with a history of heart failure, β-blockers significantly reduced both MACE, with a hazard ratio (HR) of 0.75 (95% CI, 0.70-0.87) and all-cause mortality, with HR of 0.80 (0.70-0.92). Patients with no history of heart failure but with recent myocardial infarction (MI) (<2 years before surgery) also saw a decrease in MACE with HR of 0.54 (95% CI, 0.37-0.78) with a trend toward decreased all-cause mortality (HR: 0.80, 0.53-1.21). Of note, patients on β-blockers without heart failure or recent MI showed no difference in postoperative MACE or all-cause mortality when compared with patients not taking the medication.

There is no discernable difference in perioperative outcomes based on subtype of β blocker used, with one notable exception. A recent retrospective cohort study with

**TABLE 8.1 • Applying Classification of Recommendations and Level of Evidence**

|  |  | Size of Treatment Effect | | | |
|---|---|---|---|---|---|
|  |  | **Class I**<br>Benefit strongly outweighs risk | **Class IIa**<br>Benefit outweighs risk | **Class IIb**<br>Benefit may outweigh risk | **Class III**<br>No benefit or possible harm |
| Multiple populations studied | Level A<br>Randomized control trails (RCTs or meta-analyses) | Recommendation that procedure/treatment is valuable<br>Evidence from RCTs or meta-analyses | Recommendation in favor of procedure/treatment being valuable<br>Conflicting evidence from RCTs or meta-analyses | Recommendation of procedure/treatment's value less well established<br>More conflicting evidence from RCTs or meta-analyses | Recommendation that procedure/treatment is not valuable or may be harmful<br>Evidence from RCTs or meta-analyses |
| Limited populations studied | Level B<br>Single RCT or nonrandomized studies | Recommendation that procedure/treatment is valuable<br>Evidence from single RCT or nonrandomized studies | Recommendation in favor of procedure/treatment being valuable<br>Conflicting evidence from single RCT or nonrandomized studies | Recommendation's value less well established<br>More conflicting evidence from single RCT or nonrandomized studies | Recommendation that procedure/treatment is not valuable or may be harmful<br>Evidence from single RCT or nonrandomized studies |
| Very limited populations studied | Level C<br>Only expert opinion, case studies, or standard of care | Recommendation that procedure/treatment is valuable<br>Evidence from opinion, case studies, standard of care | Recommendation in favor of procedure/treatment being valuable<br>Only diverging expert opinion, case studies, standard of care | Recommendation's value less well established<br>Only diverging expert opinion, case studies, standard of care | Recommendation that procedure/treatment is not valuable or may be harmful<br>Evidence from opinion, case studies, standard of care |

Precision of treatment effect

From Jacobs A, Kushner FG, Ettinger SM, et al. ACCF/AHA clinical practice guideline methodology summit report: a report of the American College of Cardiology Foundation/American Heart Association Task Force on Practice Guidelines. *Circulation.* 2013;127:268-310.

**TABLE 8.2 • Recommendations, Potential Changes, and New Data by Medication Class**

| Medication | Recommendation | Class/Evidence | Potential Changes/New Data |
|---|---|---|---|
| Beta-blockers | Continue beta-blockers if started >30 d before surgery | Class I, Level B | Unlikely, although no robust prospective studies as of yet |
| | Postoperative beta-blocker management should be guided by clinical circumstances (ie, hypotension) | Class IIa, Level B | No new data |
| | Consider starting periopera-tive beta-blockers in high-risk patients >I d before surgery | Class IIb, Level B | No new data |
| | Do not start beta-blockers on the day of surgery | Class III, Level B | 2017 meta-analysis on vascular surgery patients showed no difference in mortality or stroke |
| Statins | Continue statins periopera-tively for any patient already on the medication | Class I, Level B | Possible increase in Level of Evidence to A, given recent prospective study confirming benefit |
| | Initiate statins in patients un-dergoing vascular surgery | Class IIa, Level B | May expand to all surgeries due to recent data on universal clinical benefit |
| Antiplatelet Agents | Nonurgent, noncardiac surgeries should be delayed >I y following stent placement | Class I, Level B | 2016 retrospective study with increased mortality within I y of stent placement (all types) |
| | Continue DAPT for 4-6 wk after stent placement, even if patient is undergoing urgent surgery | Class I, Level C | Disproportionately high rates of in-stent thrombosis in the first month after stent placement |
| | Minimum duration of DAPT is 6 mo for DES and I mo for BMS | Class IIb, Level B | Second-generation DES may have less complications when interrupting DAPT after 6 wk for surgery |
| | In patients without prior PCI, consider continuing aspirin if risk of cardiovascular events outweighs bleeding risk | Class IIb, Level B | For geriatric patients over 70, insufficient evidence to use aspirin for primary prevention; consider holding |
| | Do not initiate aspirin before noncardiac, nonvascular surgery | Class III, Level B | No new data |

*(continued)*

**TABLE 8.2 • Recommendations, Potential Changes, and New Data by Medication Class (continued)**

| Medication | Recommendation | Class/Evidence | Potential Changes/New Data |
|---|---|---|---|
| ACE Inhibitors/ARBs | It is reasonable to continue ACE-I and ARBs perioperatively | Class IIa, Level B | 2017 prospective cohort study showed decreased mortality and hypotension in patients where medications were held >24 h before surgery |
| | Restart ACE-I and ARBs postoperatively as soon as reasonably possible | Class IIa, Level C | 2015 retrospective study showed increased mortality in patients >75 years old when not restarting ARB postoperatively. Level of evidence should increase |
| Anticoagulants | No recommendation in 2014 | N/A | 2015 study showed no difference in mortality for patients with atrial fibrillation when comparing bridging anticoagulation vs. placebo. Current ongoing trial aims to answer same question in patients with mechanical valves |
| Alpha-1 antagonists | No recommendation in 2014 | N/A | 2015 study showed initiating medication may decrease postoperative urinary retention |

Abbreviations: ACE, angiotensin-converting enzyme; ARB, angiotensin receptor blocker; BMS, bare metal stents; DAPT, dual antiplatelet therapy; DES, drug-eluting stents; PCI, percutaneous coronary intervention.

61 660 patients compared patients on atenolol, metoprolol, and carvedilol and found no significant difference in MACE or all-cause mortality between the three **medications**.[14] However, a subgroup analysis showed patients with prior MI that were treated with carvedilol had a significantly lower rate of all-cause mortality (odds ratio [OR]: 0.62; 95% CI, 0.43-0.87). This study examined a subgroup of geriatric patients that confirmed similar results.

These studies provided evidence that continuing chronic β-blocker therapy was beneficial in patients with elevated RCRI scores and significant cardiovascular disease, but did not decrease mortality in patients without these comorbidities. A variety of retrospective studies have also investigated effects of β-blocker withdrawal with respect to postoperative mortality. A 2001 study with 140 patients undergoing vascular **surgery** showed an increase in cardiovascular mortality (0% vs 29%, $P = 0.005$) and postoperative MI (OR: 17.7, $P = 0.003$) in patients where β-blocker therapy was discontinued.[15] The largest retrospective analysis addressing postoperative β-blocker withdrawal was published in 2010, analyzing more than 38 000 patients at the San Francisco VA hospital over a 10-year period. **Perioperative** discontinuation of β-blocker therapy was associated with a significant increase in both 30-day mortality (OR: 3.93; 95% CI, 2.57-6.01; $P < 0.0001$) and 1-year mortality (OR, 1.96; 95% CI, 1.49-2.58; $P = 0.0001$).[16]

Taken in concert, these retrospective studies show significant benefit of continuing chronic β-blocker therapy in patients using them based on guideline directed medical therapy (ie, heart failure or recent MI) and significant risk in discontinuing β-blocker therapy perioperatively for all patients on β-blocker therapy. The lack of randomized controlled trials explains the ACC/AHA level B recommendation.

The question regarding initiation of β-blocker therapy preoperatively is a far more contentious topic, particularly in the geriatric population. Numerous small trials addressing this question have been published over the past 20 years, starting with the 1996 study of 200 patients started on atenolol on the day of noncardiac surgery. Overall mortality was decreased at 6-month (0% vs 8%, $P < 0.001$), 1-year (3% vs 14%, $P = 0.005$), and 2-year (10% vs 21%, $P = 0.019$) follow-up.[17] Follow-up randomized controlled studies showed similar results with minimal adverse events, and initiating β-blockers perioperatively became the standard of care. Some of these recommendations were based on results from the DECREASE-IV trial, which showed significant decrease in cardiovascular death and MI postoperatively in patients treated with β-blockers without increase in adverse events.[18] However, this trial was subsequently retracted because of data falsification.

The largest randomized controlled trial addressing perioperative β-blocker use, the POISE trial, was published in 2008, with 8351 patients from 190 medical centers with an average age of 69 years. Significant results at 30-day follow-up included decreased rate of MI (4.2% vs 5.7%, with HR: 0.73; 95% CI, 0.60-0.89; $P = 0.0017$) but increased all-cause mortality (3.1% vs 2.3%, with HR: 1.33; 95% CI, 1.03-1.74; $P = 0.0317$) and stroke (1% vs 0.5%, with HR: 2.17; 95% CI, 1.26-3.74; $P = 0.0053$).[19] There was no age subgroup analysis to more specifically address adverse outcomes in geriatric patients. However, other clinically significant results included increased rates of hypotension and bradycardia in the β-blocker group. Criticism of the trial included high medication dosing (β-blocker naive patients were given metoprolol 200 mg) and initiation of therapy on the day of surgery.

Follow-up systematic reviews, however, confirmed the POISE trial results. A 2014 review including 16 randomized controlled trials similarly demonstrated decreased risk of postoperative MI but increased mortality and stroke, even with exclusion of the POISE and DECREASE-IV trials.[20] A 2014 Cochrane Review drew similar conclusions, cautioning that potential decrease in postoperative MI and arrhythmias may be offset by increased risk of stroke and mortality and that available evidence is low to moderate in quality.[21] With these data, the ACC/AHA issued a class III, level of Evidence B recommendation to initiating β-blocker therapy for patients on the day of surgery. Research into this topic is ongoing. For example, a recent 2017 meta-analysis on 32 602 vascular surgery patients showed no change in mortality, stroke, or MI with perioperative β-blocker use.[22]

The only clear recommendation on β-blocker therapy at this time is to continue patients on the medication perioperatively if they have used them chronically and to not start therapy on the day of **surgery**. There are conflicting data on whether to start β-blockers on patients perioperatively more than 1 day before **surgery**. Clinicians must weigh the risks and benefits of this decision, and using the RCRI score and assessing **perioperative** risk of hypotension and bradycardia may help stratify patients. There is a dearth of data regarding this patient population, however, so decisions on **perioperative** β-blocker therapy must be made on a case-by-case basis depending on individual risk.

## Statins

Statin use has increased tremendously in the past few decades because of multiple robust randomized controlled trials showing mortality benefit in patients with a history of coronary artery disease (CAD),[23] MI,[24] or elevated cardiovascular disease risk.[25] Not surprisingly, the ACC/AHA issued a class I, level B recommendation to continue statin therapy perioperatively for all patients who were previously on the medication. Most of the data supporting this recommendation are based on observational studies. The largest retrospective cohort study from 2004 analyzed 780 591 patients who underwent noncardiac **surgery**.[26] Patients on statin therapy had a significantly lower rate of in-hospital mortality (adjusted OR: 0.62; 95% CI, 0.58-0.67), with a more significant difference in patients with an RCRI score of at least 4. A 2010 observational trial analyzed 577 patients (with average age of 74 years) undergoing vascular **surgery**.[27] Patients with **perioperative** statin use exhibited significantly decreased 2-year mortality (6% vs 16%, $P = 0.0002$) and **perioperative** mortality and MI (11% vs 27%, $P < 0.0001$).

For patients not previously on statins, it is reasonable to initiate therapy in patients undergoing vascular procedures, earning a class IIb, level B ACC/AHA recommendation. This is largely based on a 2013 Cochrane review pooling three earlier randomized controlled trials.[28] The review showed significantly lower 30-day mortality in patients with **perioperative** statin use (6.7% vs 13.7%). In addition, statin withdrawal in vascular **surgery** patients may pose a risk. A 2007 study reviewed 298 consecutive vascular **surgery** patients on the basis of postoperative statin discontinuation.[29] Patients with statin discontinuation had significantly higher rates of cardiovascular death and MI (HR: 7.5; 95% CI, 2.8-20.1).

More recent data since the publication of the 2014 ACC/AHA guidelines further support **perioperative** statin use. A meta-analysis of four randomized controlled trials with 675 total patients and 20 observational studies with 22 861 total patients who had undergone vascular **surgery** was published in 2015.[30] Statin therapy was associated with significantly lower rates of all-cause mortality, MI, and stroke. The VISION trial, a 2016 prospective cohort study, enrolled 15 478 total patients undergoing noncardiac **surgery**.[31] Impressively, the preoperative use of statins was associated with a significant decrease in all-cause mortality (relative risk [RR], 0.58; 95% CI, 0.40-0.83; $P = 0.003$) and cardiovascular mortality (RR, 0.42; 95% CI, 0.23-0.76; $P = 0.004$).

A 2017 retrospective, observational cohort analysis with 96 486 patients (96% men, average age of 66 years) analyzed a multitude of postsurgical complications with respect to **perioperative** statin use.[32] Statins showed the greatest risk reduction for cardiac complications (RR, 0.73; 95% CI, 0.64-0.83). Thirty-day all-cause mortality was also significantly decreased with a number needed to treat of 244 ($P < 0.001$). In addition, there was a significantly decreased risk of various other complications, such as renal failure, sepsis, and respiratory failure.

More recently, a 2018 systematic review examined a hypothesized decrease in risk of postoperative cognitive dysfunction for patients on **perioperative** statin therapy.[33] Eight relevant studies were included with a mean age of 67. Statin use before **surgery** was associated with a decreased risk of postoperative cognitive dysfunction (RR, 0.81; 95% CI, 0.67-0.98; $P = 0.03$). The study was limited by significant heterogeneity in follow-up times and statin treatment duration, however.

These recent studies on statins confirm the most recent ACC/AHA recommendations to continue statin use perioperatively and initiate use for patients undergoing vascular procedures or those with increased risk of adverse cardiovascular events. However, anti-inflammatory properties of statins may provide further **perioperative** benefits beyond cardiovascular protection. Future randomized controlled trials are needed to investigate these findings, but there may be potential benefit for all geriatric patients to use **perioperative** statins.

## Antiplatelet Agents

One of the most commonly encountered **medications** in the elderly, aspirin is an irreversible platelet cyclooxygenase inhibitor. Recommendations for aspirin management perioperatively depend on the type of **surgery** and the patient's underlying bleeding risk.

In patients undergoing coronary artery bypass grafting (CABG) already taking aspirin, it is currently recommended to continue the medication up until **surgery** and postoperatively, as per the 2015 AHA recommendations.[34] A case-control study from 2000 matched 8641 consecutive patients undergoing CABG. Patients with preoperative aspirin use were less likely than nonusers to experience in-hospital mortality, with an OR of 0.73 (95% CI, 0.54-0.97), without significant difference in adverse events like postoperative transfusion or hemorrhage.[35] A 2002 prospective observation study with 5065 patients at 17 medical centers compared patients started on aspirin within 48 hours postoperatively with those who did not. Early aspirin use was associated with a significant decrease in MI (2.8% vs 5.4%, $P < 0.001$) and mortality (1.3% vs 4%, $P < 0.001$).[36]

Controversy remained, however, regarding whether to start aspirin preoperatively in patients with newly diagnosed CAD at the time of planned CABG. The ATACUS trial, published in 2016, was a randomized controlled trial that assigned 2100 patients to either aspirin 100 mg or placebo to be administered 1 hour before surgery. There was no significant difference in the primary outcome of death or thrombotic complication (19.3% in the aspirin group vs 20.4% in the placebo group with RR, 0.94; 95% CI, 0.8-1.12; $P = 0.55$) or in major hemorrhage (1.8% vs 2.1%, $P = 0.75$). There was no significant difference in overall mortality (1.3% vs 0.9%; RR, 1.56; 95% CI, 0.68-3.60).[37] Given the inconclusive nature of this study, the decision to dose aspirin preoperatively or to wait until a few hours postoperatively should be made on a case-by-case basis depending on bleeding risk.

Aspirin therapy in noncardiac surgery is more complicated. The strongest evidence for crafting recommendations is based on the 2014 POISE-2 trial, which randomized 10 010 patients with elevated risk of cardiovascular events (ie, history of CAD or stroke, but excluding patients with previous percutaneous coronary intervention [PCI] or CABG) to either starting perioperative aspirin 7 days before noncardiac surgery or placebo.[38] Patients previously on aspirin who were randomized to the placebo group discontinued the medication 1 week before surgery and did not restart it for at least 30 days postoperatively. Patients randomized to the aspirin group underwent a further subgroup analysis comparing perioperative initiation of aspirin versus continuation of the medication. Average age of participants was 69 years, but there was no subgroup analysis dedicated to geriatric patients. There was no difference in the primary outcome of all-cause mortality or nonfatal MI at 30 days (7% in aspirin vs 7.1% in placebo, HR: 0.99; 95% CI, 0.86-1.15; $P = 0.92$). Within the subgroup analysis, there was no difference in the primary outcome for patients who started or continued aspirin, and no significant difference when stratified on the basis of RCRI score. There was, however, an increase in major bleeding requiring transfusion (4.6% vs 3.8%; HR: 1.23; 95% CI, 1.01-1.49; $P = 0.04$), which was driven by an increased risk of bleeding in the subgroup of patients that initiated aspirin. Notably, there was no change in bleeding risk in patients who were previously on aspirin before randomization.

Given these findings, the ACC/AHA issued a class IIb, level B recommendation that it may be reasonable to continue aspirin in patients without previous PCI only if the risk potential perioperative cardiac events outweigh the risk of bleeding. However, many patients are prescribed aspirin for primary prevention for both cardiovascular disease and colorectal cancer, even though this is only a grade C recommendation for patients aged 65 to 69 years and a grade I recommendation for patients older than 70 years, as per U.S. Preventive Services Task Force guidelines.[39] Given these data, it is reasonable to hold aspirin in geriatric patients for 5 to 7 days before noncardiac surgery provided there are no recent cardiac stents. In addition, it is a class III, level B recommendation from the ACC/AHA to not start aspirin before elective noncardiac, noncarotid surgery.

Recommendations are somewhat more specific in relation to patients with recent coronary stents, although much of the evidence is not ideal. In general, perioperative management of dual antiplatelet therapy (DAPT) must be determined by weighing the risk of in-stent thrombosis with the RR of bleeding. Relevant factors include stent type and timing, patient age, type of surgery, and patient comorbidities. A consensus should be reached after discussion between the cardiologist, surgeon, anesthesiologist, and patient.

The 2014 ACC/AHA guidelines issued a class I, level C recommendation to continue DAPT for at least 4 to 6 weeks after stent placement, even if a patient is undergoing urgent surgery. These recommendations are based on numerous studies, which have shown disproportionately high rates of in-stent thrombosis in the first month after placement.[40,41] Nonurgent, noncardiac surgeries should preferably be delayed at least 1 year, an ACC/AHA class I, level B recommendation, regardless of stent type. A recent retrospective analysis from 2016 included 24 313 patients who underwent noncardiac surgery, 1120 patients of whom had a history of a cardiac stent.[42] The study found significantly increased rates of mortality for patients with stent placement within 1 year (adjusted OR: 2.59; 95% CI, 1.26-4.94) and increased rates of bleeding, but no difference in the two outcomes for patients more than 1 year removed from coronary stent placement. Notably, a subgroup analysis demonstrated similarly increased risk for both drug-eluting stents (DES) and bare metal stents (BMS) within 1 year.

If surgery cannot be delayed for a full year, the minimum duration of DAPT is 1 month for BMS and 6 months for DES, a class IIb, level B recommendation. Although there is no definitive evidence from randomized controlled trials, a recent observational study with more than 4000 patients showed no difference in in-stent thrombosis rates in patients with short-term interruptions in DAPT therapy 6 months after stent placement.[43]

If DAPT must be interrupted before 1 year, aspirin should be continued perioperatively and clopidogrel should be resumed immediately postoperatively, preferably with a loading dose if there is no bleeding. It is unclear what the optimal type of stent is for patients requiring PCI before surgery. The recent NORSTENT trial from 2016 randomized 9013 to contemporary DES or BMS with the primary outcome all-cause mortality or nonfatal MI at 6-year follow-up.[44] There was no difference in the death or nonfatal MI, but BMS were associated with an increased need for revascularization (16.5% vs 19.8%; HR: 0.76; 95% CI, 0.69-0.85; $P < 0.001$) and stent thrombosis (HR: 0.64; 95% CI, 0.41-1; $P = 0.0498$). For geriatric patients who may require more urgent surgery, BMS placement may be optimal because of decreased time needed for DAPT. However, given the increased association with stent thrombosis, DES may be preferred for geriatric patients awaiting nonurgent, noncardiac surgery.

## Anticoagulants

For many years, standard of care perioperative management for patients on anticoagulation involved discontinuing warfarin and initiating preoperative bridging with low-molecular-weight heparin (LMWH) to minimize the risk of thromboembolic events. This was particularly relevant to the geriatric population, who has an increased risk of atrial fibrillation and inherently elevated CHADS2-VASc score because of age older than 65 years. However, this practice has been recently altered because of results from the BRIDGE trial. This 2015 study randomized 1884 preoperative patients with atrial fibrillation on warfarin to either bridging anticoagulation with LMWH or placebo.[45] Patients with mechanical heart valves, planned cardiac **surgery**, or stroke within the previous 3 months were excluded from the study. There was no significant difference between the two study populations with regard to stroke, transient ischemic attack (TIA), or all-cause mortality at 30-day follow-up. However, patients who underwent bridging anticoagulation had a significantly higher rate of major bleeding (3.2% vs 1.3%, $P = 0.005$; number needed to harm = 50).

Only 3% of the patients in the BRIDGE trial had a CHADS2-VASc score greater than 4, meaning there may be limited applicability to patients with atrial fibrillation with higher risk of stroke. In addition, the results cannot be applied to patients on novel anticoagulant therapy. For patients with atrial fibrillation and low to moderate risk of stroke, which represents a sizable portion of geriatric patients, it is recommended to hold warfarin perioperatively for major noncardiac surgeries. These data are also supported by a large systematic review from 2012 with 7118 patients on warfarin therapy perioperatively.[46] The study similarly found no statistically significant difference in rate of **perioperative** thromboembolic events, but did see significantly increased risk of major bleeding in patients treating with bridging therapy.

Currently, it is still recommended that patients with mechanical mitral valves be bridged with LMWH until **surgery**. However, the ongoing PERIOP-2 trial is randomizing patients with mechanical mitral valves to bridging therapy versus placebo.[47] Its results should provide an important answer in guiding the management of these patients, many of whom are older than 65 years.

## Angiotensin-Converting Enzyme Inhibitors/Angiotensin Receptor Blockers

**Perioperative** angiotensin-converting enzyme (ACE) inhibitor and angiotensin receptor blocker (ARB) therapy is surrounded in controversy. In 2014, the ACC/AHA issued a class IIa, level B recommendation that continuation of these **medications** perioperatively is reasonable. Similar to other recommendations, this is based on numerous observational analyses and a dearth of geriatric specific data. One recent study focused on 18 056 matched patients undergoing noncardiac **surgery**, comparing users of ACE inhibitors to nonusers.[48] The authors found no difference in 30-day all-cause mortality or respiratory complications. However, a meta-analysis of five observational studies showed an RR of postoperative hypotension requiring vasopressors of 1.50 (95% CI, 1.15-1.96) when comparing patients who received preoperative ACE inhibitor or ARB dosing to those who had the medication held.[49] There was no significant difference in mortality or cardiovascular outcomes. Older trials with limited sample size yielded similar results, finding that patients treated perioperatively with ACE inhibitors or ARBs had increased episodes of postoperative hypotension without an increase in mortality.[50,51] Given the limited amount of data on these **medications**, decisions should be made individually for each patient. Patients with comorbidities like systolic heart failure may have increased benefit with **perioperative** ACE inhibitor and ARB therapy. However, they should be used in caution with geriatric patients, who have an increased risk of postural hypotension and are often on other antihypertensive **medications** that should not be stopped (ie, β-blockers or clonidine) at the time of **surgery**.

New literature continues to challenge the established guidelines for **perioperative** ACE inhibitor and ARB use. A large prospective cohort study from 2017 analyzed 14 687 patients undergoing noncardiac **surgery**, 4802 of whom were on ACE inhibitors or ARBs preoperatively.[52] Twenty-six percent of these patients had their **medications** held at least 24 hours before **surgery**. This group was found to have a lower composite rate of all-cause mortality, stroke, or myocardial injury when compared with patients who continued ACE inhibitors and ARBs on the day of **surgery** (12.0% vs 12.9%; adjusted RR, 0.82; 95% CI, 0.70-0.96; $P = 0.01$). These patients also showed decreased rates of intraoperative hypotension, although the risk of postoperative hypotension was insignificant. The study highlights the need for a well-conducted randomized controlled trial to establish higher quality evidence for **perioperative** guidance on these **medications**.

A recent retrospective, matched cohort study of 1351 patients further complicated the decision of whether to hold ACE inhibitors or ARBs before **surgery**.[53] However, the study focused on a relatively narrow patient population with metabolic syndrome undergoing CABG. The primary outcome was a composite of adverse events observed 30 days after procedure: new onset atrial fibrillation, arrhythmia requiring cardioversion, MI, acute respiratory failure, acute renal failure, cerebrovascular accidents, and **perioperative** death. Surprisingly, patients that continued ARBs had a lower incidence of adverse events than patients taken off **medications** (OR: 0.43; 95% CI, 0.19-0.99) or on ACE inhibitors (OR: 0.38; 95% CI, 0.16-0.86). However, the study did not have an adequately powered geriatric cohort to make similar conclusions about this population.

Although debate will continue regarding preoperative management of ACE inhibitors and ARBs, two recent retrospective cohort studies have highlighted the importance of restarting these **medications** postoperatively in a timely manner. A 2015 study analyzed 30 173 patients in the VA Health System over a 12-year period.[54] With respect to 30-day mortality, patients who restarted ARBs postoperatively versus those who did not had an outcome rate of 1.3% versus 3.2% (adjust HR: 1.74; 95% CI, 1.47-2.06; $P < 0.001$). Younger patients (those younger than 60 years) had an increased mortality risk. However, a geriatric-specific cohort of patients older than 75 years still had an increased 30-day mortality rate when not restarting ARB therapy postoperatively (HR: 1.42; 95% CI, 1.09-1.85; $P = 0.01$). A similarly designed study was published in 2014 analyzing 30-day mortality for 240 978 patients on ACE inhibitor therapy.[55] Patients who did not restart the medication within 2 weeks postoperatively had a significantly increased mortality risk (HR: 3.44; 95% CI, 3.30-3.60; $P < 0.001$). This study did not have specific data on geriatric patients. The data reinforce the class IIa ACC/AHA recommendation to restart these **medications** as soon as possible postoperatively and likely will increase from their current level of evidence of C during the next guideline updates.

## Alpha-1 Antagonists

The prevalence of BPH approaches 80% in patients older than 70 years, making it one of the most common problems in geriatric men.[56] Consequently, alpha-1 antagonists, including terazosin and tamsulosin, are frequently found on these patients' medication lists. General consensus is that these **medications** pose minimal cardiovascular risk for preoperative hypotension and that they can be continued safely in most procedures. Ophthalmologic procedures such as cataract removal, however, pose a unique risk. A 2005 retrospective study of 511 patients taking tamsulosin at the time of cataract **surgery** showed that 2% of patients developed floppy iris syndrome (IFIS), a condition involving intractable iris prolapse with progressive pupillary constriction.[57] Despite this infrequent complication, most ophthalmologic surgeons do not require that these agents be discontinued.[58] Certain intraoperative techniques can reduce the incidence of IFIS to 0.6%.[59] In addition, despite a half-life of only 15 hours, the long-term effect of alpha-1 antagonists with respect to the risk of IFIS is unclear, possibly extending from months to years. Given this, holding these **medications** for a few days preoperatively likely provides minimal benefit.

Interestingly, starting alpha-1 antagonists perioperatively may benefit a select group of geriatric patients. A recent 2015 retrospective review analyzed the possible benefit of starting tamsulosin 3 days preoperatively in patients undergoing pelvic **surgery** with respect to postoperative urinary retention.[60]) In a study population of 185 patients, the authors found a rate of urinary retention of 6.7% in the tamsulosin group versus 25% in the control group ($P = 0.029$). These findings have not yet been duplicated in a randomized controlled trial.

# SUMMARY

As the population of the United States continues to grow, particularly that of those older than 65 years, the number of geriatric patients undergoing **surgery** will also increase. The inpatient **perioperative** care of this segment of the population has unique challenges that are not currently well studied or outlined.

There have been encouraging data on preoperative risk assessments and screening for geriatric patients in recent years. Although younger patients may not have improved outcomes from a full preoperative evaluation, there are potential benefits for elderly population. However, this must be weighed against the risks of overscreening, unnecessary testing, and potentially dangerous delays in time to **surgery**. The ACC/AHA **perioperative** guidelines should continue to be used in preoperative evaluation of older adults, as it decreases unnecessary testing. Frailty screening should be completed in all geriatric patients to help predict postoperative complications and quality of life. In regard to **perioperative** medication management, some recommendations are strong and based on high-quality evidence (ie, continuation of β-blockers) and should be followed in the geriatric population. However, high-quality evidence is lacking for many medication classes, particularly in the geriatric patient population.

Older adults pose a unique set of challenges during the **perioperative** period. Therapeutic advances continue to rapidly evolve in the field and should be used in conjunction with a robust individualized risk assessment to help optimize geriatric patients' postoperative outcomes.

## References

1. Ortman JM, Velkoff VA, Hogan H. *An Aging Nation: The Older Population in the United States*. Washington, DC: U.S. Census Bureau; 2014. Report No.: Current Population Reports, P25-1140.
2. Fleisher LA, Fleischmann KE, Auerbach AD, et al. 2014 ACC/AHA guideline on perioperative cardiovascular evaluation and management of patients undergoing noncardiac surgery. *J Am Coll Cardiol*. 2014;64:e77-137.
3. Mohanty S, Rosenthal RA, Russell MM, et al. Optimal perioperative management of the geriatric patient: a best practices guideline from the American College of Surgeons NSQIP and the American Geriatrics Society. *J Am Coll Surg*. 2016;222:930-947.
4. Dakik HA, Kobrossi S, Tamim H. The yield of routine pre-operative cardiovascular evaluation in stable patients scheduled for elective non-cardiac surgery. *Int J Cardiol*. 2015;186:325-327.
5. Sheffield KM, Stone PS, Benarroch-Gampel J, et al. Overuse of preoperative cardiac stress testing in medicare patients undergoing elective noncardiac surgery. *Ann Surg*. 2013;257:73-80.
6. Smeets SJ, Poeze M, Verbruggen JP. Preoperative cardiac evaluation of geriatric patients with hip fracture. *Injury*. 2012;43:2146-2152.
7. Stitgen A, Poludnianyk K, Dulaney-Cripe E, et al. Adherence to preoperative cardiac clearance guidelines in hip fracture patients. *J Orthop Trauma*. 2015;9:500-503.
8. Koh AS, Flores JL, Keng FY, et al. Correlation between clinical outcomes and appropriateness grading for referral to myocardial perfusion imaging for preoperative evaluation prior to non-cardiac surgery. *J Nucl Cardiol*. 2012;19:277-284.
9. Lin HS, Watt JS, Peel NM, et al. Frailty and postoperative outcomes in older surgical patients: a systematic review. *BMC Geriatr*. 2016;16:157.
10. Robinson TN, Wu DS, Pointer L, et al. Simple frailty score predicts post-operative complications across surgical specialties. *Am J Surg*. 2013;206:544-550.
11. Afilalo J, Eisenberg MJ, Morin JF, et al. Gait speed as an incremental predictor of mortality and major morbidity in elderly patients undergoing cardiac surgery. *J Am Coll Cardiol*. 2010;56:1668-1676.
12. Lindenauer PK, Pekow P, Wang K, et al. Perioperative beta-blocker therapy and mortality after major noncardiac surgery. *N Engl J Med*. 2005;353:349-361.
13. Andersson C, Merie C, Jorgensen M, et al. Association of β-blocker therapy with risks of adverse cardiovascular events and deaths in patients with ischemic heart disease undergoing noncardiac surgery: a Danish nationwide cohort study. *JAMA Intern Med*. 2014;174:336-344.
14. Jorgensen ME, Sanders RD, Kober L, et al. Beta-blocker subtype and risks of perioperative adverse events following non-cardiac surgery; a nationwide cohort study. *Eur Heart J*. 2017;38(31):2421-2428.

15. Shammash JB, Trost JC, Gold JM, et al. Perioperative beta-blocker withdrawal and mortality in vascular surgical patients. *Am Heart J*. 2001;141:148-153.

16. Wallace AW, Au S, Cason BA. Association of the pattern of use of perioperative beta-blockade and postoperative mortality. *Anesthesiology*. 2010;113:794-805.

17. Mangano DT, Layug EL, Wallace A, Tateo I. Effect of atenolol on mortality and cardiovascular morbidity after noncardiac surgery. Multicenter Study of Perioperative Ischemia Research Group. *N Engl J Med*. 1996;335:1713-1720.

18. Dunkelgrun M, Boersma E, Schouten O, et al. Bisoprolol and fluvastatin for the reduction of perioperative cardiac mortality and myocardial infarction in intermediate-risk patients undergoing noncardiovascular surgery: a randomized controlled trial (DECREASE-IV). *Ann Surg*. 2009;249:921-926.

19. Devereaux PJ, Yang H, Yusuf S, et al. Effects of extendedrelease metoprolol succinate in patients undergoing noncardiac surgery: a randomised controlled trial. *Lancet*. 2008;371:1839-1847.

20. Wijeysundera DN, Duncan D, Nkonde-Price C, et al. Perioperative beta blockade in noncardiac surgery: a systematic review for the 2014 ACC/AHA guideline on perioperative cardiovascular evaluation and management of patients undergoing noncardiac surgery: a report of the American College of Cardiology/American Heart Association Task Force on practice guidelines. *J Am Coll Cardiol*. 2014;64:2406-2425.

21. Blessberger H, Kammler J, Domanovits H, et al. Perioperative beta-blockers for preventing surgery related mortality and morbidity. *Cochrane Database Syst Rev*. 2014;(9):CD004476.

22. Hajibandeh S, Hajibandeh S, Antoniou SA, et al. Effect of beta-blockers on perioperative outcomes in vascular and endovascular surgery: a systematic review and metaanalysis. *Br J Anaesth*. 2017;118:11-21.

23. LaRosa JC, Grundy SM, Waters DD, et al. Intensive lipid lowering with atorvastatin in patients with stable coronary disease. *N Eng J Med*. 2005;352:1425-1435.

24. Cannon CP, Braunwald E, McCabe CH, et al. Intensive versus moderate lipid lowering with statins after acute coronary syndromes. *N Eng J Med*. 2004;350:1495-1504.

25. Ridker PM, Danielson E, Fonseco FA, et al. Rosuvastatin to prevent vascular events in men and women with elevated C-reactive protein. *N Eng J Med*. 2008;359:2195-2207.

26. Lindenauer PK, Pekow P, Wang K, et al. Lipid-lowering therapy and in-hospital mortality following major noncardiac surgery. *JAMA*. 2004;291:2092-2099.

27. Desai H, Aronow WS, Ahn C, et al. Incidence of perioperative myocardial infarction and of 2-year mortality in 577 elderly patients undergoing noncardiac vascular surgery treated with and without statins. *Arch Gerontol Geriatr*. 2010;51:149-151.

28. Sanders RD, Nicholson A, Lewis SR, et al. Perioperative statin therapy for improving outcomes during and after noncardiac vascular surgery. *Cochrane Database Syst Rev*. 2013;(7):CD009971.

29. Schouten O, Hoeks SE, Welten GM, et al. Effect of statin withdrawal on frequency of cardiac events after vascular surgery. *Am J Cardiol*. 2007;100:316.

30. Antoniou GA, Hajibandeh S, Hajibandeh S, et al. Metaanalysis of the effects of statins on perioperative outcomes in vascular and endovascular surgery. *J Vasc Surg*. 2015;61:519-532.

31. Berwanger O, Manach YL, Suzumura EA, et al. Association between pre-operative statin use and major cardiovascular complications among patients undergoing non-cardiac surgery: the VISION study. *Eur Heart J*. 2016;37:177-185.

32. London MJ, Schwartz GG, Hur K, et al. Association of perioperative statin use with mortality and morbidity after major non noncardiac surgery. *JAMA Intern Med*. 2017;177:231-242.

33. Feinkohl I, Winterer G, Pischon T. Associations of dyslipidaemia and lipid-lowering treatment with risk of postoperative cognitive dysfunction: a systematic review and meta-analysis. *J Epidemiol Community Health*. 2018;76(2):499-506. doi:10.1136/jech-2017-210338

34. Kulik A, Ruel M, Jneid H, et al. Secondary prevention after coronary artery bypass graft surgery: a scientific statement from the American Heart Association. *Circulation*. 2015;131:927.

35. Dacey LJ, Munoz JJ, Johnson ER, et al. Effect of preoperative aspirin use on mortality in coronary artery bypass grafting patients. *Ann Thorac Surg*. 2000;70:1986.

36. Mangano DT. Aspirin and mortality from coronary bypass surgery. *N Engl J Med*. 2002;347:1309.

37. Myles PS, Smith JA, Forbes A, et al. Stopping vs. continuing aspirin before coronary artery surgery. *N Engl J Med*. 2016;374:728.

38. Devereaux PJ, Mrkobrada M, Sessler DI, et al. Aspirin in patients undergoing noncardiac surgery. *N Engl J Med*. 2014;370:1494-1503.

39. Bibbins-Domingo K. Aspirin use for the primary prevention of cardiovascular disease and colorectal cancer: U.S. Preventive Services Task Force Recommendation Statement. *Ann Intern Med.* 2016;21:836-845.

40. Wijeysundera DN, Wijeysundera HC, Yun L, et al. Risk of elective major noncardiac surgery after coronary stent insertion: a population-based study. *Circulation.* 2012;126:1355-1362.

41. Hawn MT, Graham LA, Richman JS, et al. Risk of major adverse cardiac events following noncardiac surgery in patients with coronary stents. *JAMA.* 2013;310:1462-1472.

42. Mahmoud K, Sanon S, Habermann EB, et al. Perioperative cardiovascular risk of prior coronary stent implantation among patients undergoing noncardiac surgery. *J Am Coll Cardiol.* 2016;67:1038-1049.

43. Silber S, Kirtane AJ, Belardi JA, et al. Lack of association between dual antiplatelet therapy use and stent thrombosis between 1 and 12 months following resolute zotarolimus-eluting stent implantation. *Eur Heart J.* 2014;35:1949.

44. Bonaa KH, Mannsverk J, Wiseth R, et al. Drug-eluting or bare-metal stents for coronary artery disease. *N Eng J Med.* 2016;375:1242-1252.

45. Douketis JD, Spyropoulos AC, Kaatz S, et al. Perioperative bridging anticoagulation in patients with atrial fibrillation. *N Eng J Med.* 2015;373:823-833.

46. Siegal D, Yudin J, Kaatz S, et al. Periprocedural heparin bridging in patients receiving vitamin K antagonists: systematic review and meta-analysis of bleeding and thromboembolic rates. *Circulation.* 2012;126:1630.

47. ClinicalTrials.gov: PERIOP2 - A safety and effectiveness of LMWH vs placebo bridging therapy for patients on long term warfarin requiring temporary interruption of warfarin. https://www.clinicaltrials.gov/ct2/show/NCT00432796. Accessed March 1, 2017.

48. Turan A, You J, Shiba A, Kurz A, Saager L, Sessler DI. Angiotensin converting enzyme inhibitors are not associated with respiratory complications or mortality after noncardiac surgery. *Anesth Analg.* 2012;114:552-560.

49. Rosenman DJ, McDonald FS, Ebbert JO, et al. Clinical consequences of withholding versus administering renin-angiotensin-aldosterone system antagonists in the preoperative period. *J Hosp Med.* 2008;3:319-325.

50. Coriat P, Richer C, Douraki T, et al. Influence of chronic angiotensin-converting enzyme inhibition on anesthetic induction. *Anesthesiology.* 1994;81:299.

51. Bertrand M, Godet G, Meersshaert K, et al. Should the angiotensin II antagonists be discontinued before surgery? *Anesth Analg.* 2001;92:26.

52. Roshanov PS, Rochwerg B, Patel A, et al. Withholding versus continuing angiotensin-converting enzyme inhibitors or angiotensin II receptor blockers before noncardiac surgery: an analysis of the vascular events in noncardiac surgery patients cohort evaluation prospective cohort. *Anesthesiology.* 2017;126:16.

53. Manning MW, Cooter M, Mathew J, et al. Angiotensin receptor blockade improves cardiac surgical outcomes in patients with metabolic syndrome. *Ann Thorac Surg.* 2017;104(1):98-105.

54. Lee SM, Takemoto S, Wallace AW. Association between withholding angiotensin receptor blockers in the early postoperative period and 30-day mortality: a cohort study of the veterans affairs healthcare system. *Anesthesiology.* 2015;123:288-306.

55. Mudumbai SC, Takemoto S, Cason BA, et al. Thirtyday mortality risk associated with the postoperative nonresumption of angiotensin-converting enzyme inhibitors: a retrospective study of the Veterans Affairs Healthcare System. *J Hosp Med.* 2014;9:289-296.

56. Berry SJ, Coffey DS, Walsh PC, et al. The development of human benign prostatic hyperplasia with age. *J Urol.* 1984;132:474.

57. Chang DF, Campbell JR. Intraoperative floppy iris syndrome associated with tamsulosin. *J Cataract Refract Surg.* 2005;31:664-673.

58. Yaycioglu O, Altan-Yaycioglu R. Intraoperative floppy iris syndrome: facts for the urologist. *Urology.* 2010;76:272-276.

59. Chang DF, Osher RH, Wang L, et al. Prospective multicenter evaluation of cataract surgery in patients taking tamsulosin (Flomax). *Ophthalmology.* 2007;144:957.

60. Poylin V, Curran T, Cataldo T, et al. Perioperative use of tamsulosin significantly decreases rates of urinary retention in men undergoing pelvic surgery. *Int J Colorectal Dis.* 2015;30:1223-1228.

# Therapeutic Advances in the Management of Common Geriatric Conditions

# CHAPTER 9

# Therapeutic Advances in the Prevention and Treatment of Delirium

Courtney Kluger, MD, Pooja Vyas, DO, Sutapa Maiti, MD, Olawumi Babalola, MD, Colm Mulvany, BS, and Liron Sinvani, MD

## BACKGROUND

**Delirium** is a common, costly, and devastating condition affecting nearly one-third of hospitalized older patients, with an associated hospital mortality rate of up to 33%, and annual health care expenditures exceeding $152 billion.[1-4] Although it has been described in the literature for many centuries, **delirium** remains poorly understood.[1,5] **Delirium** is characterized by acute disruptions in cognition, attention, wakefulness, and behavior with fluctuations in the ability to perform and complete basic daily tasks.[2,6]

Although it may occur in all settings, the majority of **delirium** is seen in acute care, with prevalence in the elderly ranging from 30% to 40% on medical units and as high as 80% in the intensive care unit (ICU).[2,5,7-13] In addition, postoperative **delirium** is a common complication occurring in up to 60% of older adults.[14] As the number of surgical procedures in older adults increases, optimizing, preventing, and treating postoperative cognitive dysfunction is of critical importance.[15] According to the American **Delirium** Society, more than 7 million hospitalized patients suffer from **delirium** annually in the United States.[6,16] Indeed, **delirium** is one of the six foremost causes of preventable medical conditions in hospitalized older adults and has been associated with lengthy hospitalizations, acute care readmissions, significant patient suffering with reduced quality of life, residual long-term cognitive impairment, and need for institutionalization.[6-8] Studies have shown that patients who experience **delirium** while hospitalized have a 62% increased risk of mortality within the first 12 months of discharge.[17] **Delirium** is a neurobehavioral syndrome caused by the interplay of predisposing (cognitive impairment and polypharmacy) and precipitating (infection and metabolic derangements) factors.[2,5,6] Although a number of theories have been proposed to explain the pathophysiology of **delirium**, the underlying mechanism involves the dysregulation of neuronal activity secondary to systemic disturbances.[18] **Delirium** is unlikely the result of a single hypothesis but instead develops as a function of multiple interacting pathways.

The central features of **delirium** include acute onset and fluctuating course, inattention, as well as a disturbance in sleep-wake cycle, disorientation, altered level of consciousness, disorganized thoughts with perceptual disturbances, and incoherent speech. **Delirium** can present as hyperactive, hypoactive, or in mixed forms. Hyperactive **delirium** is usually characterized by hypervigilance and agitation, which is often readily recognized by caregivers and providers.[5] Conversely, hypoactive **delirium** often goes undiagnosed because it usually presents with lethargy and psychomotor slowing that may not be evident without formal **delirium** screening. It is important to note that hypoactive **delirium** occurs three times more often than hyperactive **delirium** and carries a worse prognosis. The mixed form of **delirium** occurs with the presence and fluctuation of both hypoactive and hyperactive features.

**Delirium** is a clinical diagnosis that requires a formal cognitive assessment.[1] Studies have demonstrated that routine assessment techniques without the use of standardized tools may miss **delirium** in 32% to 66% of older adults.[19-21] Of the many instruments described in the literature for the diagnosis of **delirium**, the Confusion Assessment Method (CAM) is the most commonly studied and used. A 2010 systematic review of 11 bedside **delirium** instruments revealed that the CAM has the best available evidence as a bedside **delirium** tool.[22] The CAM has been validated in many languages and across numerous settings. When used by trained professionals, the CAM-ICU has been found to have a sensitivity of 95% and specificity of 89%.[23] However, the sensitivity and specificity of the CAM may decrease when used by untrained providers.[1] Recently, the three-dimensional CAM was found to improve accuracy without requiring specialized training.[24] Other validated **delirium** instruments include the **Delirium** Rating Scale (DRS-R-98)[25] and the Memorial **Delirium** Assessment Scale,[26] whereas symptom-based tools that are more commonly used by nurses include the Nursing **Delirium** Screening Scale (Nu-DESC),[27] Neelon and Champagne Confusion Scale (NEECHAM),[28] and the **Delirium** Observation Screening.[29] Finally, in the ICU setting, the CAM-ICU and the Intensive Care **Delirium** Screening Checklist are designed for patients who may be intubated and under sedation.[23,30]

In addition, innovative screening modalities such as the 4A test (4AT) and the Ultra-Brief **Delirium** Assessment, may offer brief, easy-to-administer alternatives. The 4AT is validated as a simple and quick **delirium** screen, with a sensitivity of 89.7% and specificity 84.1%, that does not require additional training.[31-33] The two-question Ultra-Brief **Delirium** Assessment, consisting of naming the months of the year backward and naming the day of the week, has a sensitivity of 93%; however, these results are yet to be validated in a large sample.[34] This ultra-brief assessment should be considered a screen that necessitates a formal test, such as the CAM, for diagnosis.

Once **delirium** is suspected or diagnosed, a thorough review of the patient's history and physical examination should be performed to assess for the potential causes of **delirium**. Family, caregivers, and hospital staff should be interviewed to determine the patient's baseline mental status before performing a targeted workup, as noted in Table 9.1. The presentation of **delirium** should alarm providers of "acute brain failure" and a comprehensive assessment must follow to identify and treat any contributing underlying conditions (infections, acute exacerbations of chronic conditions, metabolic abnormalities, and adverse drug reactions).

**TABLE 9.1 • Key Components of Delirium Workup and Management**

| Vital Element | Specific Concerns | Recommended Actions |
|---|---|---|
| Medical/surgical history | Adrenal insufficiency, B12 deficiency, CAD, CHF, cirrhosis, pulmonary disease, diabetes mellitus, hypo- or hyperthyroidism, renal disease, seizure disorder, neurologic disorders | Check electrolytes, glucose, renal, and hepatic function Consider cardiac enzymes, ABG, ammonia level, cortisol, TSH level in at-risk patients |
| Medication history and review | Benzodiazepines, opioids, histamine receptor blockers, tricyclic antidepressants, neuroleptics | Discontinue unnecessary medications Consider drug screen, serum drug levels of high-risk medications |
| Substance abuse history | Alcohol, benzodiazepines, opioids, associated high-risk behaviors | Initiation of CIWA, symptomatic management of withdrawal Consider drug screen, thiamine level, HIV, RPR, ammonia level |
| Complete review of systems | Last bowel and bladder movements | Work up for any abnormal answers Consider urinalysis, urine culture, abdominal X-ray, bowel regimen |
| Complete set of vital signs | Infection, hypoxia | Consider sepsis workup with blood cultures, urinalysis, urine culture, sputum culture, CXR, lumbar puncture |
| General observation | Dehydration, uncontrolled pain, IV lines, physical restraints, Foley catheters | Consider IV hydration or encouragement of po hydration Improve pain control Remove unnecessary lines, catheters, or tethering devices |
| Complete skin exam | Skin breakdown, occult infection, DVT | Treat any abnormal findings |
| Complete neurologic and mental status exam | New focal findings on exam, signs of head trauma | Consider neuroimaging Consider EEG |

The workup for the cause of delirium should include a complete history and physical examination with particular emphasis placed on the above elements. Not all of the above testing should be performed for every patient who develops delirium but rather the history and physical examination findings should guide any further testing.

Abbreviations: ABG, arterial blood gas; CAD, coronary artery disease; CHF, congestive heart failure; CIWA, Clinical Institute Withdrawal Assessment for Alcohol; CXR, chest X-ray; DVT, deep vein thrombosis; EEG, electroencephalogram; HIV, human immunodeficiency virus; IV, intravenous; po, orally; RPR, rapid plasma reagin; TSH, thyrotropin.

# AREAS OF UNCERTAINTY

The approach to the prevention and treatment of **delirium** differs across disciplines and health care settings. Although there is no evidence to support the use of antipsychotics in the prevention and treatment of **delirium** in medical patients, the evidence has been mixed for patients undergoing surgical procedures. Furthermore, in the ICU setting, the 2013 "Clinical Practice Guidelines for the Management of Pain, Agitation, and **Delirium** in Adult Patients in the Intensive Care Unit" did not recommend for or against the use of antipsychotics for the treatment of **delirium**.[35] Current recommendations from the American Geriatric Society do not support the use of antipsychotics for the prevention and first-line treatment of **delirium**. Indeed, the Beers List of Potentially Inappropriate Medications strongly recommends that antipsychotics be avoided unless nonpharmacologic efforts have failed and the older adult is threatening self-harm.[36] Given that **delirium** can be highly distressing for patients and for caregivers and providers, in addition to the associated poor clinical outcomes, understanding the evidence behind therapeutic interventions used for its prevention and treatment is of critical importance. This chapter will review advances across the hospital setting.

# THERAPEUTIC ADVANCES

## Nonpharmacologic Interventions

Multiple risk factors have previously been identified and described for the development of **delirium**, including increased age, prior cognitive impairment, increased number of comorbidities, sleep deprivation, social isolation, visual or hearing impairment (sensory deprivation), hospitalization for fractures, stroke, or infection, physical restraint use, addition of more than three new drugs or use of psychoactive drugs, use of indwelling Foley catheters, uncontrolled pain, hypoxia, dehydration, temperature abnormalities, and malnutrition/low serum albumin.[37,38] Identifying and avoiding these risk factors can reduce **delirium** by 30% to 40%.[38-40]

## The Hospital Elder Life Program

The **Hospital Elder Life Program (HELP)** is a comprehensive multidisciplinary program, targeting six of the above risk factors.[40] The HELP has demonstrated success in both decreasing the incidence and the number of **delirium** episodes. However, it does not seem to reduce the severity of **delirium** once it has occurred. In the original prospective study, 862 hospitalized patients older than 70 years were assigned to either a usual care unit located on a general medicine floor or to the intervention unit also on a general medicine floor. Before their "unit" assignment, participants were individually matched by age, sex, and the number of nonmodifiable risk factors for

**delirium**. Participants on the "intervention unit" were visited throughout the day by an interdisciplinary team of a geriatric nurse specialist, two elder life specialists, a therapeutic recreation specialist, a physical therapist, a geriatrician, and trained hospital volunteers.[40,41] The six components of the HELP are described in Table 9.2.

Since the advent of the HELP in 1999, it has been implemented in roughly 200 hospitals across the world, including in 11 different countries and 32 states.[42] The program has been successful in academic medical centers and community hospitals.[40,43] Since the initial HELP study, multiple other studies have demonstrated that many of these interventions do not require trained professionals but rather can be performed with hospital volunteers or patient's family members or caregivers.[44,45] A more recent study has shown that implementation of HELP is associated with a lower rate of hospital readmission within 30 days.[46]

A recent Cochrane review of nonpharmacologic multicomponent prevention interventions revealed that the overall incidence of **delirium** had a risk ratio of 0.69

| TABLE 9.2 • Interventions of HELP | |
|---|---|
| **Delirium Risk Factor** | **HELP Intervention** |
| Cognitive impairment (MMSE < 20) | • Visitation by HELP team member 1–3 times per day to provide patient with frequent reorientation to his or her hospital caregivers, the date, and the day's events as well as to discuss current events, to assist patient with reminiscing, and to play word games |
| Sleep deprivation | • Bedtime warm milk, herbal tea, relaxation tapes, music, and back massages provided to patients<br>• Implementation of "Sleep Enhancement Protocol," which included rescheduling of medications and procedures at night to allow for continuous sleep as well as use of vibrating beepers on IV poles |
| Immobility | • Encouragement of early mobilization with ambulation as able<br>• Assistance with active range of motion exercises 3×/d for bed- and wheelchair-bound patients |
| Visual impairment (Visual acuity <20/70) | • Visual screening performed on admission to unit<br>• Visually impaired patients given large print books, magnifying glasses, and glasses as needed<br>• Large illuminated telephone keypads and fluorescent tape on call bells given to such patients |
| Hearing impairment | • Earwax disimpaction performed as needed<br>• Portable amplifying devices provided for hearing-impaired patients |
| Dehydration (BUN/Cr > 18) | • Aggressive encouragement of oral intake provided<br>• Assistance with meals and fluid intake provided to dehydrated patients |

The six modifiable delirium risk factors and the associated interventions addressed in the HELP.
Abbreviations: BUN/Cr, blood urea nitrogen-creatinine level; HELP, Hospital Elder Life Program; IV, intravenous; MMSE, Mini–Mental State Exam.

(95% confidence interval, 0.59-0.81) when comparing multicomponent nonpharmacologic interventions to usual hospital care.[47] The review rated this as moderate-quality evidence. Furthermore, in a 2016 meta-analysis of nonpharmacologic **delirium** interventions, the experimental groups had an odds ratio of 0.47 (95% confidence interval, 0.38-0.58) for developing **delirium** compared with control; however, the findings were limited by study heterogeneity.[39] The use of multicomponent nonpharmacologic interventions should be first line in the prevention of **delirium**.

## Pharmacologic Approach to Delirium Management

Multiple medications have been investigated in terms of their ability to prevent and treat **delirium**.

## Typical Antipsychotics

Haloperidol studies evaluating the role of **typical antipsychotics** for **delirium** prevention have not shown benefit in decreasing the incidence of **delirium**. A meta-analysis evaluating both adult surgical and medical patients found that there is currently no evidence supporting the use of antipsychotics for the prevention of **delirium**.[48] In contrast, one randomized controlled trial (RCT) of 457 patients older than 65 years, comparing haloperidol to placebo as prophylaxis to prevent **delirium** after noncardiac surgery, found a decrease in **delirium** in the intervention group. In this study, haloperidol 0.5 mg given by an intravenous push, followed by continuous infusion at a rate of 0.1 mg/h for 12 hours, was used in the intervention group. The incidence of **delirium** during the first 7 days after the surgery was 15.3% in the haloperidol group versus 23.2% in the control group ($P = 0.031$).[49] Hospital length of stay was also decreased in patients who received haloperidol.

In addition, haloperidol may be useful in reducing the duration and severity of **delirium** once it develops in the postoperative period. A Cochrane Systematic Review evaluating the use of antipsychotics in the treatment of **delirium** found that "low-dose haloperidol decreased the severity and duration of **delirium** in postoperative patients, although not the incidence of **delirium**."[50] Likewise, a randomized, double-blind, placebo-controlled trial with a total of 430 postoperative hip surgery patients demonstrated that low-dose haloperidol of 1.5 mg/d as prophylactic treatment demonstrated no efficacy in reducing the incidence of postoperative **delirium**, but it did reduce duration and severity of **delirium**, as measured by the **Delirium** Rating Scale.[51] However, a more recent RCT using haloperidol in the early treatment of **delirium** in critically ill patients admitted to the mixed medical–surgical ICU found no evidence that haloperidol modifies the duration of **delirium**.[52]

The use of haloperidol, however, has been shown to be better than the use of benzodiazepines for the treatment of **delirium**. Benzodiazepines have been shown to result in more side effects, including worsening of **delirium** symptoms. One trial randomly assigned 300 individuals admitted to the hospital with advanced acquired immunodeficiency syndrome and subsequent development of **delirium** to haloperidol, lorazepam, or chlorpromazine.[53] The use of lorazepam did not decrease the incidence of **delirium**, but demonstrated increased complications from adverse effects and therefore was discontinued.

Once **delirium** develops, the use of haloperidol in the postoperative period may decrease the duration and severity of **delirium**, especially situations in which nonpharmacologic strategies are ineffective. Controversy remains as to whether the decrease in the duration and severity of **delirium** relates to the conversion of hyperactive **delirium** to a hypoactive **delirium**.[52] In addition, a systemic review of 12 studies in which **delirium** was treated with haloperidol found that haloperidol was associated with side effects well after treatment termination.[54] Haloperidol nonselectively blocks postsynaptic dopaminergic D2 receptors in the brain. The use of haloperidol has been associated with QTc prolongation, cardiac arrhythmias, extrapyramidal reactions, pancytopenia, and visual disturbances. Given its significant side-effect profile, including a black-box warning of cardiovascular mortality, and the inconclusive evidence as to its treatment effect, haloperidol is not currently recommended for the prevention and treatment of **delirium**. Treatment of **delirium** with haloperidol should be restricted for patients with severe agitation and psychosis who present a risk to themselves or others.

## Atypical Antipsychotics

Although haloperidol is the most studied antipsychotic, **atypical antipsychotics** may have a slightly superior adverse risk profile.[55] One large study of patients prescribed a typical antipsychotic showed a 32% dose-dependent increased risk of death within 180 days as compared with those given an atypical antipsychotic.[56] Another Medicare-based study found that in the first 180 days of use, 17.9% of patients who began using conventional antipsychotic medications died, as compared with 14.6% of those who began using atypical agents.[57] Although **atypical antipsychotics** are less likely to cause extrapyramidal adverse effects, they have been labeled with a black-box warning for increased risk of stroke, sudden death, decreased respiratory drive, increased risk of psychosis, hyperglycemia, and overdose/postsedation syndromes.[56,58,59] The black-box warning specifically describes increased mortality that applies to all **atypical antipsychotics** when used for dementia-related psychosis. In June 2008, the Food and Drug Administration extended this warning to cover "typical" antipsychotics.[56,59] The warning has been applied to the use of antipsychotics in the management of **delirium**. Table 9.3 summarizes typical and **atypical antipsychotics**.

### Olanzapine

Olanzapine is an atypical antipsychotic with antagonistic effects on dopamine and serotonin receptors. A prospective, randomized trial of a mixed medical–surgical critical care unit, comparing olanzapine and haloperidol, found that there were no notable side effects in the olanzapine group, whereas those in the haloperidol group were noted to have extrapyramidal side effects.[60]

**TABLE 9.3 • Antipsychotics and Usage in Delirium Treatment**

| Medication | Population | Study Dose | Evidence | Side Effects |
|---|---|---|---|---|
| Haloperidol | ICU,[52] surgery,[49,50,51] medicine (AIDS),[53] mixed[48] | po, IM, IV | No effect on incidence of delirium.[48,50,51] May have some effect on severity and duration[50,51,53] | Extrapyramidal effects, QTc prolongation, cardiac arrhythmias, pancytopenia, visual disturbances, and oversedation.[54] May convert hyperactive to hypoactive delirium[52] |
| Olanzapine | Mixed ICU,[60] surgery[61] | po, IM | May have some effect on incidence of delirium but also increased duration and severity[60] | Lowers calcium and albumin levels, associated with obesity, abnormal lipid and glucose metabolism, and increased prolactin levels[61] |
| Risperidone | Cardiac surgery,[62] Neuropsychiatric[63] | po, IM | Reduced incidence of delirium,[62] reduced incidence of adverse effects compared with other medications[63] | Tardive dyskinesia, neuroleptic malignant syndrome, increase in suicidal ideation, hyperglycemia, sleepiness, weight gain, and constipation |
| Quetiapine | ICU[64] | po | Shortened duration and fewer doses of symptom triggered haloperidol[64,65] | Lethargy, constipation, weight gain, dry mouth, orthostatic hypotension, decreased seizure threshold, hyperglycemia, and neuroleptic malignant syndrome |
| Ziprasidone | Mechanically ventilated ICU[66] | po, IM | No difference between ziprasidone, haloperidol, and placebo[66] | EPS, tremor, parkinsonism, muscle rigidity, and hyperglycemia |

All antipsychotics have a black-box warning for an increased mortality due to cardiovascular or infectious events when used for dementia-related psychosis.

Abbreviations: AIDS, acquired immunodeficiency syndrome; EPS, extrapyramidal symptoms; ICU, intensive care unit; IM, intramuscular; IV, intravenous; po, orally.

A study comparing olanzapine with placebo for the prevention of postoperative **delirium**, in patients with joint replacement surgeries, found that although the incidence of **delirium** was lower in the group that received olanzapine, **delirium** in the intervention group lasted longer and was more severe. In addition, they demonstrated that patients treated with olanzapine had lower calcium and albumin levels, obesity, abnormal lipid and glucose metabolism, and increased prolactin levels.[61]

### Risperidone

Risperidone, another second-generation atypical antipsychotic, is sometimes preferred because it is less sedating. One randomized controlled study evaluating the use of risperidone for **delirium** prevention in patients undergoing cardiac surgery found that a single dose of risperidone (1 mg) decreased postoperative **delirium** incidence by 20%.[62] Another study compared the use of risperidone, oral haloperidol, and intravenous or intramuscular haloperidol and found that the incidence of adverse events was significantly lower for risperidone, and the incidence of death during **delirium** was significantly higher for intravenous or intramuscular haloperidol.[63] Although these two studies highlight the possible safety profile of risperidone, more rigorous trials are needed.

### Quetiapine

Quetiapine is an atypical antipsychotic that has higher sedative properties with less extrapyramidal symptoms. In a systematic review, the time to **delirium** improvement was significantly shorter with quetiapine compared with haloperidol.[64] In a study of three academic medical centers, a standing dose of quetiapine 50 mg every 12 hours resulted in faster **delirium** resolution and less agitation compared with the placebo. The group receiving quetiapine required fewer symptom-triggered ("as needed") doses for agitation as compared with haloperidol.[65] However, it is important to note that mortality did not differ between the quetiapine and haloperidol groups.

### Ziprasidone

The atypical antipsychotic ziprasidone is one of the least studied medications in the treatment of **delirium**. In a randomized, double-blind, placebo-controlled trial, 100 intubated, medical and surgical ICU patients from six tertiary care centers in the United States were randomized to receive ziprasidone, haloperidol, or placebo for the treatment of **delirium**. The study found no significant difference between patients who received ziprasidone, haloperidol, and placebo. In addition, there was no difference in the length of hospitalization or the number of ventilator-free days.[66]

In evaluating antipsychotic use in **delirium**, the benefits and risks discussed thus far indicate the need for careful consideration of the intervention's appropriateness to the specificities of the patient population. Although **atypical antipsychotics** seem to have fewer side effects than **typical antipsychotics**, data regarding their effectiveness are currently limited. Given their adverse event profile and limited evidence for efficacy, the use of antipsychotics should be done judiciously. Furthermore, it is imperative to stress a "start low and go slow" approach when prescribing these medications for the treatment of **delirium**.

## Cholinesterase Inhibitors

Acetylcholine is an important neurotransmitter that has been implicated in the pathophysiology of acute and chronic cognitive impairment. By inhibiting its degradation, these medications increase the level of acetylcholine, slowing the progression of dementia and possibly preventing **delirium**. The use of **cholinesterase inhibitors** has been evaluated in several double-blind RCTs.

### Rivastigmine

Rivastigmine is one such cholinesterase inhibitor that has been investigated in the treatment of **delirium**. Two double-blind, placebo-controlled, randomized trials yielded no evidence in favor of rivastigmine.[67,68] In a 2009 trial of patients older than 65 years undergoing cardiac surgery, the use of rivastigmine to placebo was compared.[67] The intervention group received daily doses of 1.5 mg of rivastigmine on the day before the surgery and daily through postoperative day 6. The study revealed no difference in the Mini–Mental State Exam (MMSE) and clock drawing test between patients who received rivastigmine and placebo. In addition, adverse events limited the completion of the study. Similarly, a 2012 multicenter trial of ICU patients was halted because the rivastigmine group was found to have a higher mortality rate without decreasing the duration of **delirium**.[68] Accordingly, the "Clinical Practice Guidelines for the Management of Pain, Agitation, and **Delirium** in Adult Patients in the Intensive Care Unit" recommend against the use of rivastigmine for **delirium** treatment.[35]

### Donepezil

Donepezil, another cholinesterase inhibitor, has been studied in several postoperative patient populations. Since 2005, there have been three randomized, double-blind, placebo-controlled trials, and all three have failed to demonstrate a clear benefit to the use of donepezil.[69-71] A 2005 study of older patients undergoing joint replacement surgery did not demonstrate a difference between donepezil and placebo in the incidence or duration of **delirium**.[69] In a 2007 study of patients recovering from hip surgery, the intervention group was given 5 mg of donepezil after hip surgery and every 24 hours for 3 days as compared with placebo.[70] Donepezil was well tolerated, but the incidence of **delirium** was not significantly different compared with placebo and did not reduce hospital length of stay. A similar study conducted in 2011 again compared donepezil with placebo in patients after hip fracture, which likewise did not show significant benefit in the treatment of **delirium**.[71] At this time, there is a recommendation against the use of **cholinesterase inhibitors** for the prevention and treatment of **delirium** across medical/surgical and ICU settings.

## Melatonin and Ramelteon

There is a strong link between poor sleep quality and the development of **delirium**. Therefore, interventions aimed at enhancing sleep are of particular interest in preventing and treating **delirium**. Sedatives, although decreasing sleep latency, often cause a decrease in slow-wave sleep and rapid eye movement sleep and therefore may not provide the same restorative properties as natural sleep.[72] With this theory in mind, **melatonin** has been a promising drug studied for the prevention of **delirium**. **Melatonin** readily passes through the blood-brain barrier and accumulates in the central nervous system, exhibiting neuroprotective effects.[73]

Melatonin and its agonist, **ramelteon**, have shown promising results in medical, surgical, and ICU populations. In a randomized study of 145 patients admitted to a medical unit, low-dose **melatonin** was compared with placebo and found to lower the incidence of **delirium**.[74] In another, large, double-blind, RCT of patients who underwent hip arthroplasty, patients received prophylactic, preoperative doses of **melatonin**, midazolam, and clonidine[75]; patients who subsequently developed postoperative **delirium** in all three groups were given a further dose of **melatonin** for three nights. The prophylactic **melatonin** group showed a statistically significant decrease (9.43%) in the percentage of postoperative **delirium**. Of those who developed postoperative **delirium** (58%), **melatonin** was successful in treating **delirium** in more than half of the patients, demonstrating both prophylactic and treatment potential. Conversely, a more recent, multicenter, double-blind, RCT of elderly hip fracture patients showed that **melatonin** had no effect in the incidence of **delirium**.[76]

**Ramelteon**, a **melatonin** agonist, was studied in trial of 67 patients admitted to the hospital with a medical illness. Among older adults with chronic insomnia, **ramelteon** at both 4 and 8 mg reportedly produced significant sleep-promoting activity, as indicated by polysomnographically recorded reductions of latency to persistent sleep, prolongation of total sleep time, and improvements in sleep efficiency.[77] The medication did not help with sleep parameters but did show lower risk of **delirium** compared with placebo.[78] Although there are currently no recommendations for or against the use of **melatonin**, **melatonin**'s low potential for abuse, relatively fewer side effects, and avoidance of other sedatives makes it an interesting topic for further study.[79]

## Psychostimulants

Hypoactive **delirium** may not warrant the same urgency for symptom control; however, studies have suggested that it carries a worse prognosis. The use of psychostimulants has been explored in the treatment of hypoactive **delirium**. Methylphenidate has been associated with improved alertness and cognition. In a population of terminally ill cancer patients with hypoactive **delirium**, methylphenidate demonstrated an improvement in the patient's ability to communicate.[80] In another study, 14 patients with advanced cancer and hypoactive **delirium** were evaluated using the MMSE and for sleep-wake patterns, psychomotor retardation, and hallucinations. Patients treated with methylphenidate were found to have improved cognitive function via MMSE assessment and showed decrease in disturbance in their sleep-wake pattern and delusions/hallucinations.[81] Given the significant side-effect profile of these medications, more rigorous studies are needed to assess the use of psychostimulants in treating hypoactive **delirium**.

## Dexmedetomidine

**Dexmedetomidine** is used mostly in the critical care setting for its sedative effects and works by activating adrenoceptors in the brain stem. The use of **dexmedetomidine** seems to offer an advantage over the use of benzodiazepines for patients with ICU **delirium**. Two double-blind, randomized control studies in the

ICU setting demonstrated the potential benefits of **dexmedetomidine** for managing agitation during weaning from mechanical ventilation.[82,83] Subjects who received **dexmedetomidine** had fewer ventilator days compared with those receiving benzodiazepines. The study did not reveal a difference in the number of ICU days. Furthermore, two additional studies evaluated the effects of **dexmedetomidine** compared with haloperidol or placebo in the management of mechanically ventilated patients in the ICU, with agitated **delirium**.[84,85] In both studies, the median time to extubation was lower in the **dexmedetomidine** group, although, once again, there was no difference in ICU length of stay. It remains unclear whether **dexmedetomidine** has an antidelirium effect or if it is associated with decreased use of medications prone to cause **delirium** such as benzodiazepines.[86]

Although there is some evidence to support the use of **dexmedetomidine** in critically ill older adults, the evidence is mixed in regard to postoperative **delirium**. A single-blinded, prospective, RCT evaluating the use of **dexmedetomidine** versus propofol for older adults undergoing cardiac surgery found that **dexmedetomidine** sedation was associated with reduced incidence, delayed onset, and shortened duration of postoperative **delirium**.[87] A meta-analysis of RCTs evaluating the use of **dexmedetomidine** versus propofol in patients with cardiac surgery found that **dexmedetomidine** sedation could reduce postoperative **delirium** and was associated with less ventilator days but may also increase the incidence of bradycardia.[88] On the other hand, a multicenter, double-blind, randomized, placebo-controlled trial of 404 patients, that infused **dexmedetomidine** versus saline placebo during surgery and for 2 hours in the recovery room, found that **dexmedetomidine** given during surgery did not significantly reduce the incidence of **delirium** (12.2% vs 11.4%).[89]

## General Anesthetics

Postoperative **delirium** is strongly associated with a reduction in intraoperative cerebral blood flow.[90,91] Cerebral blood flow has been shown to be decreased in both propofol and general anesthesia. In addition to **dexmedetomidine**, propofol use has been compared with general anesthetics, such as sevoflurane and desflurane.[87,88] In a double-blind, prospective study comparing propofol with sevoflurane in elderly patients undergoing surgery, there was a statistically lower incidence of postoperative **delirium** in elderly patients who received propofol as compared with sevoflurane.[92] An additional study comparing sevoflurane to propofol suggests that the faster emergence time and fewer adverse effects may both contribute to a reduction in the incidence of postoperative days in elderly patients in this study.[93] In a prospective randomized trial of 100 obese elderly patients undergoing elective total knee replacement, there was no difference in the incidence of postoperative **delirium** between desflurane and propofol.[94] A Cochrane review of the use of intravenous versus inhalational maintenance of anesthesia for postoperative cognitive outcomes in elderly surgical patients is currently underway.[95] Table 9.4 summarizes therapeutic interventions for the prevention and treatment of **delirium**.

| TABLE 9.4 • Medication Categories and Usage in Delirium Treatment | | | |
|---|---|---|---|
| **Medication** | **Population** | **Evidence** | **Side Effects** |
| Typical antipsychotics | ICU,[52] surgery,[49-51] medicine (AIDS),[53] mixed[48] | No effect on incidence; some evidence for positive effect on severity and duration of delirium in postoperative setting; preferred over benzodiazepines | Extrapyramidal side effects, over sedation, and QTc elongation Black-box warning for increased mortality |
| Atypical antipsychotics | ICU,[60,64,66] medicine,[63] surgery[61,62] | No effect on incidence; some evidence for positive effect on severity and duration of delirium | Extrapyramidal side effects, oversedation, and QTc elongation Black-box warning for increased mortality |
| Cholinesterase inhibitors | ICU,[68] surgery[67,69-71] | No evidence of benefit | Studies were ended due to increased mortality |
| Melatonin and ramelton | Medicine,[74] surgery[75] | Some evidence for positive effect on incidence of delirium | Dizziness |
| Dexmedetomidine | Mechanically ventilated ICU patients,[81,82] surgery[87-89] | Some evidence for positive effect on incidence and duration of delirium | Increased risk of bradycardia |
| General anesthetics | Surgery[92-97] | Some evidence for positive effect on incidence and duration; fewer side effects | Reduced cerebral blood flow |

Abbreviations: AIDS, acquired immunodeficiency syndrome; ICU, intensive care unit.

# SUMMARY

**Delirium** is one of the most common, costly, and devastating complications affecting up to 56% of hospitalized older patients, with an associated hospital mortality rate of 25% to 33%, and annual health care expenditures exceeding $152 billion. Despite its high prevalence and poor outcomes, there is a significant gap in therapeutic interventions for the prevention and treatment of **delirium**. Nonpharmacologic multicomponent prevention interventions such as the HELP and early mobilization and reorientation remain first line as they have consistently demonstrated a reduction in the incidence of **delirium**. There is currently no evidence to support the use of antipsychotics, **cholinesterase inhibitors**, or psychostimulants for the prevention of **delirium** across all health care settings, including the ICU. Avoiding sedation, and specifically benzodiazepines, is an important modality to prevent **delirium**. Given the lack of evidence to support the use of antipsychotics along with the adverse event profile, including a black-box warning for an increase in cardiovascular mortality, these medications should only be used for the treatment of **delirium** with features of severe agitation and psychosis. In the ICU setting, **dexmedetomidine** in lieu of propofol or other classic sedatives may prevent and shorten the duration of **delirium**. Finally, **dexmedetomidine** and general anesthetics, such as sevoflurane and desflurane, are being evaluated in the prevention and treatment of postoperative **delirium**. Multicomponent nonpharmacologic interventions are currently the most effective modality for the prevention and treatment of **delirium**.

## References

1. Inouye SK, Westendorp RG, Saczynski JS. Delirium in elderly people. *Lancet*. 2014;383:911-922.
2. Inouye SK. Delirium in older persons. *N Engl J Med*. 2006;354:1157-1165.
3. Witlox J, Eurelings LS, De Jonghe JF. Delirium in elderly patients and the risk of postdischarge mortality, institutionalization, and dementia a meta-analysis. *JAMA*. 2010;304:443-451.
4. Leslie DL, Marcantonio ER, Zhang Y, et al. One-year health care costs associated with delirium in the elderly population. *Arch Intern Med*. 2008;168:27-32.
5. Martins S, Fernandes L. Delirium in elderly people: a review. *Front Neurol*. 2012;3:101.
6. Harrington CJ, Vardi K. Delirium: presentation, epidemiology, and diagnostic evaluation (part 1). *R I Med J (2013)*. 2014;97:18-23.
7. Ryan DJ, O'Regan NA, Caoimh RÓ, et al. Delirium in an adult acute hospital population: predictors, prevalence and detection. *BMJ Open*. 2014;3:e001772.
8. Wass S, Webster PJ, Nair BR. Delirium in the elderly: a review. *Oman Med J*. 2008;23:150-157.
9. Inouye SK, Viscoli CM, Horwitz RI, et al. A predictive model for delirium in hospitalized elderly medical patients based on admission characteristics. *Ann Int Med*. 1993;119:474-481.
10. Marcantonio ER, Goldman L, Mangione CM, et al. A clinical prediction rule for delirium after elective noncardiac surgery. *JAMA*. 1994;271:134-139.
11. Marcantonio ER, Flacker JM, Michaels M, et al. Delirium is independently associated with poor functional recovery after hip fracture. *J Am Geriatr Soc*. 2000;48:618-624.
12. Ely EW, Shintani A, Truman B, et al. Delirium as a predictor of mortality in mechanically ventilated patients in the intensive care unit. *JAMA*. 2004;291:1753-1762.
13. Ansaloni L, Catena F, Chattat R, et al. Risk factors and incidence of postoperative delirium in elderly patients after elective and emergency surgery. *Br J Surg*. 2010;97:273-280.
14. Schenning KJ, Deiner SG. Postoperative delirium in the geriatric patient. *Anesthesiol Clin*. 2015;33:505-516.
15. Berger M, Nadler J, Browndyke J, et al. Postoperative cognitive dysfunction: minding the gaps in our knowledge of a common postoperative complication in the elderly. *Anesthesiol Clin*.2015;33:517-550.
16. American Delirium Society. https://www.americandeliriumsociety.org/. Accessed July 18, 2017.
17. Leslie DL, Zhang Y, Holford TR, et al. Premature death associated with delirium at 1-year follow-up. *Arch Intern Med*. 2005;165:1657-1662.
18. Maldonado JR. Neuropathogenesis of delirium: review of current etiologic theories and common pathways. *Am J Geriatr Psychiatry*. 2013;21:1190-1222.
19. Rice KL, Bennett M, Gomez M, et al. Nurses' recognition of delirium in the hospitalized older adult. *Clin Nurse Spec*. 2011;25:299-311.
20. Inouye SK, Foreman MD, Mion LC, et al. Nurses' recognition of delirium and its symptoms: comparison of nurse and researcher ratings. *Arch Intern Med*. 2001;161: 2467-2473.
21. Girard TD, Pandharipande PP, Ely EW. Delirium in the intensive care unit. *Crit Care*. 2008; 12(suppl 3):428.
22. Wong C, Holroyd-Leduc J, Simel DL, et al. Does this patient have delirium?: value of bedside instruments. *JAMA*. 2010;304:779-786.

23. Ely EW, Inouye SK, Bernard GR, et al. Delirium in mechanically ventilated patients: validity and reliability of the confusion assessment method for the intensive care unit (CAM-ICU). *JAMA.* 2001;286:2703-2710.

24. Marcantonio ER, Ngo LH, O'Connor M, et al. 3D-CAM: derivation and validation of a 3-minute diagnostic interview for CAM-defined delirium: a cross-sectional diagnostic test study. *Ann Intern Med.* 2014;161:554.

25. Trzepacz PT, Mittal D, Torres R, et al. Validation of the delirium rating scale-revised-98: comparison with the delirium rating scale and the cognitive test for delirium. *J Neuropsychiatry Clin Neurosci.* 2001;13:229-242.

26. Breitbart W, Rosenfeld B, Roth A, et al. The memorial delirium assessment scale. *J Pain Symptom Manag.* 1997;13:128-137.

27. Gaudreau JD, Gagnon P, Harel F, et al. Fast, systematic, and continuous delirium assessment in hospitalized patients: the nursing delirium screening scale. *J Pain Symptom Manag.* 2005;29:368-375.

28. Neelon VJ, Champagne MT, Carlson JR, et al. The NEECHAM confusion scale: construction, validation, and clinical testing. *Nurs Res.* 1996;45:324-330.

29. Schuurmans MJ, Shortridge-Baggett LM, Duursma SA. The delirium observation screening scale: a screening instrument for delirium. *Res Theor Nurs Pract.* 2003;17:31.

30. Radtke FM, Franck M, Oppermann S, et al. The intensive care delirium screening checklist (ICDSC)–translation and validation of intensive care delirium checklist in accordance with guidelines [in German]. *Anasthesiol Intensivmed Notfallmed Schmerzther.* 2009;44:80-86.

31. Bellelli G, Morandi A, Davis DH, et al. Validation of the 4AT, a new instrument for rapid delirium screening: a study in 234 hospitalised older people. *Age Ageing.* 2014;43:496-502.

32. De J, Wand AP, Smerdely PL, Hunt GE. Validating the 4A's test in screening for delirium in a culturally diverse geriatric inpatient population. *Int J Geriatr Psychiatry.* 2017;32(12):1322-1329.

33. Hendry K, Quinn TJ, Evans J, et al. Evaluation of delirium screening tools in geriatric medical inpatients: a diagnostic test accuracy study. *Age Ageing.* 2016;45:832-837.

34. Jin HH, Vasilevskis EE. Ultra-brief delirium assessments–are they ready for primetime? *J Hosp Med.* 2015;10:694.

35. Barr J, Fraser GL, Puntillo K, et al. Clinical practice guidelines for the management of pain, agitation, and delirium in adult patients in the intensive care unit. *Crit Care Med.* 2013;41:263-306.

36. American Geriatrics Society 2015 Beers Criteria Update Expert Panel. American geriatrics society 2015 updated beers criteria for potentially inappropriate medication use in older adults. *J Am Geriatr Soc.* 2015;63:2227-2246.

37. Inouye SK. Delirium in hospitalized older patients. *Clin Geriatr Med.* 1998;14:745.

38. Inouye SK, Bogardus STJ, Charpentier PA, et al. A multicomponent intervention to prevent delirium in hospitalized older patients. *N Engl J Med.* 1999;340:669-676.

39. Hshieh T, Yue J, Oh E, et al. Effectiveness of multicomponent nonpharmacological delirium interventions: a meta-analysis. *JAMA Intern Med.* 2015;175:512-520.

40. Marcantonio ER, Flacker JM, Wright RJ, et al. Reducing delirium after hip fracture: a randomized trial. *J Am Geriatr Soc.* 2001;49:516-522.

41. Reuben DB, Inouye SK, Bogardus ST, et al. Models of geriatrics practice; the Hospital Elder Life Program: a model of care to prevent cognitive and functional decline in older hospitalized patients. *J Am Geriatr Soc.* 2000;48:1697-1706.

42. Chen CC, Li H, Liang J, et al. Effect of a modified Hospital Elder Life Program on delirium and length of hospital stay in patients undergoing abdominal surgery: a cluster randomized clinical trial. *JAMA Surg.* 2017;152(9):827-834. doi:10.1001/jamasurg.2017.1083

43. Rubin FH, Williams JT, Lescisin DA, et al. Replicating the Hospital Elder Life Program in a community hospital and demonstrating effectiveness using quality improvement methodology. *J Am Geriatr Soc.* 2006;54:969-974.

44. Caplan GA, Harper EL. Recruitment of volunteers to improve vitality in the elderly: the REVIVE* study. *Intern Med J.* 2007;37:95-100.

45. Martinez FT, Tobar C, Beddings, et al. Preventing delirium in an acute hospital using a non-pharmacological intervention. *Age Ageing.* 2012;41:629-634.

46. Rubin FH, Bellon J, Bilderback A, et al. Effect of the Hospital Elder Life Program on risk of 30-day readmission. *J Am Geriatr Soc.* 2018;66:145-149.

47. Siddqi N, Harrison JK, Clegg A, et al. Interventions for preventing delirium in hospitalised non-ICU patients. *Cochrane Database Syst Rev.* 2016;(3):CD005563.

48. Serafim RB, Bozza FA, Soares M, et al. Pharmacologic prevention and treatment of delirium in intensive care patients: a systematic review. *J Crit Care.* 2015;30:799-807.

49. Wang W, Li HL, Wang DX, et al. Haloperidol prophylaxis decreases delirium incidence in elderly patients after noncardiac surgery: a randomized controlled trial. *Crit Care Med.* 2012;40:731–739.

50. Lonergan E, Britton AM, Luxenberg J. Antipsychotics for delirium. *Cochrane Database Sys Rev.* 2007;(18):CD005594.

51. Kalisvaart KJ, De Jonghe JF, BogaardsMJ, et al. Haloperidol prophylaxis for elderly hip-surgery patients at risk for delirium: a randomized placebo-controlled study. *J Am Geriatr Soc.* 2005;53:1658-1666.

52. Page VJ, Ely EW, Gates S, et al. Effect of intravenous haloperidol on the duration of delirium and coma in critically ill patients (hope-ICU): a randomised, double-blind, placebo-controlled trial. *Lancet Respir Med.* 2013;1:515-523.

53. Breitbart W, Marotta R, Platt MM, et al. A double-blind trial of haloperidol, chlorpromazine, and lorazepam in the treatment of delirium in hospitalized AIDS patients. *Am J Psychiatry.* 1996;153:231.

54. Schrijver EJM, de Graaf K, de Vries OJ, et al. Efficacy and safety of haloperidol for in-hospital delirium prevention and treatment: a systematic review of current evidence. *Eur J Intern Med.* 2016; 27:14-23.

55. Gilchrist NA, Asoh I, Greenberg B. Atypical antipsychotics for the treatment of ICU delirium. *J Intensive Care Med.* 2012;27:354-361.

56. Schneeweiss S, Setoguchi S, Brookhart A, Dormuth C, Wang PS. Risk of death associated with the use of conventional versus atypical antipsychotic drugs among elderly patients. *CMAJ.* 2007;176:627-632.

57. Wang PS, Schneeweiss S, Avorn J, et al. Risk of death in elderly users of conventional vs. atypical antipsychotic medications. *N Engl J Med.* 2005;353:2335-2341.

58. Dorsey ER, Rabbani A, Gallagher SA, et al. Impact of FDA black box advisory on antipsychotic medication use. *Arch Intern Med.* 2010;170:96-103.

59. Gill SS, Bronskill SE, Normand SLT, et al. Antipsychotic drug use and mortality in older adults with dementia. *Ann Intern Med.* 2007;146:775-786.

60. Skrobik YK, Bergeron N, Dumont M, et al. Olanzapine vs haloperidol: treating delirium in a critical care setting. *Intensive Care Med.* 2004;30:444-449.

61. Larsen KA, Kelly SE, Stern TA, et al. Administration of olanzapine to prevent postoperative delirium in elderly joint-replacement patients: a randomized, controlled trial. *Psychosomatics.* 2010;51:409-418.

62. Prakanrattana U, Prapaitrakool S. Efficacy of risperidone for prevention of postoperative delirium in cardiac surgery. *Anaesth Intensive Care.* 2007;35:714.

63. Miyaji S, Yamamoto K, Hoshino S, et al. Comparison of the risk of adverse events between risperidone and haloperidol in delirium patients. *Psychiatry Clin Neurosci.* 2007;61:275-282.

64. Hawkins SB, Bucklin M, Muzyk AJ. Quetiapine for the treatment of delirium. *J Hosp Med.* 2013;8:215-220.

65. Devlin JW, Roberts RJ, Fong JJ, et al. Efficacy and safety of quetiapine in critically ill patients with delirium: a prospective, multicenter, randomized, double-blind, placebo-controlled pilot study. *Crit Care Med.* 2010;38:419-427.

66. Girard TD, Pandharipande PP, Carson SS, et al. Feasibility, efficacy, and safety of antipsychotics for intensive care unit delirium: the MIND randomized, placebo controlled trial. *Crit Care Med.* 2010;38:428.

67. Gamberini M, Bolliger D, Buse GAL, et al. Rivastigmine for the prevention of postoperative delirium in elderly patients undergoing elective cardiac surgery—a randomized controlled trial. *Crit Care Med.* 2009;37:1762-1768.

68. Zaslavsky A, Haile M, Kline R, et al. Rivastigmine in the treatment of postoperative delirium: a pilot clinical trial. *Int J Geriatr Psychiatry.* 2012;27:986-988.

69. Liptzin B, Laki A, Garb JL, et al. Donepezil in the prevention and treatment of post-surgical delirium. *Am J Geriatr Psychiatry.* 2005;13:1100-1106.

70. Sampson EL, Raven PR, Ndhlovu PN, et al. A randomized, double-blind, placebo-controlled trial of donepezil hydrochloride (aricept) for reducing the incidence of postoperative delirium after elective total hip replacement. *Int J Geriatr Psychiatry.* 2007;22:343-349.

71. Marcantonio ER, Palihnich K, Appleton P, et al. Pilot randomized trial of donepezil hydrochloride for delirium after hip fracture. *J Am Geriatr Soc.* 2011;59:S282-S288.

72. Watson PL, Ceriana P, Fanfulla F. Delirium: is sleep important? *Best Pract Res Clin Anaesthesiol.* 2012;26:355-366.

73. Tan DX. Melatonin and brain. *Curr Neuropharmac.* 2010;8:161.

74. Al-Aama T, Brymer C, Gutmanis I, et al. Melatonin decreases delirium in elderly patients: a randomized, placebo-controlled trial. *Int J Geriatr Psychiatry.* 2011;26:687-694.

75. Sultan SS. Assessment of role of perioperative melatonin in prevention and treatment of postoperative delirium after hip arthroplasty under spinal anesthesia in the elderly. *Saudi J Anaesth.* 2010;4:169-173.

76. de Jonghe A, van Munster BC, Goslings JC, et al. Effect of melatonin on incidence of delirium among patients with hip fracture: a multicentre, double-blind randomized controlled trial. *Can Med Assoc J.* 2014;186:E547-E556.

77. Roth T, Seiden D, Sainati S, et al. Effects of ramelteon on patient-reported sleep latency in older adults with chronic insomnia. *Sleep Med.* 2006;7:312-318.

78. Hatta K, Kishi Y, Wada K, et al. Preventive effects of ramelteon on delirium: a randomized placebo-controlled trial. *JAMA Psychiatry.* 2014;71:397-403.

79. Mo Y, Scheer CE, Abdallah GT. Emerging role of melatonin and melatonin receptor agonists in sleep and delirium in intensive care unit patients. *J Intensive Care Med.* 2016;31:451-455.

80. Morita T, Otani H, Tsunoda J, Inoue S, Chihara S. Successful palliation of hypoactive delirium due to multi-organ failure by oral methylphenidate. *Support Care Cancer.* 2000;8:134-137.

81. Gagnon B, Low G, Schreier G. Methylphenidate hydrochloride improves cognitive function in patients with advanced cancer and hypoactive delirium: a prospective clinical study. *J Psychiatry Neurosci.* 2005;30:100.

82. Pandharipande PP, Pun BT, Herr DL, et al. Effect of sedation with dexmedetomidine vs. lorazepam on acute brain dysfunction in mechanically ventilated patients. *JAMA.* 2007;298:2644-2653.

83. Riker RR, Shehabi Y, Bokesch PM, et al. Dexmedetomidine vs. midazolam for sedation of critically ill patients: a randomized trial. *JAMA.* 2009;301:489-499.

84. Reade MC, O'Sullivan K, Bates S, et al. Dexmedetomidine vs. haloperidol in delirious, agitated, intubated patients: a randomised open-label trial. *Crit Care.* 2009;13:R75.

85. Reade MC, Eastwood GM, Bellomo R, et al. Effect of dexmedetomidine added to standard care on ventilator-free time in patients with agitated delirium. *JAMA.* 2016;315:1460-1468.

86. Conti G, Ranieri, VM, Costa R, et al. Effects of dexmedetomidine and propofol on patient-ventilator interaction in difficult-to-wean, mechanically ventilated patients: a prospective, open-label, randomised, multicentre study. *Crit Care.* 2016;20:206.

87. Djaiani G, Silverton N, Fedorko, L, et al. Dexmedetomidine versus propofol sedation reduces delirium after cardiac surgery: a randomized controlled trial. *Anesthesiology.* 2016;124:362-368.

88. Liu Xu, Xie G, Zhang K, et al. Dexmedetomidine vs propofol sedation reduces delirium in patients after cardiac surgery: a meta-analysis with trial sequential analysis of randomized controlled trials. *J Crit Care.* 2017;38:190-196.

89. Deiner S, Luo X, Sessler DI, et al. Intraoperative infusion of dexmedetomidine for prevention of postoperative delirium and cognitive dysfunction in elderly patients undergoing major elective noncardiac surgery: a randomized clinical trial. *JAMA Surg.* 2017:e171505.

90. Yokota H, Ogawa S, Kurokawa A, et al. Regional cerebral blood flow in delirium patients. *Psychiatry Clin Neurosci.* 2003;57:337-339.

91. Jones SC, Radinsky CR, Furlan AJ, et al. Variability in the magnitude of the cerebral blood flow response and the shape of the cerebral blood flow-pressure autoregulation curve during hypotension in normal rats. *Anesthesiology.* 2002;97:488-496.

92. Ishii K, Makita T, Yamashita H, et al. Total intravenous anesthesia with propofol is associated with a lower rate of postoperative delirium in comparison with sevoflurane anesthesia in elderly patients. *J Clin Anesth.* 2016;33:428-431.

93. Conti A, Lacopino DG, Fodale V, et al. Cerebral haemodynamic changes during popofol-remifentanyl or sevoflurane anaesthesia: transcranial doppler study under bispectral index monitoring. *Br J Anaesth*. 2006;97:333-339.

94. Tanaka P, Goodman S, Sommer BR, et al. The effect of desflurane versus propofol anesthesia on postoperative delirium in elderly obese patients undergoing total knee replacement: a randomized, controlled, double-blinded clinical trial. *J Clin Anesth*. 2017;39:17-22.

95. Miller ID, Shelton CL, Lewis SR, et al. Intravenous versus inhalational maintenance of anaesthesia for postoperative cognitive outcomes in elderly surgical patients. *Cochrane Database Sys Rev*. 2016;(8):cd012317.

# Management of Chronic Pain in the Elderly

# CHAPTER 10

Neal Murphy, MD, Corey Karlin-Zysman, MD,
and Sam Anandan, MD

## BACKGROUND

Pain plays a significant role in the lives of older adults. Up to 50% of community-dwelling older adults report pain that interferes with normal function, and half of nursing home patients report pain daily.[1] The term "**chronic pain**" has been used to describe pain that continues longer than expected for healing or pain lasting longer than 3 to 6 months.[2] The reasons for increased pain in the elderly are numerous. One proposed reason is homeostenosis, which is the loss of homeostatic reserve of organ systems that come with aging. This loss of reserve is manifested as liver and renal function decline, decreased muscle mass and increased frailty that can lead to falls, decreased appetite, sleep disturbances, depression, delirium, agitation, and overall debility.[3] In addition, physiologic changes occur in the elderly, which impact their ability to sense pain compared with younger adults. Some contributing factors include a decrease in the number of peripheral nociceptive neurons, increased pain thresholds, reduced endogenous analgesic responses, and a decrease in neurotransmitters, such as gamma-aminobutyric acid, serotonin, noradrenaline, and acetylcholine. Despite the logical assumption that a decrease in neurotransmitters would decrease pain in the elderly, often the opposite is seen.[1]

Several treatments for **chronic pain** are available for use in the elderly, as in their younger adult counterparts. These consist of nonpharmacologic measures, nonopioid medications, opioid medications, pain modulating drugs, topical medications, and the **novel therapeutics**, which are shown in Table 10.1.

When deciding on treatment of **chronic pain** in the elderly, some general principles apply.[2] First, the least invasive method of drug administration should be used. The oral route is preferable because of steadier blood concentrations and convenience. Second, as with younger adults, shorter acting medications should be used for episodic pain, with scheduled doses before events that incite pain. Third, least toxic medications should

**TABLE 10.1 • List of New and Current Therapeutics**

| Current Therapeutics | Novel Therapeutics |
| --- | --- |
| Acetaminophen | Micronized NSAIDs |
| NSAIDs: oral and topical | Targeted opioids: TRV130 |
| Lidocaine patches | Mixed MOP/NOP agonists: SR16435, BU08028 |
| Capsaicin | Cannabinoids |
| Weak opioids: tapentadol, tramadol | |
| Strong opioids: morphine, hydromorphone, oxycodone, fentanyl, buprenorphine | |
| Coanalgesics: TCAs, SNRIs | |
| Antiepileptics: carbamazepine, gabapentin, pregabalin | |
| Muscle spasm: baclofen, benzodiazepines, cyclobenzaprine, methocarbamol | |
| Bone pain: calcitonin, bisphosphonates | |

Abbreviations: MOP, mu opioid peptide; NOP, nociceptin opioid peptide; NSAID, nonsteroidal anti-inflammatory drug; SNRI, serotonin–norepinephrine reuptake inhibitor; TCA, tricyclic antidepressant.

be used first, starting with nonpharmacologic treatments if possible. Fourth, "rational polypharmacy" should be considered, which consists of combining drugs with complementary mechanisms of actions to cause greater relief when one single agent cannot accomplish this goal without adverse side effects. This is especially important for providers to be cognizant of in geriatrics, where polypharmacy is an important consideration.[4]

A comprehensive treatment program should also include functional restoration and psychosocial support. Often, providers follow the World Health Organization's analgesic ladder (Table 10.2), although there is little evidence to support this approach.[1]

Furthermore, **opioids** prompt concern about addiction, even when given for the intent of pain control. The American Geriatrics Society (AGS) has two sets of questions to help guide opioid therapy in the elderly (Table 10.3).[2]

Although older people have increased sensitivity to **opioids**, they are a heterogeneous population, and optimal dosing and side-effect profiles are not easy to delineate. It is important to remember that completely stopping pain is often an unachievable goal. Clinical trials often consider a 50% reduction in pain to be significant, along with an increase in functional status and decrease in occurrence of adverse effects.[1] Some chronic diseases, such as dementia, make a reliable pain diagnosis difficult; certain scales, such as PAINAD (Pain Assessment in Advanced Dementia Scale) and CNPI (Checklist of Nonverbal Pain Indicators), can help by assessing nonverbal signs of pain. Despite patients' self-report being the best indicator for pain, these simple screening tools have proven to be effective.[5]

### TABLE 10.2 • WHO Pain Relief Ladder

| | |
|---|---|
| 3 | Freedom from Cancer Pain |
| | Opioid for mild-to-moderate pain |
| | ±nonopioid |
| | ±adjuvant |
| 2 | Pain Persisting or Increasing |
| | Opioid for mild-to-moderate pain |
| | ±nonopioid |
| | ±adjuvant |
| 1 | Pain Persisting or Increasing |
| | Use a nonopioid ±an adjuvant |

Abbreviation: WHO, World Health Organization.
Adapted from http://www.who.int/cancer/palliative/painladder/en/.

### TABLE 10.3 • Question to Guide Opioid Therapy

| Initial Evaluation | Role of Consultant/Specialist |
|---|---|
| 1. What is the conventional practice for this type of pain or patient? | 1. Am I able to treat this patient without help? |
| 2. Is there an alternative therapy that may offer a better therapeutic index for pain control, functional restoration, and improvement in quality of life? | 2. Do I need the help of a pain specialist or other consultant to comanage this patient? |
| 3. Does the patient have medical problems that may increase the risk of opioid adverse effects? | 3. Are there appropriate specialists and resources available to help me comanage this patient? |
| 4. Is the patient likely to manage the opioid therapy responsibly? | 4. Are the patient's medical, behavioral, or social circumstances so complex as to warrant referral to a pain medicine specialist for treatment? |

# AREAS OF UNCERTAINTY

Many medications are used for **chronic pain**, but a challenge in older adults is identifying the best agents for this specific patient population. Unfortunately, the amount of studies involving elderly patients is limited, as well as studies involving diverse populations of elderly patients.[6] In addition to the lack of a comprehensive evidence base, additional challenges arise in treating pain among the elderly. Some patients or providers may feel that pain is "natural," and thus pain is often undertreated. Managing pain alongside multiple chronic, comorbid conditions presents therapeutic and appropriate drug dosing challenges, whereas the fears of addiction and polypharmacy affect both doctors and patients alike. New therapeutic advances have attempted to address some of these concerns.

# THERAPEUTIC ADVANCES

## Acetaminophen

Nonopioid analgesics are often the first medications used in pain treatment in the elderly. **Acetaminophen** has been used for many years as the first-choice agent for **chronic pain**, given its good side-effect profile when used in therapeutic doses. However, it is not a potent analgesic, and recent studies have raised concerns about its safety because of small increases in mortality as well as cardiovascular, gastrointestinal (GI), and renal adverse effects.[7] These studies, however, included patients concurrently using **nonsteroidal anti-inflammatory drugs (NSAIDs)**, for which the side effects are known. As of now, **acetaminophen** can be continued with a goal of up to 4 g/d, with dose reductions in patients with liver failure or those who are severely malnourished.[8] Of note, our literature review is in concordance with the literature review from the British Geriatrics Society (BGS), which did not find any studies primarily investigating the effectiveness of Tylenol in a geriatric population.[9] However, both the AGS and the BGS recommend it as the first-line agent for pain in the elderly.[2]

## Nonsteroidal Anti-inflammatory Drugs

NSAIDs are not recommended in older adults for long-term pain management, given the increased risk of GI, cardiovascular, and renal side effects. NSAIDs should be used for the shortest time possible and only used for flare-like inflammatory pain.[1] NSAIDs are often better for short-term pain in certain conditions, such as osteoarthritis (OA). A study of adverse drug reactions leading to hospitalizations in the elderly (age 65 or older) showed NSAIDS to be the culprit in 23.5% of cases, obviating the need for caution in dosing and usage.[10] Common side effects in the elderly include GI toxicity, especially when patients are on cardioprotective doses of aspirin. Prescribing a gastroprotective agent, such as a proton pump inhibitor, H2 blocker, or misoprostol, can reduce GI ulcer risk in chronic NSAID users.[11] Selective cyclooxygenase 2–inhibiting NSAIDs have fewer GI side effects, but can lead to renal failure and thrombosis, warranting caution for use in the elderly.[12] Overall, NSAIDs should be used with caution if **acetaminophen** is ineffective in the older patient. An individual decision needs to be made, based on their comorbidities, medications, and risk factors. The AGS and the BGS and the Beers List recommend cautious use in the elderly given the side-effect profile of this class of medications.[2,9,13]

## Topical Agents

Topical NSAIDs have been studied and systemic absorption seems to be minimal, leading to a lower rate of adverse effects when compared with oral NSAIDs. Two topical NSAID formulations are approved for OA and are available in the United States: diclofenac sodium topical solution 1.5% in 45.5% dimethyl sulfoxide solution and diclofenac sodium 1% gel. There are few prospective, head-to-head comparisons of oral and topical NSAIDs. One randomized controlled trial found that topical diclofenac sodium had similar efficacy to that of oral NSAIDs when treating knee OA.[14] More research is needed to compare the effectiveness of topical application to single versus multiple joints, and the risk of serious adverse events such as GI bleed or myocardial infarction. Currently, the American College of Rheumatology recommends using topical instead of oral NSAID therapy for hand OA in persons aged 75 years or older. Other topical agents include rubefacients that contain salicylate or nicotinate esters and are available for musculoskeletal pain relief without the need for a prescription. However, topical rubefacients are not as effective when compared with topical NSAIDs for **chronic pain**, and salicylate toxicity may occur.[15]

Lidocaine patches are often used for a broad array of conditions, although they are only Food and Drug Administration (FDA) approved for postherpetic neuralgia. This broad use is due to ease of application and low side-effect profile. The most common adverse effect is skin irritation to the applied area. A review article concluded that lidocaine 5% patches are safe, effective, and tolerable when used for postherpetic neuralgia and other neuropathic pain conditions. The authors also reported minimal drug-drug interactions and systemic toxicity.[16] Capsaicin is another topical treatment proven to be of some benefit for neuropathic and non-neuropathic pain. The mechanism of action involves depletion of substance P and attenuation of cutaneous hypersensitivity nociceptive fibers. Capsaicin patches have been associated with an initial burning sensation that is intolerable to nearly a third of patients. The initial burning sensation can be overcome by multiple administrations of low-concentration capsaicin or a one-time administration of high-concentration capsaicin to desensitize the area of application.[17] A high-concentration capsaicin 8% patch approved by the FDA, Qutenza, has been shown to provide neuropathic pain relief for up to 12 weeks after a single 60-minute application.[17]

## Opioids

Opioid analgesics can be divided into weak and strong categories. Weak **opioids**, such as tapentadol and tramadol, have a dual mechanism of action as mu-opioid agonists and norepinephrine reuptake inhibitors. Tapentadol was approved for use by the FDA in 2008. Unlike tramadol, tapentadol has only weak effects on serotonin reuptake and has no active metabolites. One study has been performed evaluating the tolerability and analgesic efficacy of tapentadol extended release (ER) compared with oxycodone controlled release. Elderly patients older than 75 years with chronic severe lower back pain or knee OA were included. The authors pooled data from three randomized, double-blind, placebo-, and active-controlled phase 3 studies over a 15-week treatment period. Tolerability was evaluated by assessing the number of adverse events and efficacy using an 11-point numerical pain intensity rating scale. For change in pain intensity, the authors found no significant statistical difference between the tapentadol ER and oxycodone controlled-release groups. In addition, tapentadol had fewer reported GI adverse effects compared with oxycodone.[18] Another meta-analysis of three randomized controlled trials reached similar conclusions for tapentadol versus oxycodone.[19] Therefore, tapentadol use before oxycodone may represent a reasonable choice in the elderly. However, use in the elderly may prove to be limited because of the risk of causing severe hypotension and respiratory and central nervous system sedation.[20]

Tramadol was approved by the FDA in 1995 and an ER formulation in 2005.[21] One prospective cohort, age group–controlled study explored the effectiveness and safety profile of tramadol instant release and sustained release. Patients were stratified into similarly sized age groups: <75, 65-75, and >65. The authors concluded that tramadol instant release and sustained release were both generally well tolerated and effective for all three age groups, with the eldest group consuming 20% less tramadol on average.[22] However, given tramadol's serotonin reuptake inhibition, the drug must be prescribed cautiously to avoid serotonin syndrome in elderly patients taking selective serotonin reuptake inhibitors. Overall, like tapentadol, the current literature on tramadol use in the elderly is promising, but tramadol use may be more limited secondary to risk over sedation, cognitive impairment, and interaction with other medications. Therefore, tapentadol and tramadol should be used cautiously and with close follow-up. Other weak **opioids** that also include codeine and dextropropoxyphene are also generally avoided secondary to intolerable adverse effects.[1]

Strong **opioids**, such as morphine, hydromorphone, oxycodone, fentanyl, and buprenorphine, are widely used for pain, but also pose many issues for use in the elderly. Buprenorphine is the only opioid without an increase in half-life of the active drug and metabolites. Therefore, for all **opioids** except buprenorphine, doses should be reduced with longer time intervals between doses. Starting low and titrating the dose slowly upward is essential in elderly patients.[23] One review article analyzed the literature on short- versus long-acting **opioids**. The authors found both forms of **opioids** to be efficacious, with neither being more effective than the other. The main takeaway was that **opioids** need to be tailored to the patient and their state of pain. Some patients prefer the immediate pain relief of short-acting agents, whereas others prefer the convenience of sustained pain relief with long-acting agents.[24] When comparing long-acting agents, a randomized crossover study found that transdermal fentanyl was preferred to sustained-release morphine. Of 212 patients (age 26-82 years), 138 (65%) preferred transdermal fentanyl, 59 (28%) preferred sustained-release morphine, and 15 (7%) had no preference. Transdermal fentanyl was preferred because of better pain relief. Adverse effect incidence was similar between the two groups, with more constipation reported in the morphine group.[25] Overall, the literature on opioid therapy in the elderly consists mainly of uncontrolled case series, which show that patients can achieve acceptable levels of analgesia without significant impairment of cognitive or psychomotor function.[23] However, evidence on improvement in functional status and quality of life is inconclusive, with different outcomes for patients secondary to different levels of pain relief or adverse effects.[26]

Adverse effects of **opioids** are important to recognize. Respiratory depression is a significant concern, although tolerance develops quickly. Caution is especially advised with methadone, given its variable pharmacokinetics. In addition, awareness of respiratory depression is also important when other central nervous system depressants are used in combination with **opioids**, such as benzodiazepines. Long-term opioid therapy may also suppress the production of several hypothalamic, pituitary, gonadal, and adrenal hormones, with symptoms including depression, fatigue, and decreased libido.[2] Various tools are available to assess the risk of problematic drug use, including the Opioid Risk Tool (ORT) and the SOAPP-R (Screener and Opioid Assessment for Patients with Pain—Revised), the use of which is beyond the scope of this chapter.[27]

## Adjuvant Analgesics

Several coanalgesics are also used in the treatment of pain. Tricyclic antidepressants (TCAs), which affect serotonin and noradrenergic reuptake, are not often recommended for the elderly because of increased risk of confusion or delirium. However, small doses of TCAs, such as amitriptyline or nortriptyline, are often used for neuropathic pain. Other commonly used coanalgesics are the serotonin–norepinephrine reuptake inhibitors (SNRIs), particularly venlafaxine and duloxetine. Both drugs are commonly used for neuropathic pain secondary to diabetes or fibromyalgia. However, a Cochrane review in 2015 noted that venlafaxine does not have enough compelling evidence to be recommended for neuropathic pain.[28] One randomized controlled trial showed that 56% of patients receiving venlafaxine 150 to 225 mg had a 50% reduction in pain, when compared with a group receiving placebo.[29] Despite this benefit, the authors noted increased hypertensive episodes at the above doses, which in light of the Cochrane review earlier and these findings may limit the use of venlafaxine in the elderly.[30] Duloxetine, however, does not have cardiovascular effects and has been shown to reduce diabetic peripheral neuropathic pain by 50% compared with placebo.[31] Given the risk of dose-dependent side effects mentioned previously, coanalgesics (SNRIs, TCAs, etc.) should be titrated carefully and monitored frequently.

Antiepileptic drugs are also used, mainly for neuropathic pain. Carbamazepine is first-line for facial neuropathic pain, seen in trigeminal neuralgia. Gabapentin and pregabalin have been well studied in short courses (2-4 months) and in certain conditions, such as postherpetic neuralgia, diabetic neuropathy, central neuropathic pain after spinal cord injury, and fibromyalgia.[32] One meta-analysis assessed the efficacy of using pregabalin daily for neuropathic pain caused by postherpetic neuralgia. The authors found that a dose of at least 300 mg daily could achieve 50% or more in pain reduction on an 11-point pain scale.[33] Furthermore, pregabalin has proven to have a small benefit compared with placebo when used in fibromyalgia.[34] The antiepileptics have significant adverse effects, including eyesight, balance, cognitive function, and weight gain. Other agents used have limited evidence to support them, including phenytoin, lamotrigine, topiramate, and valproate.[1]

Agents used for muscle pain include benzodiazepines and baclofen. Caution should be advised because of their propensity to cause falls in the elderly, especially for benzodiazepines, which have high-risk profiles that often preclude any potential benefit for pain relief. Use should be justified on an individual basis for anxiety or muscle spasms. Benzodiazepines are on the Beers List, including both long- and short-acting agents.[13] About a third of those aged 65 years or older living in the community are estimated to fall at least once per year.[35] Among these community-dwelling elders, about 10% to 12% use benzodiazepines,[36] despite evidence that both long- and short-acting benzodiazepines have been shown to increase the fall risk in the elderly. One observational study assessed the fall risk of both short- and long-acting agents. Both short- and long-acting agents increased the risk of falls (adjusted odds ratio 1.32; 95% confidence interval, 1.02-1.72, and adjusted odds ratio 1.45; 95% confidence interval, 1.00-2.19, respectively).[37] Other muscle relaxants available include cyclobenzaprine, methocarbamol, and others. These do not specifically relieve muscle spasms, despite their name, and should not be given for this purpose specifically.[38]

# NEW THERAPIES

## Micronized NSAIDs

Nanoformulations of low-dose NSAIDs are currently being developed and tested in clinical trials. These new formulations have similar efficacy when compared with traditional oral NSAIDs, while minimizing adverse effects. This is achieved by optimizing the pharmacokinetic profile. Nanotechnology increases drug surface area, which increases absorption with lower doses to generate the same clinical effect.[39] Currently, there are two FDA-approved micronized NSAIDs, diclofenac (Zorvolex)[40] and indomethacin (Tivorbex),[41] for the use of mild-to-moderate pain. Although these new formulations show promise given their comparable efficacy and potential for lower adverse effects, more clinical data will be needed over time to assess how these new formulations will fit into current pain medication regimens. As more elderly patients continue to use them without serious GI or cardiac events, these new formulations may become a mainstay medicine that could limit the utilization of **opioids** in this population.

## Targeted Opioids

Currently, there is growing interest in developing **opioids** that target specific pathways of known opioid receptors. Since the delta opioid receptor (DOR) and mu opioid receptor (MOR) receptors were cloned in 1992 and 1993, respectively, there has been an increased understanding of how these receptors work at the molecular level.[42] Specifically, the MOR activation has two signaling pathways, a G-protein pathway responsible for analgesic affects and a β-arrestin recruitment pathway responsible for the respiratory depression and GI adverse effects. TRV130 is a new agonist that targets the G-protein signaling pathway. In a phase 2 study, the drug has proven to have similar analgesic effects as morphine with less opioid-induced adverse effects.[43] PZM21, another drug targeting the G-protein pathway, has similar therapeutic potential as TRV130 and has shown promise in animal models.[44]

In addition to targeting specific pathways, mixed opioid agonists that target combinations of the mu (mu-opioid peptide [MOP]), delta opioid peptide (DOP), and opioid receptor-like 1 (nociceptin opioid peptide [NOP]) receptors are currently being tested. Most of the traditional **opioids** are MOP agonists.[45] Animal studies of NOP agonists have shown effective analgesia with decreased abuse potential in comparison with traditional **opioids**.[46,47] Therefore, derivatives of buprenorphine became an area of interest, given that the drug is an MOP agonist and a weak NOP agonist.[48] Furthermore, unlike MOP selective agents, MOP/NOP agonists have been shown to treat neuropathic pain.[45] Two novel mixed MOP/NOP ligands that have been developed, SR16435 and BU08028, effectively decreased neuropathic pain in mouse models.[49,50] One study tested the safety and efficacy of BU08028 in nonhuman primates. BU08028 was found to provide long-lasting analgesia. After self-administering the drug on a progressive ratio schedule, the reinforcing strength of BU08028 was lower compared with buprenorphine, remifentanil, and cocaine. When compared with traditional MOP agonists, BU08028 at 10- to 30-fold higher doses did not cause adverse cardiologic events or respiratory depression. When studying withdrawal, determined by changes in vitals such as increase in heart rate and respiratory rate, the nonhuman primates ended up withdrawing after repeated administration of morphine. No withdrawal or vital sign changes were seen after discontinuing BU08028.[51] Overall, the current data available regarding efficacy, tolerance, and abuse-free potential of MOP/NOP agonists are promising, and further studies are needed to validate the therapeutic profiles of these dual agonists.

Modulating opioid kinetics is another therapeutic approach that has shown significant potential. The abuse of mu-opioid agonists appears to be dependent on their interaction with dopaminergic pathways achieved through rapid entry into the central nervous system. In contrast, analgesia depends on exposure alone and, as such, is not rate dependent. NKTR-181 takes advantage of this physiologic property and has been designed to have low permeability across the blood-brain barrier, slowing entry into the brain and attenuating dopamine release.[52] The novel drug recently showed promise in a phase 3 study including over 600 patients with chronic back pain who reported their pain scores dropped by an average of 65% when taking the drug twice daily.[53] NKTR-181 has been granted fast track designation by the FDA because of these results.[54]

Another opioid that has shown promise, NFEPP, binds MORs under acidic conditions, which are a hallmark for inflammation and the origin of pain signals. Two research teams in Germany used computer modeling to modify the structure of fentanyl and create this peripherally acting opioid. NFEPP produced injury-restricted analgesia in rats with inflammatory pain without exhibiting respiratory depression, constipation, sedation, or addiction.[55] How this drug performs in human clinical trials, and treating pain not primarily generated by acidic conditions, will need to be assessed.

## Cannabinoids

Cannabinoids are now more widely used legally for medical reasons, but their use has proven to be more beneficial for nausea, spasticity, and neuropathic pain. Dronabinol and nabilone, synthetic tetrahydrocannabinoid analogs, have shown minimal analgesic benefits and have been mostly used for chemotherapy-induced nausea and vomiting. Sativex, an oral spray consisting of cannabinoid plant extract with a 1:1 ratio of tetrahydrocannabinoids and cannabinoids, is licensed in the United Kingdom for multiple sclerosis–related spasticity.[32] Of the two classic cannabinoid receptors, CB1r and CB2r, central CB1r receptors are mainly responsible for the addiction and psychotomimetic adverse effects seen with cannabinoids. Current research is now focusing on the effectiveness of CB2r agonists, developing peripherally restricted cannabinoids, targeting cannabinoid metabolizing enzyme inhibitors, or activating other nonclassic receptors within the cannabinoid system.[56] For now, current data mainly support the use of cannabinoids for the treatment of spasticity and chronic neuropathic pain.[26]

# SUMMARY

A significant proportion of the elderly are affected by chronic pain, resulting in a decreased quality of life. Opiate use has become increasingly common in older adult patients. There are both well-established current and novel therapies for the management of chronic pain in older adults; however, the number of studies involving management of chronic pain in elderly patients is limited. Managing pain alongside multiple chronic, comorbid conditions presents therapeutic and appropriate drug dosing challenges.

Some of the well-established therapies include NSAIDs, acetaminophen, and opioids. Even within these categories, there are upcoming novel therapeutic agents. For instance, NSAID nanoformulations have shown promise in clinical trials, which have similar efficacy to oral NSAIDs, while minimizing adverse effects. TRV130 and PZM21, newly targeted opioids, selectively activate the analgesic pathway of the mu-opioid receptor. These drugs have been proven to have analgesic effects similar to morphine, with less opioid-induced adverse effects. Mixed opioid agonists, targeting the mu and NOP receptors, may prove superior among the opioid class given their effectiveness, improved safety profile, and low abuse potential. Modulating opioid pharmacokinetics to slow delivery across the blood-brain barrier or specifically target areas of inflammation is another potential therapeutic strategy under investigation. In addition, there is ongoing research assessing reduction of pain by targeted and peripherally restricted **cannabinoids**, attempting to limit activation of the central receptors responsible for addiction and psychotomimetic effects.

In facing the opiate epidemic, providers must use multicomponent strategies to find the most effective and safest combinations of pain medications to achieve adequate pain control. Regardless of the variety and complexity of pain medications available, prescribing physicians should start with low doses, titrate slowly, and monitor pain control frequently. Treating **chronic pain** is a complex and difficult issue that hopefully will become more manageable as pain medication regimens improve and new therapeutics are developed.

## References

1. Hall T. Management of persistent pain in older people. *J Pharm Pract Res*. 2016;46:60-67.
2. American Geriatrics Society Panel. Pharmacological management of persistent pain in older persons: pharmacological management of persistent pain in older persons. *J Am Geriatr Soc*. 2009;57:1331-1346.
3. Shega JW, Dale W, Andrew M, et al. Persistent pain and frailty: a case for homeostenosis. *J Am Geriatr Soc*. 2012;60:113-117.
4. Maher RL, Hanlon J, Hajjar ER. Clinical consequences of polypharmacy in elderly. *Expert Opin Drug Saf*. 2014;13:57-65.
5. Lints-Martindale AC, Hadjistavropoulos T, Lix LM, et al. A comparative investigation of observational pain assessment tools for older adults with dementia. *Clin J Pain*. 2012;28:226-237.
6. Reid MC, Eccleston C, Pillemer K. Management of chronic pain in older adults. *BMJ*. 2015;350:h532.
7. Roberts E, Delgado Nunes V, Buckner S, et al. Paracetamol: not as safe as we thought? A systematic literature review of observational studies. *Ann Rheum Dis*. 2016;75:552-559.
8. Hayward KL, Powell EE, Irvine KM, et al. Can paracetamol (acetaminophen) be administered to patients with liver impairment? *Br J Clin Pharmacol*. 2016;81:210-222.
9. Abdulla A, Adams N, Bone M, et al. Guidance on the management of pain in older people. *Age Ageing*. 2013;42(suppl 1):i1-i57.
10. Franceschi M, Scarcelli C, Niro V, et al. Prevalence, clinical features and avoidability of adverse drug reactions as cause of admission to a geriatric unit: a prospective study of 1756 patients. *Drug Saf*. 2008;31:545-556.
11. Rostom A, Dube C, Wells G, et al. Prevention of NSAID induced gastroduodenal ulcers. *Cochrane Database Syst Rev*. 2002;CD002296.
12. Savage R. Cyclo-oxygenase-2 inhibitors: when should they be used in the elderly? *Drugs Aging*. 2005;22:185-200.
13. American Geriatrics Society 2015 Beers Criteria Update Expert Panel. American geriatrics society 2015 updated beers criteria for potentially inappropriate medication use in older adults. *J Am Geriatr Soc*. 2015;63:2227-2246.
14. Tugwell PS, Wells GA, Shainhouse JZ. Equivalence study of a topical diclofenac solution (pennsaid) compared with oral diclofenac in symptomatic treatment of osteoarthritis of the knee: a randomized controlled trial. *J Rheumatol*. 2004;31:2002-2012.
15. Arnstein PM. Evolution of topical NSAIDs in the guidelines for treatment of osteoarthritis in elderly patients. *Drugs Aging*. 2012;29:523-531.
16. Gammaitoni AR, Alvarez NA, Galer BS. Safety and tolerability of the lidocaine patch 5%, a targeted peripheral analgesic: a review of the literature. *J Clin Pharmacol*. 2003;43:111-117.
17. Anand P, Bley K. Topical capsaicin for pain management: therapeutic potential and mechanisms of action of the new high-concentration capsaicin 8% patch. *Br J Anaesth*. 2011;107:490-502.

18. Biondi DM, Xiang J, Etropolski M, et al. Tolerability and efficacy of tapentadol extended release in elderly patients ≥75 years of age with chronic osteoarthritis knee or low back pain. *J Opioid Manag.* 2015;1:393-403.

19. Merchant S, Provenzano D, Mody S, et al. Composite measure to assess efficacy/gastrointestinal tolerability of tapentadol ER versus oxycodone CR for chronic pain: pooled analysis of randomized studies. *J Opioid Manag.* 2013;9:51-61.

20. UpToDate. Tapentadol: drug information. https://www.uptodate.com/contents/tapentadol-drug-information?search=tapentadol%20drug%20information&source=panel_search_result&selectedTitle=1~10&usage_type=panel&kp_tab=drug_general&display_rank=1. Accessed January 17, 2017.

21. McCarberg B. Tramadol extended-release in the management of chronic pain. *Ther Clin Risk Manag.* 2007;3:401-410.

22. Likar R, Wittels M, Molnar M, et al. Pharmacokinetic and pharmacodynamic properties of tramadol IR and SR in elderly patients: a prospective, age-group-controlled study. *Clin Ther.* 2006;28:2022-2039.

23. Pergolizzi J, Böger RH, Budd K, et al. Opioids and the management of chronic severe pain in the elderly: consensus statement of an international expert panel with focus on the six clinically most often used World Health Organization step III opioids (buprenorphine, fentanyl, hydromorphone, methadone, morphine, oxycodone). *Pain Pract.* 2008;8:287-313.

24. Argoff CE, Silvershein DI. A comparison of long- and short-acting opioids for the treatment of chronic noncancer pain: tailoring therapy to meet patient needs. *Mayo Clinic Proc.* 2009;84:602-612.

25. Allan L, Hays H, Jensen NH, et al. Randomised crossover trial of transdermal fentanyl and sustained release oral morphine for treating chronic non-cancer pain. *BMJ.* 2001;322:1154.

26. Noble M, Treadwell JR, Tregear SJ, et al. Long-term opioid management for chronic noncancer pain. *Cochrane Database Syst Rev.* 2010;CD006605.

27. Henrie-Barrus P, Averill LA, Sudweeks RR, et al. Development and preliminary validation of the opioid abuse risk screener. *Health Psychol Open.* 2016;3: 2055102916648995. doi:10.1177/2055102916648995

28. Gallagher HC, Gallagher RM, Butler M, et al. Venlafaxine for neuropathic pain in adults. *Cochrane Database Syst Rev.* 2015;CD011091.

29. Rowbotham MC, Goli V, Kunz NR, et al. Venlafaxine extended release in the treatment of painful diabetic neuropathy: a double-blind, placebo-controlled study. *Pain.* 2004;110:697-706.

30. Marcum ZA, Duncan NA, Makris UE. Pharmacotherapies in geriatric chronic pain management. *Clin Geriatr Med.* 2016;32:705-724.

31. Peltier A, Goutman SA, Callaghan BC. Painful diabetic neuropathy. *BMJ.* 2014;348:g1799.

32. Schug SA, Goddard C. Recent advances in the pharmacological management of acute and chronic pain. *Ann Palliat Med.* 2014;3:263-275.

33. Snedecor SJ, Sudharshan L, Cappelleri JC, et al. Systematic review and meta-analysis of pharmacological therapies for pain associated with postherpetic neuralgia and less common neuropathic conditions. *Int J Clin Pract.* 2014;68:900-918.

34. Üçeyler N, Sommer C, Walitt B, et al. Anticonvulsants for fibromyalgia. *Cochrane Database Syst Rev.* 2013;CD010782.

35. Stel VS, Smit JH, Pluijm SMF, et al. Consequences of falling in older men and women and risk factors for health service use and functional decline. *Age Ageing.* 2004;33:58-65.

36. Blazer D, Hybels C, Simonsick E, et al. Sedative, hypnotic, and antianxiety medication use in an aging cohort over ten years: a racial comparison. *J Am Geriatr Soc.* 2000;48:1073-1079.

37. Landi F, Onder G, Cesari M, et al. Psychotropic medications and risk for falls among community-dwelling frail older people: an observational study. *J Gerontol A Biol Sci Med Sci.* 2015;60:622-626.

38. Billups SJ, Delate T, Hoover B. Injury in an elderly population before and after initiating a skeletal muscle relaxant. *Ann Pharmacother.* 2011;45:485-491.

39. Manvelian G, Daniels S, Altman R. A phase I study evaluating the pharmacokinetic profile of a novel, proprietary, nano-formulated, lower-dose oral indomethacin. *Postgrad Med.* 2012;124:197-205.

40. U.S. Food and Drug Administration. ZORVOLEX (diclofenac) capsules for oral use. http://www.accessdata.fda.gov/drugsatfda_docs/label/2013/204592s000lbl.pdf. Accessed January 17, 2017.

41. U.S. Food and Drug Administration. TIVORBEX (indomethacin) capsules for oral use. https://www.accessdata.fda.gov/ drugsatfda_docs/label/2014/204768s000lbl.pdf. Accessed January 17, 2017.

42. Chen Y, Mestek A, Liu J, Hurley JA, Yu L. Molecular cloning and functional expression of a mu-opioid receptor from rat brain. *Mol Pharmacol.* 1993;44:8-12.

43. Viscusi ER, Webster L, Kuss M, et al. A randomized, phase 2 study investigating TRV130, a biased ligand of the m-opioid receptor, for the intravenous treatment of acute pain. *Pain.* 2016;157:264-272.

44. Manglik, A, Lin H, Aryal DK, et al. Structure-based discovery of opioid analgesics with reduced side effects. *Nature.* 2016;537:185-190.

45. Bird MF, Lambert DG. Simultaneous targeting of multiple opioid receptor types. *Curr Opin Support Palliat Care.* 2015;9:98-102.

46. Kiguchi N, Ding H, Ko MC. Central N/OFQ-NOP receptor system in pain modulation. *Adv Pharmacol.* 2016;75:217-243.

47. Ko MC, Woods JH, Fantegrossi WE, et al. Behavioral effects of a synthetic agonist selective for nociceptin/orphanin FQ peptide receptors in monkeys. *Neuropsychopharmacology.* 2009;34:2088-2096.

48. Lutfy K, Cowan A. Buprenorphine: a unique drug with complex pharmacology. *Curr Neuropharmacology.* 2004;2:395-402.

49. Sobczak M, Cami-Kobeci G, Salaga M, et al. Novel mixed NOP/MOP agonist BU08070 alleviates pain and inhibits gastrointestinal motility in mouse models mimicking diarrhea-predominant irritable bowel syndrome symptoms. *Eur J Pharmacol.* 2014;736:63-69.

50. Sukhtankar DD, Zaveri NT, Husbands SM, et al. Effects of spinally administered bifunctional nociceptin/orphanin FQ peptide receptor/m-opioid receptor ligands in mouse models of neuropathic and inflammatory pain. *J Pharmacol Exp Ther.* 2013;346:11-22.

51. Ding H, Czoty PW, Kiguchi N, et al. A novel orvinol analog, BU08028, as a safe opioid analgesic without abuse liability in primates. *Proc Natl Acad Sci.* 2016;113:E5511-E5518.

52. Miyazaki, T, Choi IY, Rubas W, et al. NKTR-181: A novel mu-opioid analgesic with inherently low abuse potential. *J Pharmacol Exp Ther.* 2017;363:104-113.

53. Martin, J. New opioid analgesic NKTR-181 safe, efficacious for low back pain. *Clinical Pain Advisor.* 2017. https://www.clinicalpainadvisor.com/chronic-pain/low-back-pain-relief-opioid-analgesic-nkrt-181/article/697880/.

54. Healio. FDA grants fast track designation to opioid analgesic NKTR-181. March 20, 2017. https://www.healio.com/family-medicine/pain-management/news/online/%7Bab9a6e15-09f3-4136-9db9-d612f3690625%7D/fda-grants-fast-track-designation-to-opioid-analgesic-nktr-181.

55. Spahn, V, Del Vecchio G, Labuz D, et al. A nontoxic pain killer designed by modeling of pathological receptor conformations. *Science.* 2017;355:966-969.

56. Davis MP. Cannabinoids in pain management: CB1, CB2 and non-classic receptor ligands. *Expert Opin Investig Drugs.* 2014;23:1123-1140.

# CHAPTER 11

# Advancements in the Treatment of Constipation in Hospitalized Older Adults

Jacqueline Moore, MD, Sheila Firoozan, MD, and Nichol Martinez, MD

## BACKGROUND

**Constipation** is a widespread condition encountered across all health care settings. The prevalence of **constipation** in North America is between 2% and 27%, with average estimates at 15%,[1-3] and higher rates among female population, the elderly, nonwhites, and those of lower socioeconomic status.[1,2] Other identified risk factors for **constipation** include the use of medication, low physical activity,[4] low fiber consumption,[5] and institutionalization.[6] The prevalence of **constipation** among individuals older than 65 years in some reports is estimated to be between 50% and 74%.[7] A systematic review examining 13 studies of predominantly adults determined that the negative impact of **constipation** on quality of life is significant and comparable to other chronic conditions such as inflammatory bowel disease, allergies, and rheumatologic conditions, highlighting **constipation** as a problem warranting greater attention.[8]

The rising health care costs associated with the diagnosis and treatment of **constipation** are staggering. Approximately 2.5 million individuals visit a physician for **constipation**,[9] and more than $800 million per year is spent on over-the-counter laxatives alone.[9,10] Although relatively benign in most patients, **constipation** in the elderly can result in complications that can increase the length of stay at hospitals and result in additional morbidity and even death.[11] In the United States, the aggregate cost of hospitalization for **constipation** was nearly $4.25 billion in 2010.[12] In comparison, all **constipation**-related direct costs totaled $1.6 billion in 2004.[13] **Constipation**-related emergency department visits have jumped by 41.5% between 2006 and 2011, particularly in those older than 85 years.[14] Hospital discharges of all age groups with a diagnosis of **constipation** increased from around 300 000 in 1997 to more than 1.3 million in 2010, with the elderly comprising the largest group of patients with **constipation**-related hospitalizations.[12] Medicare has been particularly affected, with **constipation**-related discharges more than doubling from 7.9/10 000 in 1997 to 15.8/10 000 in 2010.[12] Despite the majority of treatment for **constipation** taking place in ambulatory settings, total costs associated with inpatient treatment of **constipation** actually supersede ambulatory costs.[15] **Constipation** affects patients in intensive care as well, with an incidence measured as high as 72%.[16]

Numerous factors likely play a role in the increasing cost associated with **constipation**. For instance, prescription opioid sales have increased 4-fold between 1999 and 2010, contributing to a higher incidence of opioid-induced **constipation** (OIC).[17] A systematic review of 11 double-blind, randomized controlled trials (RCTs) found that 41% individuals taking oral opioids for chronic noncancer pain for up to 8 weeks experienced OIC or bowel dysfunction, with the number needed to harm of 3.4.[18] Furthermore, **constipation** can be poorly evaluated and treated when addressing more complicated medical concerns, as seen in a study of 100 advanced cancer patients with only one-third self-reporting **constipation**, whereas 50% met the diagnostic criteria.[19]

The Rome III diagnostic criteria for **constipation** are a tool that can be used to identify patients suffering from functional **constipation**, particularly those with chronic symptoms. The criteria are defined as two or more of the following present for at least 12 weeks in the past year: straining, hard stools, sensation of incomplete evacuation or anorectal blockage, requiring use of manual maneuvers, having three or fewer bowel movements per week, without meeting criteria for irritable bowel syndrome (IBS).[20]

Given the high prevalence, associated inpatient costs, impact on the quality of life, and potential for complications in geriatric patients, additional guidance is needed for medical practitioners as to the treatment options for **constipation** available in this population in the hospital. The tremendous impact that **constipation** has on health care costs and quality of life highlights the importance of treating this condition with therapies that are evidence based.

# AREAS OF UNCERTAINTY

An underrecognized problem besides choosing the optimal therapeutic agent(s), barriers to treating **constipation** effectively include identifying the affected population, determining the underlying cause, and deciding when to initiate therapy. **Constipation** is often unrecognized in the inpatient. The Rome III diagnostic criteria[20] are not typically used in the hospitalized patient, but it could help to identify patients experiencing significant symptoms in need of treatment. Improvement in diagnosis is necessary as **constipation** in the elderly can result in complications such as delirium, colonic pseudo-obstruction (Ogilvie syndrome), fecal impaction, fecal incontinence, stercoral colitis, and even fatal stercoral perforation.[11] Fecal impaction can lead to colonic dilation and reduced anal sphincter tone, causing anal incontinence and diarrhea. A systematic review of stercoral perforation found that those at the highest risk of complications are the elderly, the institutionalized, and those with neuropsychiatric disease or chronic renal failure.[11]

With prevalence as high as 39% in acutely hospitalized patients, an additional 43% developed signs of constipation within the first 3 days of admission.[21] Bowel habits are frequently not reviewed by providers, despite improvements in documentation.[22] Recognition of patients at risk of OIC is also suboptimal. In patients older than 65 years receiving hospice care and opioid pain management, approximately half of the patients did not have laxatives available to them during their last 7 days of life.[23] Rates of laxative use tend to be lower in inpatient hospice settings compared with long-term and nursing facilities. Furthermore, nonwhite patients were significantly less likely to receive laxatives than their white counterparts.[23] A systematic review of 130 RCTs of pharmacologic treatments of constipation noted that only 10 studies analyzed efficacy data in patients receiving palliative care.[24] There is urgent need to assess the efficacy of traditional and newer agents for both geriatric and palliative patients who are often hospitalized, given the high rates of constipation among these populations.

## Identifying Etiology

Identifying the cause of constipation in elderly patients can often be challenging because of a multitude of potential contributing factors. Assessment of constipation in hospitalized older adults begins with a detailed history and physical examination, including a rectal examination, which can reveal hardened or impacted stool, rectal masses, hemorrhoids, fissures, prolapse, or sphincter dysfunction. Weight loss, acute severe constipation, change in stool caliber, hematochezia or fecal occult blood, and unresponsiveness to treatment are red flags and should elicit prompt additional evaluation.

The etiology of constipation in the geriatric population may be related to primary colorectal dysfunction or secondary factors and is frequently multifactorial. Primary constipation disorders include IBS, slow transit constipation, and dyssynergic defecation. Secondary constipation may be associated with other medical conditions, the use of chronic opioids, and other contributing factors such as weakened musculature, decreased mobility, and dehydration.[25,26] Well-known potential secondary causes include medication side effects (such as opioids, tricyclic antidepressants), neurologic disorders (including multiple sclerosis, Parkinson disease, autonomic neuropathy), diabetes mellitus, hypothyroidism, hypercalcemia, iron deficiency anemia, and gastrointestinal masses and obstruction. Elimination or optimization of these possible underlying causes should be undertaken at the same time as the initiation of treatment for constipation in hospitalized geriatric patients. Age-specific considerations for elderly patients should also be examined. These may include decreased mobility, poor caloric intake, poor hydration, decreased rectal sensation, dementia, and encephalopathy related to acute illness.[27] The presence of "tethers" such as urinary catheters or intravenous lines can limit patient mobility and contribute to the development of constipation.

Polypharmacy in the elderly is a well-documented problem,[28] and it is associated with increased adverse drug events,[29] medication interactions,[30] functional decline,[31] and falls.[32] However, it is unclear whether polypharmacy in and of itself causes **constipation** in the elderly. Retrospective evaluation of 250 nursing home residents (mean age, 85.4 years) did not find a correlation with polypharmacy and **constipation** rates in general, but rather a trend toward **constipation** in residents using certain drug classes including anticholinergics, antidepressants, and benzodiazepines.[33] Many medication classes, including common analgesics, tricyclic antidepressants, anticholinergic drugs, calcium channel blockers, dopaminergic agents, antipsychotics, antacids, bile acid resin, iron supplements, antihistamines, diuretics, and anticonvulsants, have **constipation** and other gastrointestinal side effects listed in their known side-effect profiles.[7] Both planned and unplanned hospitalizations pose opportunities for clinicians to evaluate prescribed medications for necessity and adverse effects. Although the evidence is mixed as to whether deprescribing medications has mortality benefit as seen in a systematic review and meta-analysis of 132 deprescribing studies with more than 34 000 adults (median age, 73.8 ± 5.4 years),[34] the potential to decrease both adverse effects and medication noncompliance could be substantial.

## Evaluation and Initiation of Therapy

Although most inpatients have routine laboratory work readily available, there is limited evidence to show that routine laboratory testing is required during the initial evaluation of **constipation**.[35,36] A systematic review found no studies that have assessed the utility of routine hematologic, metabolic, or thyroid studies in the diagnosis of chronic **constipation**, yet these studies are frequently obtained with initial workup.[37]

Most imaging studies employed in the assessment of **constipation** also lack clinic evidence to support their use.[35] Abdominal x-rays are frequently ordered because they are inexpensive, readily obtainable, and offer limited radiation exposure; however, they are limited in their ability to assess severity of **constipation**.[38] A single film can have a wide range of interpretations by different radiologists.[39] Contrarily, in the appropriate clinical context, diagnostic studies including imaging such as computed tomography should be promptly utilized if suspicion for small bowel obstruction, ileus, or perforation exists.

Inpatient endoscopic evaluation of **constipation** should be limited to those with red flag symptoms as described earlier, in those planned to undergo surgery for **constipation**, and in a limited number of patients without prior colorectal cancer screening.[40] More specialized physiologic testing including anorectal and colonic manometry, balloon expulsion, and colonic transit studies can be useful in diagnosing the subtype of **constipation** by assessing abnormalities in rectal hyposensitivity, pelvic floor dysfunction, and colonic transit time. These studies are unlikely to be used in the hospitalized setting because of decreased availability of specialized equipment, time involvement, and limited data yield, and thus, they are typically performed in the ambulatory setting. Differentiating between **constipation** subtypes in admitted patients may be difficult without these studies; however, attention should be paid to a prior diagnosis of a specific primary etiology to help direct therapy.

In many patients, treatment is often initiated without precisely identifying the underlying cause of **constipation**. Many of these patients may be diagnosed with functional or chronic idiopathic **constipation** (CIC), a broad term encompassing those meeting the Rome III diagnostic criteria and not meeting the IBS criteria.[41] In addition, patients' self-reporting of chronic **constipation** far exceeds the number of affected patients identified by the Rome criteria.[26,42] Treatment in the hospital is often approached in a trial-and-error fashion by clinicians. In most cases, simply continuing an elderly patient on laxatives they are using effectively as an outpatient represents the best approach in preventing **constipation** during hospitalization. A retrospective cohort analysis of 600 patients hospitalized with congestive heart failure found that failure to continue patients on their outpatient laxatives increased the length of stay by approximately 2 days compared with those receiving a prophylactic regimen.[43] No reduced length of stay was observed in the use of bowel prophylaxis in patients not previously using laxatives at home. Unfortunately, up to half of patients older than 65 years are not prescribed their previously used home laxatives upon hospitalization.[44] Unless otherwise contraindicated, it is imperative that elderly patients receive their outpatient regimen to prevent inpatient **constipation**.

Little is known regarding prophylactic bowel regimens in patients not using laxatives or other agents at home. Most studies supporting empiric bowel regimen use involve surgical patients; implementing postoperative bowel regimens following major arthroplasty ($N = 331$; age $> 18$ years)[45] or pelvic reconstructive surgery[46] reduced the length of time to first bowel movement and reduced rates of postoperative ileus and **constipation** ($N = 1223$).[47] Data from these studies involved adults of all ages, and more studies evaluating the utility of perioperative use of laxatives for **constipation** prevention in the elderly are necessary. The effectiveness of starting **constipation** prophylaxis regimen for elderly patients admitted to general medical and other services is essentially unknown, with available recommendations predominantly based on expert opinion and anecdotal evidence.[44] Furthermore, determining specific medication regimens to be utilized on a large scale for **constipation** prophylaxis is another area requiring further investigation.

# TRADITIONAL THERAPEUTICS

## Fiber and Osmotic Laxatives

The beneficial effect of increased dietary fiber on **constipation** in all patients is well supported by evidence.[7,48] Furthermore, dietary fiber has few contraindications, has limited adverse effects, and is generally well tolerated. Fiber draws water into the colon to increase fecal mass. Many hospitalized patients, particularly the elderly, fail to reach the recommended daily consumption of 20 to 30 g.[35] Familiar agents include natural fibers, such as psyllium and wheat dextrin, and semisynthetic fibers, such as methylcellulose and polycarbophil. One controlled, blinded trial of 30 frail nursing home residents found that those served oat bran in their diet were able to discontinue laxative use by 59% compared with the control group.[49] Fiber is a first-line choice for most individuals with **constipation**, particularly if the goal is to avoid additional medications. Adverse effects include worsened bloating and abdominal pain, which can sometimes be mitigated by increasing the amount of fiber supplementation slowly. Patients with slow transit **constipation** or dyssynergic defecation do not benefit from increased fiber.[50]

Osmotic laxatives also increase the luminal content of intestinal water, leading to softer and looser stools. Commonly used agents include polyethylene glycol (PEG), magnesium salts, lactulose, and sorbitol. PEG is an osmotic laxative found to be superior to other osmotic laxatives in several studies.[51,52] A meta-analysis including 10 RCTs, six of which were performed on adults, found that PEG outperforms lactulose in increasing stool frequency and stool form and relieving abdominal pain.[53] The evidence supporting the use of PEG as well-tolerated treatment for **constipation** is extensive,[54,55] although it should be noted that most available literature utilizes younger patient populations. In one multicenter study where 37% of the subjects were aged 65 to 89 years, 115 patients with chronic **constipation** were randomized to receive either PEG or lactulose, and patients treated with PEG noted higher number of stools, lower score of straining, and less flatus. Neither group experienced serious adverse effects.[56] Furthermore, in a placebo-controlled, double-blinded RCT of 304 subjects, PEG was shown to be safe and effective for prolonged periods of treatment, including in the elderly subgroup of 75 patients with no increased adverse events except statistically insignificant diarrhea, flatulence, and nausea.[57]

There is strong evidence supporting the use of lactulose in the elderly, in particular with two placebo-controlled RCTs, one involving more than 100 patients older than 60 years and a smaller study with nursing home residents (mean age, 84 years).[58,59] Some patients did experience increased loose stools, flatulence, and bloating, side effects well known to be related to lactulose. These studies were conducted several decades ago, and new comparisons to more recently available medication are warranted, but lactulose remains a safe and efficacious option in the hospitalized geriatric patient.

In the critical care setting, PEG is effective in prophylactic use in mechanically ventilated patients receiving nasogastric tube feeds and is effective but somewhat less so for the treatment of **constipation** and ileus[60]; however, mean age in the groups studied ranged from 51 to 59 years. Both PEG and lactulose were shown to reduce time to first bowel movements in patients receiving mechanical ventilation, and use of both laxatives was associated with shortened duration of stay in the intensive care unit. Notably, lactulose had higher rates of acute colonic pseudo-obstruction compared with PEG (mean age, 65.3 ± 16.5 years).[61]

Fewer studies exist to support the use of other commonly used osmotic laxative, such as sorbitol and magnesium salts. Sorbitol is a nonabsorbable carbohydrate, which is cheaper than lactulose. A double-blind, crossover RCT of 30 men (age, 65-86 years) with chronic **constipation** treated with either lactulose or sorbitol found that there were no significant differences in the number of bowel movements per week or adverse effects.[62] A separate study of 41 nursing home residents with dementia showed no difference in the efficacy of sorbitol when compared with lactulose.[63] In a similar population, milk of magnesia produced a higher number of bowel movements with more normal consistency compared with bulk-forming laxatives.[64] Overall, osmotic laxatives, particularly PEG and lactulose, are safe and effective for use in hospitalized, geriatric patients in acute **constipation** but particularly in the treatment of chronic **constipation**. Depending on individual patient circumstances and clinical situations, however, a different therapy within this class should be attempted if the patient has poor response to the initial choice agent.[7]

## Stimulant Laxatives

Stimulant laxatives promote bowel movements by stimulating peristalsis and inhibiting water reabsorption. Senna and bisacodyl are the most frequently prescribed drugs in this class in the hospital; most of the evidence supporting their utility in the elderly, hospitalized population stems from relatively small studies conducted several decades ago. Senna alters transportation of electrolytes across the colonic lumen, thereby promoting intraluminal fluid secretion and causing mucosal irritation. Both effects result in increased peristalsis and reduced stool transit time. In two RCTs with 107 patients (mean age, 82 years), combination therapy with senna and a bulking agent produced significantly more bowel movements per week and improved stool consistency compared with lactulose, although with a somewhat greater frequency of loose stools[65,66]; however, there are limited data available regarding bisacodyl exclusively. In an older study of 164 elderly patients in long-term care, lactulose resulted in a greater proportion of patients with chronic **constipation** having normal bowel movements than in those receiving senna, bisacodyl, or other anthraquinone derivatives.[67] Sometimes used alone or in combination with bisacodyl, sodium picosulfate is another stimulant laxative shown to produce similar numbers of bowel movements as senna, although with an increase in minor side effects such as diarrhea and cramping.[68]

## Stool Softeners and Lubricants

Stool softeners and lubricants such as docusate sodium (or calcium) and mineral oil are often utilized individually or added to a combination of senna, bisacodyl, and PEG in the management of inpatient and outpatient **constipation**. These agents promote secretion of water, sodium, and chloride into the bowel lumen to facilitate stool passage.[69] Docusate has been given grade B evidence as treatment for **constipation**. A double-blind, placebo-controlled RCT found that docusate was no more effective than placebo when added to sennoside for the management of **constipation** of hospice patients.[70] The mean age of patients in the study was 71.9 years in the placebo group and 75.3 years in the docusate group. The addition of docusate to sennosides actually produced less bowel movements than using sennosides exclusively in a separate study of hospitalized patients with cancer, but this result was not statistically significant.[71] Given that the study involved a nonblinded, nonrandomized cohort and excluded patients declining a trial of a different bowel regimen, further studies will be needed to validate these findings. Current evidence is insufficient to support the claim that docusate is more effective than placebo in treating **constipation**.[72] Despite evidence against its utility, docusate is routinely continued and even started in the hospital for constipated elderly patients, in up to half of admitted patients in some institutions.[73] Deprescribing docusate should be a goal for practitioners in efforts to promote high-value, cost-conscious care; reduce polypharmacy in the elderly; and ensure that patients are on optimal available therapies for **constipation**.

There is a paucity of studies on the value of using mineral oil for the treatment of **constipation** in adults; the majority of recent literature comprised small studies focused on children with functional **constipation**. The use of mineral oil is contraindicated in patients with dysphagia or other conditions with a high risk of aspiration because of its known complication of lipoid pneumonia. Anecdotal beliefs also persist maintaining that prolonged mineral oil use may decrease the absorption of lipid-soluble vitamins. Regardless, the wide availability of alternative evidence-supported treatments of **constipation** should limit the use of these agents in the hospital.

## Suppositories and Enemas

In hospitalized and long-term institutionalized elderly patients, clinicians often turn to rectally administered methods when managing **constipation**. Suppositories and enemas are typically employed in cases to prevent and relieve obstructed defecation.[27] Use in patients receiving palliative care is frequent because such patients may have limited ability to use oral medications. [69] The most commonly utilized suppositories include bisacodyl and glycerin. There are very limited data regarding use of these agents, with most literature on glycerin suppositories investigating use in pediatric populations. Suppositories can be useful tools in patients with spinal cord injuries.[74] Enemas are frequently performed with tap water, phosphate, soapsuds, mineral oil, or castor oil. In elderly patients, the use of phosphate enemas should be avoided, given the risk of causing electrolyte abnormalities. Tap water enemas are considered the most benign. Apart from cases such as spinal cord injury, prolonged use of rectally administered agents is not recommended, and oral agents should be started concomitantly.

## Miscellaneous Agents

Neostigmine is an acetylcholinesterase inhibitor that stimulates colonic motor activity by increasing cholinergic activity in the gut wall. It is not indicated for **constipation**, but instead can be used in the treatment of colonic pseudo-obstruction (Ogilvie syndrome) or postoperative ileus,[75-77] administered as a single dose either intravenously or subcutaneously. Common side effects include hypersalivation, vomiting, abdominal pain, bronchoconstriction, and transient bradycardia. Evidence supporting neostigmine use often comes from anecdotal case reports and relatively small trials typically involving less than 12 patients, the majority of whom were older than 60 years[78,79]; but in these small studies, between 50% and 75% of patients had spontaneous decompression of the colon following administration, typically within 2 hours. Other studies have shown benefit in the use of neostigmine (with glycopyrrolate) in the management of **constipation** related to spinal cord injury (Table 11.1).[80,81]

Older medications, such as colchicine, misoprostol, and bethanechol, have limited evidence supporting their use in **constipation**. Given the abundance of **constipation** treatments, use of these medications in hospitalized elderly inpatients should be limited to particular comorbidities or clinical situations. For instance, colchicine was effective in short-term treatment of slow transit **constipation** in a double-blind placebo-controlled trial of 60 patients[82], with adverse effects such as abdominal pain observed with doses greater than 1 g daily.[83] Because of the general decline in renal function in the elderly, however, use of colchicine for **constipation** treatment should be limited to those with comorbidities such as gout. Furthermore, a dearth of evidence exists for misoprostol, a prostaglandin analog, but has focused predominantly on slow transit and refractory **constipation**. Studies of 9[84] and 18 patients[85] showed improved colonic transit time with treatment, but large proportions of patients withdrew because of intolerable cramping and abdominal pain. Additionally, data supporting the use of bethanechol, a direct smooth muscle muscarinic agent, are restricted to case reports (Table 11.1).[86]

**TABLE 11.1 • Traditional Agents Available for Treatment of Constipation**

| Class | Mechanism of Action | Agents |
|---|---|---|
| Fiber | Increases water retention in lumen by increasing stool bulk | Psyllium, methylcellulose, polycarbophil, wheat dextrin |
| Osmotic laxatives | Produce osmotic gradient causing retention of water in lumen | Polyethylene glycol, lactulose, sorbitol, glycerin, magnesium sulfate, magnesium citrate |
| Stimulant laxatives | Stimulate enteric sensory nerves to promote peristalsis | Bisacodyl, senna, sodium picosulfate |
| Stool softeners and lubricants | Emulsify and lubricate stool | Docusate sodium, docusate calcium, mineral oil |
| Suppositories and enemas | Agent dependent, stimulation of rectal peristalsis, increased stool lubrication | Bisacodyl, glycerin, tap water, oil-based, phosphate, soapsuds |
| Other | | Neostigmine, colchicine, misoprostol, bethanechol |

# THERAPEUTIC ADVANCES

## Secretagogues

Lubiprostone was approved by the US Food and Drug Administration (FDA) in 2006 for CIC. This type 2 chloride channel activator increases the luminal concentration of chloride ions, resulting in a water shift down the osmotic gradient, thus increasing intraluminal fluid and promoting stool softening and motility. It has been used in the management of OIC, CIC, and **constipation**-predominant irritable bowel syndrome (IBS-C). Adverse events include nausea, abdominal pain, abdominal distention, diarrhea, dyspnea, and headache; yet, several studies have established improvement in symptoms in patients treated with lubiprostone compared with placebo.

A multicenter double-blind RCT with 242 subjects showed a statistically significant improvement in spontaneous bowel movements that continued during the treatment period of 4 weeks. Subjects experienced improvements in symptoms of stool consistency, straining, and **constipation** severity. The study was limited in generalizability because the majority of subjects were white (86%) and female (89.7%) and lacked significant systemic disease. The mean age of subjects was 48.5 years (range, 22-80 years), with only 13.2% older than 65 years. Subgroup analysis of the elderly patients did show improvement in spontaneous bowel movement frequency and statistically significant reduction in **constipation** symptoms, with only mild to moderate occurrences of adverse side effects.[87] Also, researchers completed a phase 3 randomized, double-blind, placebo-controlled trial for patients receiving chronic opioids for noncancer pain and who developed OIC, and it showed improvement in symptoms with lubiprostone.[88]

Under the same class but with a slightly different mechanism, linaclotide was approved for the treatment of IBS-C,[89] but may also be useful in treating OIC.[90] The oligopeptide activates guanylate cyclase C receptors, thereby increasing chloride secretion in the colon to increase intraluminal water and promote stool transit. Subgroup analysis of an RCT with a subpopulation of 30 geriatric patients found linaclotide to be equally effective in that subgroup when compared with the general study population in a dose-dependent fashion; the drug was well tolerated, with mild diarrhea being the most commonly reported adverse effect.[91] Lubiprostone and linaclotide have not been compared directly, but it seems that linaclotide may have a slight advantage in the reduction of abdominal pain, and the incidence of nausea seemed to be lower with linaclotide in the drugs' separate trials.

## Peripherally Acting Mu-Opioid Receptor Antagonists

Recent years have witnessed a dramatic increase in the prescription of opioids, resulting in an increased prevalence of OIC.[90] Opioids bind to receptors in the gastrointestinal tract, resulting in decreased bowel motility and increased stool transit time, leading to excess water absorption and decreased pancreatic secretions. A class of drugs known as **peripherally acting mu-opioid receptor antagonists (PAMORAs)** has been developed in response to the increase in OIC. These medications do not cross the blood-brain barrier[92] and thus do not precipitate typical opioid withdrawal effects or reverse analgesia, acting instead on mu receptors of the peripheral nervous system to minimize the constipating effects of opioids.

The first approved PAMORA was alvimopan. Early evidence supporting alvimopan use in OIC was mixed. One phase 3 trial of 518 patients demonstrated increased spontaneous bowel movements and less discomfort, incomplete evacuation, and straining,[93] whereas a concurrent trial of 485 patients did not show increased numbers of bowel movements but some reduction in symptoms and laxative use was noted.[94] Unfortunately, subsequent analyses of these phase 3 trials of alvimopan in treating OIC raised concerns regarding an increased risk of severe adverse cardiovascular events including myocardial infarction.[95] Because of this, further development of alvimopan for OIC treatment has been stopped, and it remains approved for only brief inpatient use for the indication of postoperative ileus following partial bowel resection.[96]

Shortly after, methylnaltrexone bromide was approved by the FDA and boasted a superior safety profile. Specifically approved for the treatment of OIC, it was found to be superior to placebo in a meta-analysis of 14 RCTs involving 4101 patients.[52] Regarding use in an elderly population, one such double-blind RCT with 133 patients (average age, 71 years) on stable doses of opioids demonstrated increased laxation within 4 hours of the first dose compared with placebo (48% vs 15%).[97] Common side effects include abdominal cramping, nausea, vomiting, flatulence, and dizziness. As the medication is exclusively peripherally acting, studies have confirmed no reduction in pain control with improvements in bowel function.[98] This agent has been associated with an elevated risk of worsened abdominal pain and even perforation, and thus must be used with caution. Initially limited to subcutaneous formulation, an oral version was approved in 2017 for OIC in noncancer patients.

In 2014, naloxegol was also approved for the treatment of OIC. Two double-blind, placebo-controlled trials[99] with 1352 subjects (mean age, 52 years) demonstrated improved spontaneous bowel movement rates (44.4% vs 29.4% and 39.7% vs 29.3%) when compared with placebo, with no reduction in analgesia or opioid withdrawal reported. Abdominal pain, nausea, vomiting, and diarrhea were the most common adverse events, which appeared to be dose related, transient, and disappeared after discontinuation of naloxegol.

Safety of use for 1 year was demonstrated.[100] Studies evaluating a prolonged release oxycodone/naloxone combination pill for patients with severe pain and laxative-refractory **constipation** are ongoing. Typically used for acute opioid overdose and associated respiratory depression, naloxone may be given orally, intravenously, intranasally, or intramuscularly, and it crosses the blood-brain barrier when given parenterally. Its low bioavailability (<3%) due to high first-pass effects from hepatic metabolism enables it to interfere with mu receptors in the gut when given orally, with limited effects on the central nervous system.[101] During observational study, patients (mean age, 59.8 ± 13.3 years) with OIC despite use of at least two laxatives were switched from oxycodone to prolonged release oxycodone/naloxone and subsequently demonstrated decreased symptoms, reduced laxative usage, improved quality of life, and even improved pain control.

## Serotoninergic Agonists

In recent years, a link between gastrointestinal motility and serotonin receptors (ie, 5-hydroxytryptamine [5-HT]) has been established.[102] Tegaserod, a selective partial 5-HT4 agonist, had been approved for CIC and IBS-C. A multicenter, double-blind, RCT assigned 607 patients (mean age, 35 years; only 6.6% older than 65 years) with chronic **constipation** to receive either tegaserod or placebo for a 4-week period.[103] Tegaserod was found to cause a statistically significantly increase in spontaneous bowel movements, improvement in stool form, reduced straining, and reported relief of symptoms. In 2007, tegaserod was suspended because a clinical trial demonstrated an increased risk of ischemic cardiovascular events; however, a larger cohort study, with 52 229 patients, did not show an increased risk.[104] It is now available only on a case-by-case basis requiring prior approval by the FDA.

Cisapride has dual 5-HT4 and 5-HT3 activity and was approved by the FDA for gastroesophageal reflux disease, gastroparesis, chronic idiopathic pseudo-obstruction, chronic **constipation**, and dyspepsia. Unfortunately, cisapride was found to be associated with cardiac arrhythmias and death, eventually leading to discontinuation of the drug, aside from a limited access program.[105]

## Upcoming Therapeutics

Several agents are currently under investigation or recently approved for the treatment of OIC. Naldemedine was approved in March 2017 for the treatment of OIC in adults with non–cancer-related chronic pain, although subgroup analysis in the elderly is needed.[106] Axelopran (developmental name TD-1211) is in phase 3 trials for the same indication. Both of these compounds are in the PAMORA family. A sustained release formulation of naloxone is also undergoing phase 2 trials. Velusetrag and prucalopride, 5-HT4 receptor agonists, are also being studied toward the improvement of bowel motility. Lower doses of prucalopride have been shown to have improved bowel movements in patients older than 65 years at 1- and 4-week intervals in a double-blind, placebo-controlled RCT.[107] Plecanatide, a guanylate cyclase C agonist (similar to linaclotide), has shown promise in the treatment of CIC and became FDA approved in January 2017 following trials supporting its safety and effectiveness with limited side-effect profile.[108,109] With an average age of 45 years in all study groups, future analysis is needed to determine its efficacy in older adults (Table 11.2).

| TABLE II.2 • Innovative Agents Available for Treatment of Constipation | | |
|---|---|---|
| **Class** | **Mechanism of Action** | **Agents** |
| Secretagogues | Activate apical surface gut receptors increasing intraluminal water secretion | Lubiprostone, linaclotide, plecanatide |
| Peripherally acting mu-opioid receptor antagonists | Bind gut opioid receptors to prevent opioid inhibition of bowel motility | Alvimopan, methylnaltrexone, naloxegol, naldemedine, velusetrag,[a] axelopran[a] |
| Serotonergic agonists | Stimulate gut serotonin receptors, thus increasing peristalsis | Renzapride, tegaserod,[b] cisapride,[b] prucalopride[a] |

[a]In development or approved outside the United States.
[b]FDA approval revoked.

Work also continues on alternative drug classes as novel approaches to **constipation** treatment. Research into inhibitors of ileal bile acid transporters has shown some early promise, and one drug known as elobixibat (A3309) is currently entering phase 3 trials.[110]

# CONCLUSIONS

Hospitalized elderly adult patients are at a high risk of developing **constipation**. A thorough history and physical examination are needed to distinguish primary **constipation** from secondary causes. Lifestyle modifications, including increasing dietary fiber, eliminating tethers to promote mobility, and maintaining an environment to prevent delirium, are helpful initial measures to treat and reduce the risk of developing **constipation**. Patients' medications and their side-effect profiles should be carefully reviewed, and efforts should be made to discontinue medications that can lead to **constipation** if nonessential or switch to a less offending agent. In addition, medical treatment for pathologies such as endocrinopathies, neurologic disorders, and others must be optimized to facilitate relief of secondary **constipation**. After serious and life-threatening etiologies such as bowel obstruction are ruled out, it is appropriate to begin empiric treatment for **constipation** while concurrently addressing secondary causes. Numerous frequently used therapies such as stimulant laxatives have limited published data supporting or opposing their use; furthermore, use of other agents such as docusate persists despite limited evidence supporting its use and mounting evidence demonstrating its lack of effectiveness. Strong evidence supports the efficacy of bulking fibers like psyllium, osmotic laxatives, and **secretagogues**. Recent studies also support the use of newer agents for OIC (Figure 11.1). As clinicians gain familiarity with these newer agents, they will likely be utilized more commonly. In efforts to move toward high-efficacy, cost-conscious care, clinicians should choose agents with evidence supporting their use. More studies are needed examining newer

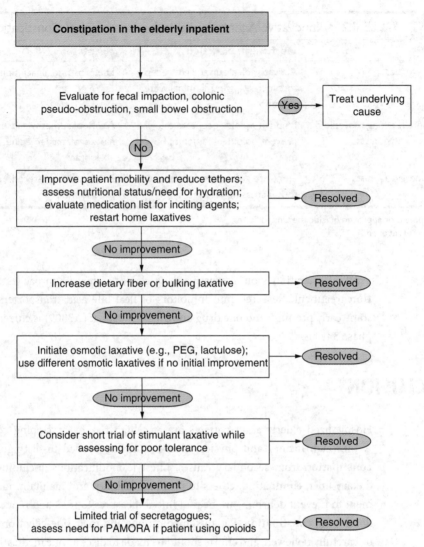

FIGURE 11.1 Algorithm for the treatment of constipation in hospitalized elderly patients. PAMORA, peripherally acting mu-opioid receptor antagonist; PEG, polyethylene glycol.

agents for treating **constipation** in the hospitalized elderly population and to determine their efficacy compared with traditional agents. Such studies would be vital to providing clinicians with more rigorous guidelines for evidence-based treatment of **constipation** and reduce the reliance on anecdotal evidence and clinician preference.

# SUMMARY

Despite its prevalence among hospitalized older adults, **constipation** is frequently treated with ineffective agents. Although data exist to support the use of bulk and osmotic laxatives in geriatric patients, commonly used medications, such as docusate sodium, have been shown to lack clear benefit. Physicians and other providers should review the evidence, or lack thereof, behind familiar and commonly employed agents. Recently, investigators have developed novel agents that rely on alternative mechanisms of action to promote bowel motility. These innovative agents are rapidly becoming powerful tools in the management of **constipation** in older adults. RCTs have demonstrated that secretory agents, including lubiprostone and linaclotide, are quite effective in the general population for the management of **constipation** as well as in geriatric subgroups. Additionally, with the widespread use of opioids to manage chronic pain in the geriatric population, new pharmacologic interventions are available to counter OIC. Compounds such as methylnaltrexone and naloxegol, known as PAMORAs based on their mechanism of action in the gastrointestinal tract, are increasingly being used in the hospital setting for elderly patients with **constipation** associated with the use of opioids; however, further studies are needed to make specific recommendations regarding use in older adults. Finally, serotonergic agents have also been extensively studied for their potential to augment gut motility, but many have been associated with an increased risk of cardiovascular events and are thus at this time not recommended as first-line therapy. Although promising new agents are becoming available for the treatment of this highly prevalent condition, both traditional and innovative therapies for **constipation** need additional study for their efficacy and safety in the elderly population.

## References

1. Suares NC, Ford AC. Prevalence of, and risk factors for, chronic idiopathic constipation in the community: systematic review and meta-analysis. *Am J Gastroenterol.* 2011;106:1582-1591; quiz 1581, 1592.

2. Sandler RS, Jordan MC, Shelton BJ. Demographic and dietary determinants of constipation in the US population. *Am J Public Health.* 1990;80:185-189.

3. Stewart WF, Liberman JN, Sandler RS, et al. Epidemiology of constipation (EPOC) study in the United States: relation of clinical subtypes to sociodemographic features. *Am J Gastroenterol.* 1999; 94:3530-3540.

4. Campbell AJ, Busby WJ, Horwath CC. Factors associated with constipation in a community based sample of people aged 70 years and over. *J Epidemiol Community Health.* 1993;47:23-26.

5. Dukas L, Willett WC, Giovannucci EL. Association between physical activity, fiber intake, and other lifestyle variables and constipation in a study of women. *Am J Gastroenterol.* 2003;98:1790-1796.

6. Bharucha AE, Pemberton JH, Locke GR III. American gastroenterological association technical review on constipation. *Gastroenterology.* 2013;144:218-238.

7. Rao SS, Go JT. Update on the management of constipation in the elderly: new treatment options. *Clin Interv Aging.* 2010;5:163-171.

8. Belsey J, Greenfield S, Candy D, et al. Systematic review: impact of constipation on quality of life in adults and children. *Aliment Pharmacol Ther.* 2010;31:938-949.

9. Johanson JF, Sonnenberg A, Koch TR. Clinical epidemiology of chronic constipation. *J Clin Gastroenterol.* 1989;11:525-536.

10. Faigel DO. A clinical approach to constipation. *Clin Cornerstone.* 2002;4:11-21.

11. Falcon B, Barceló López M, Munoz B, et al. Fecal Impaction: a systematic review of its medical complications. *BMC Geriatr.* 2016;16:4.

12. Sethi S, Mikami S, Leclair J, et al. Inpatient burden of constipation in the United States: an analysis of national trends in the United States from 1997 to 2010. *Am J Gastroenterol.* 2014;109:250-256.

13. Everhart JE, Ruhl CE. Burden of digestive diseases in the United States Part III: liver, biliary tract, and pancreas. *Gastroenterology.* 2009;136:1134-1144.

14. Sommers T, Corban C, Sengupta N, et al. Emergency department burden of constipation in the United States from 2006 to 2011. *Am J Gastroenterol*. 2015;110:572-579.

15. Martin BC, Barghout V, Cerulli A. Direct medical costs of constipation in the United States. *Manag Care Interf*. 2006;19:43-49.

16. Guerra TL, Mendonça SS, Marshall NG. Incidence of constipation in an intensive care unit [in Portuguese]. *Rev Bras Ter Intensiva*. 2013;25:87-92.

17. Cobaugh DJ, Gainor C, Gaston CL, et al. The opioid abuse and misuse epidemic: implications for pharmacists in hospitals and health systems. *Am J Health Syst Pharm*. 2014;71:1539-1554.

18. Kalso E, Edwards JE, Moore RA, et al. Opioids in chronic non-cancer pain: systematic review of efficacy and safety. *Pain*. 2004;112:372-380.

19. Rhondali W, Nguyen L, Palmer L, et al. Self-reported constipation in patients with advanced cancer: a preliminary report. *J Pain Symptom Manage*. 2013;45:23-32.

20. Rome Foundation. Appendix A: Rome III diagnostic criteria for functional gastrointestinal disorders. https://www.theromefoundation.org/assets/pdf/19_RomeIII_apA_885-898.pdf. Accessed June 12, 2017.

21. Noiesen E, Trosborg I, Bager L, Herning M, Lyngby C, Konradsen H. Constipation–prevalence and incidence among medical patients acutely admitted to hospital with a medical condition. *J Clin Nurs*. 2014;23:2295-2302.

22. Jackson R, Cheng P, Moreman S, Davey N, Owen L. "The constipation conundrum": improving recognition of constipation on a gastroenterology ward. *BMJ Qual Improv Rep*. 2016;5:pii:u212167.

23. Lau DT, Dwyer LL, Shega JW. Concomitant opioid and laxative use in older adults in hospice care in the United States: 2007. *J Am Geriatr Soc*. 2016;64:e160-e165.

24. Bader S, Weber M, Becker G. Is the pharmacological treatment of constipation in palliative care evidence based?: a systematic literature review [in German]. *Schmerz*. 2012;26:568-586.

25. Linton A. Improving management of constipation in an inpatient setting using a care bundle. *BMJ Qual Improv Rep*. 2014;3:pii:u201903.

26. Everhart JE, Go VL, Johannes RS, et al. A longitudinal survey of self-reported bowel habits in the United States. *Dig Dis Sci*. 1989;34:1153-1162.

27. Bouras EP, Tangalos EG. Chronic constipation in the elderly. *Gastroenterol Clin North Am*. 2009; 38:463-480.

28. Maher RL, Hanlon J, Hajjar ER. Clinical consequences of polypharmacy in elderly. *Expert Opin Drug Saf*. 2014;13:57-65.

29. Bourgeois FT, Shannon MW, Valim C, et al. Adverse drug events in the outpatient setting: an 11-year national analysis. *Pharmacoepidemiol Drug Saf*. 2010;19:901-910.

30. Mallet L, Spinewine A, Huang A. The challenge of managing drug interactions in elderly people. *Lancet*. 2007;370:185-191.

31. Jyrkka J, Enlund H, Lavikainen P, et al. Association of polypharmacy with nutritional status, functional ability and cognitive capacity over a three-year period in an elderly population. *Pharmacoepidemiol Drug Saf*. 2011;20:514-522.

32. Fletcher PC, Berg K, Dalby DM, et al. Risk factors for falling among community-based seniors. *J Patient Saf*. 2009;5:61-66.

33. Fosnes GS, Lydersen S, Farup PG. Drugs and constipation in elderly in nursing homes: what is the relation? *Gastroenterol Res Pract*. 2012;2012:290231.

34. Page AT, Clifford RM, Potter K, et al. The feasibility and effect of deprescribing in older adults on mortality and health: a systematic review and meta-analysis. *Br J Clin Pharmacol*. 2016;82:583-623.

35. Gallegos-Orozco JF, Foxx-Orenstein AE, Sterler SM, et al. Chronic constipation in the elderly. *Am J Gastroenterol*. 2012;107:18-25.

36. Alame AM, Bahna H. Evaluation of constipation. *Clin Colon Rectal Surg*. 2012;25:5-11.

37. Rao SS, Ozturk R, Laine L. Clinical utility of diagnostic tests for constipation in adults: a systematic review. *Am J Gastroenterol*. 2005;100:1605-1615.

38. Moylan S, Armstrong J, Diaz-Saldano D, et al. Are abdominal x-rays a reliable way to assess for constipation? *J Urol*. 2010;184(suppl 4):1692-1698.

39. Cowlam S, Vinayagam R, Khan U, et al. Blinded comparison of faecal loading on plain radiography versus radio-opaque marker transit studies in the assessment of constipation. *Clin Radiol*. 2008; 63:1326-1331.

40. Cash BD, Acosta RD, Chandrasekhara V, et al. The role of endoscopy in the management of constipation. *Gastrointest Endosc*. 2014;80:563-565.

41. Longstreth GF, Thompson WG, Chey WD, et al. Functional bowel disorders. *Gastroenterology*. 2006;130:1480-1491.

42. Higgins PD, Johanson JF. Epidemiology of constipation in North America: a systematic review. *Am J Gastroenterol*. 2004;99:750-759.

43. Staller K, Khalili H, Kuo B. Constipation prophylaxis reduces length of stay in elderly hospitalized heart failure patients with home laxative use. *J Gastroenterol Hepatol*. 2015;30:1596-1602.

44. Cardin F, Minicuci N, Droghi AT, et al. Constipation in the acutely hospitalized older patients. *Arch Gerontol Geriatr*. 2010;50:277-281.

45. Ross-Adjie GM, Monterosso L, Bulsara M. Bowel management post major joint arthroplasty: results from a randomised controlled trial. *Int J Orthop Trauma Nurs*. 2015;19:92-101.

46. Patel M, Schimpf MO, O'Sullivan DM, et al. The use of senna with docusate for postoperative constipation after pelvic reconstructive surgery: a randomized, double-blind, placebo-controlled trial. *Am J Obstet Gynecol*. 2010;202:479 e1-479 e5.

47. Linari LR, Schofield LC, Horrom KA. Implementing a bowel program: is a bowel program an effective way of preventing constipation and ileus following elective hip and knee arthroplasty surgery? *Orthop Nurs*. 2011;30:317-321.

48. Costilla VC, Foxx-Orenstein AE. Constipation: understanding mechanisms and management. *Clin Geriatr Med*. 2014;30:107-115.

49. Sturtzel B, Elmadfa I. Intervention with dietary fiber to treat constipation and reduce laxative use in residents of nursing homes. *Ann Nutr Metab*. 2008;52(suppl 1):54-56.

50. Voderholzer WA, Schatke W, Muhldorfer BE, et al. Clinical response to dietary fiber treatment of chronic constipation. *Am J Gastroenterol*. 1997;92:95-98.

51. Ramkumar D, Rao SS. Efficacy and safety of traditional medical therapies for chronic constipation: systematic review. *Am J Gastroenterol*. 2005;100:936-971.

52. Ford AC, Suares NC. Effect of laxatives and pharmacological therapies in chronic idiopathic constipation: systematic review and meta-analysis. *Gut*. 2011;60:209-218.

53. Lee-Robichaud H, Thomas K, Morgan J, et al. Lactulose versus polyethylene glycol for chronic constipation. *Cochrane Database Syst Rev*. 2010;(7):CD007570.

54. Corazziari E, Badiali D, Bazzocchi G, et al. Long term efficacy, safety, and tolerability of low daily doses of isosmotic polyethylene glycol electrolyte balanced solution (PMF-100) in the treatment of functional chronic constipation. *Gut*. 2000;46:522-526.

55. DiPalma JA, DeRidder PH, Orlando RC, et al. A randomized, placebo-controlled, multicenter study of the safety and efficacy of a new polyethylene glycol laxative. *Am J Gastroenterol*. 2000; 95:446-450.

56. Attar A, Lemann M, Ferguson A, et al. Comparison of a low dose polyethylene glycol electrolyte solution with lactulose for treatment of chronic constipation. *Gut*. 1999;44:226-230.

57. Dipalma JA, Cleveland MV, McGowan J, et al. A randomized, multicenter, placebo-controlled trial of polyethylene glycol laxative for chronic treatment of chronic constipation. *Am J Gastroenterol*. 2007;102:1436-1441.

58. Wesselius-De Casparis A, Braadbaart S, Bergh-Bohlken GE, et al. Treatment of chronic constipation with lactulose syrup: results of a double-blind study. *Gut*. 1968;9:84-86.

59. Sanders JF. Lactulose syrup assessed in a double-blind study of elderly constipated patients. *J Am Geriatr Soc*. 1978;26:236-239.

60. Guardiola B, Llompart-Pou JA, Ibanez J, Raurich JM. Prophylaxis versus treatment use of laxative for paralysis of lower gastrointestinal tract in critically ill patients. *J Clin Gastroenterol*. 2016;50:e13-e18.

61. van der Spoel JI, Oudemans-van Straaten HM, Kuiper MA, et al. Laxation of critically ill patients with lactulose or polyethylene glycol: a two-center randomized, double-blind, placebo-controlled trial. *Crit Care Med*. 2007;35:2726-2731.

62. Lederle FA, Busch DL, Mattox KM, et al. Cost-effective treatment of constipation in the elderly: a randomized double-blind comparison of sorbitol and lactulose. *Am J Med*. 1990;89:597-601.

63. Volicer L, Lane P, Panke J, et al. Management of constipation in residents with dementia: sorbitol effectiveness and cost. *J Am Med Dir Assoc*. 2004;5:239-241.

64. Kinnunen O, Salokannel J. Constipation in elderly longstay patients: its treatment by magnesium hydroxide and bulk-laxative. *Ann Clin Res*. 1987;19:321-323.

65. Kinnunen O, Winblad I, Koistinen P, et al. Safety and efficacy of a bulk laxative containing senna versus lactulose in the treatment of chronic constipation in geriatric patients. *Pharmacology*. 1993;47 (suppl 1):253-255.

66. Passmore AP, Wilson-Davies K, Stoker C, et al. Chronic constipation in long stay elderly patients: a comparison of lactulose and a senna-fibre combination. *BMJ*. 1993;307:769-771.

67. Connolly P, Hughes IW, Ryan G. Comparison of "duphalac" and "irritant" laxatives during and after treatment of chronic constipation: a preliminary study. *Curr Med Res Opin*. 1974;2:620-625.

68. MacLennan WJ, Pooler A. A comparison of sodium picosulphate ("laxoberal") with standardised senna ("senokot") in geriatric patients. *Curr Med Res Opin*. 1974;2:641-647.

69. Fallon M, O'Neill B. ABC of palliative care. Constipation and diarrhoea. *BMJ*. 1997;315:1293-1296.

70. Tarumi Y, Wilson MP, Szafran O, et al. Randomized, double-blind, placebo-controlled trial of oral do- cusate in the management of constipation in hospice patients. *J Pain Symptom Manage*. 2013;45:2-13.

71. Hawley PH, Byeon JJ. A comparison of sennosides-based bowel protocols with and without docusate in hospitalized patients with cancer. *J Palliat Med*. 2008;11:575-581.

72. Brandt LJ, Prather CM, Quigley EM, et al. Systematic review on the management of chronic constipa- tion in North America. *Am J Gastroenterol*. 2005;100(suppl 1):S5-S21.

73. McKee KY, Widera E. Habitual prescribing of laxatives: it's time to flush outdated protocols down the drain. *JAMA Intern Med*. 2016;176:1217-1219.

74. Coggrave M, Norton C, Cody JD. Management of faecal incontinence and constipation in adults with central neurological diseases. *Cochrane Database Syst Rev*. 2014;13:CD002115.

75. Ponec RJ, Saunders MD, Kimmey MB. Neostigmine for the treatment of acute colonic pseudo-obstruction. *N Engl J Med*. 1999;341:137-141.

76. van der Spoel JI, Oudemans-van Straaten HM, Stoutenbeek CP, Bosman RJ, Zandstra DF. Neostigmine resolves critical illness-related colonic ileus in intensive care patients with multiple organ failure–a prospective, double-blind, placebo-controlled trial. *Intensive Care Med*. 2001;27:822–827.

77. Zeinali F, Stulberg JJ, Delaney CP. Pharmacological management of postoperative ileus. *Can J Surg*. 2009;52:153-157.

78. Rubiales AS, Hernansanz S, Gutierrez C, et al. Neostigmine for refractory constipation in advanced cancer patients. *J Pain Symptom Manage*. 2006;32:204-205.

79. Paran H, Silverberg D, Mayo A, et al. Treatment of acute colonic pseudo-obstruction with neostig- mine. *J Am Coll Surg*. 2000;190:315-318.

80. Korsten MA, Rosman AS, Ng A, et al. Infusion of neostigmine-glycopyrrolate for bowel evacuation in persons with spinal cord injury. *Am J Gastroenterol*. 2005;100:1560-1565.

81. Rosman AS, Chaparala G, Monga A, et al. Intramuscular neostigmine and glycopyrrolate safely ac- celerated bowel evacuation in patients with spinal cord injury and defecatory disorders. *Dig Dis Sci*. 2008;53:2710-2713.

82. Taghavi SA, Shabani S, Mehramiri A, et al. Colchicine is effective for short-term treatment of slow tran- sit constipation: a double-blind placebo-controlled clinical trial. *Int J Colorectal Dis*. 2010;25:389-394.

83. Verne GN, Davis RH, Robinson ME, et al. Treatment of chronic constipation with colchicine: ran- domized, double-blind, placebo-controlled, crossover trial. *Am J Gastroenterol*. 2003;98:1112-1116.

84. Soffer EE, Metcalf A, Launspach J. Misoprostol is effective treatment for patients with severe chronic constipation. *Dig Dis Sci*. 1994;39:929-933.

85. Roarty TP, Weber F, Soykan I, et al. Misoprostol in the treatment of chronic refractory constipation: results of a long-term open label trial. *Aliment Pharmacol Ther*. 1997;11:1059-1066.

86. Poetter CE, Stewart JT. Treatment of clozapine-induced constipation with bethanechol. *J Clin Psycho- pharmacol*. 2013;33:713-714.

87. Ueno R, Wahle A, Zhu Y, et al. Long-term safety and efficacy of lubiprostone for the treatment of chronic constipation in elderly subjects [abstract S1260]. *Gastroenterology*. 2006;130(suppl 2):188.

88. Jamal MM, Adams AB, Jansen JP, et al. A randomized, placebo-controlled trial of lubiprostone for opioid-induced constipation in chronic noncancer pain. *Am J Gastroenterol*. 2015;110:725-732.

89. Nelson AD, Camilleri M, Chirapongsathorn S, et al. Comparison of efficacy of pharmacological

treatments for chronic idiopathic constipation: a systematic review and network meta-analysis. *Gut.* 2017;66:1611-1622.

90. Nelson AD, Camilleri M. Opioid-induced constipation: advances and clinical guidance. *Ther Adv Chronic Dis.* 2016;7:121-134.

91. Lembo AJ, Kurtz CB, Macdougall JE, et al. Efficacy of linaclotide for patients with chronic constipation. *Gastroenterology.* 2010;138:886-895.e1.

92. Thomas J. Opioid-induced bowel dysfunction. *J Pain Symptom Manage.* 2008;35:103-113.

93. Jansen JP, Lorch D, Langan J, et al. A randomized, placebo-controlled phase 3 trial (study SB-767905/012) of alvimopan for opioid-induced bowel dysfunction in patients with non-cancer pain. *J Pain.* 2011;12:185-193.

94. Irving G, Penzes J, Ramjattan B, et al. A randomized, placebo-controlled phase 3 trial (study SB-767905/013) of alvimopan for opioid-induced bowel dysfunction in patients with non-cancer pain. *J Pain.* 2011;12:175–184.

95. Rodriguez RW. Off-label uses of alvimopan and methylnaltrexone. *Am J Health Syst Pharm.* 2014; 71:1450-1455.

96. Holder RM, Rhee D. Novel oral therapies for opioid-induced bowel dysfunction in patients with chronic noncancer pain. *Pharmacotherapy.* 2016;36:287-299.

97. Thomas J, Karver S, Cooney GA, et al. Methylnaltrexone for opioid-induced constipation in advanced illness. *N Engl J Med.* 2008;358:2332-2343.

98. Iyer SS, Randazzo BP, Tzanis EL, et al. Effect of subcutaneous methylnaltrexone on patient-reported constipation symptoms. *Value Health.* 2011;14:177-183.

99. Chey WD, Drossman DA, Johanson JF, et al. Safety and patient outcomes with lubiprostone for up to 52 weeks in patients with irritable bowel syndrome with constipation. *Aliment Pharmacol Ther.* 2012;35:587-599.

100. Webster L, Chey WD, Tack J, et al. Randomised clinical trial: the long-term safety and tolerability of naloxegol in patients with pain and opioid-induced constipation. *Aliment Pharmacol Ther.* 2014; 40:771-779.

101. Poelaert J, Koopmans-Klein G, Dioh A, et al. Treatment with prolonged-release oxycodone/naloxone improves pain relief and opioid-induced constipation compared with prolonged-release oxycodone in patients with chronic severe pain and laxative-refractory constipation. *Clin Ther.* 2015;37:784-792.

102. Gershon MD. Nerves, reflexes, and the enteric nervous system: pathogenesis of the irritable bowel syndrome. *J Clin Gastroenterol.* 2005;39(5)(suppl 3):S184-S193.

103. Lin SR, Ke MY, Luo JY, et al. A randomized, double blind, placebo-controlled trial assessing the efficacy and safety of tegaserod in patients from China with chronic constipation. *World J Gastroenterol.* 2007;13:732-739.

104. Loughlin J, Quinn S, Rivero E, et al. Tegaserod and the risk of cardiovascular ischemic events: an observational cohort study. *J Cardiovasc Pharmacol Ther.* 2010;15:151-157.

105. Wysowski DK, Bacsanyi J. Cisapride and fatal arrhythmia. *N Engl J Med.* 1996;335:290-291.

106. Katakami N, Harada T, Murata T, et al. Randomized phase III and extension studies of naldemedine in patients with opioid-induced constipation and cancer. *J Clin Oncol.* 2017;35:3859-3866.

107. Muller-Lissner S, Rykx A, Kerstens R, et al. A double-blind placebo-controlled study of prucalopride in elderly patients with chronic constipation. *Neurogastroenterol Motil.* 2010;22:991-998.

108. Shailubhai K, Comiskey S, Foss JA, et al. Plecanatide, an oral guanylate cyclase C agonist acting locally in the gastrointestinal tract, is safe and well-tolerated in single doses. *Dig Dis Sci.* 2013;58:2580-2586.

109. Miner PB Jr, Koltun WD, Wiener GJ, et al. A randomized phase III clinical trial of plecanatide, a uroguanylin analog, in patients with chronic idiopathic constipation. *Am J Gastroenterol.* 2017;112:613-621.

110. Acosta A, Camileleri M. Elobixibat and its potential role in chronic idiopathic constipation. *Therap Adv Gastroenterol.* 2014;7:167-175.

# CHAPTER 12

# Innovations in Insomnia Management: A Review of Current Approaches and Novel Targets

Ryann Quinn, MD, Raj Patel, MD, and Jonathan Silver, MD

## BACKGROUND

**Insomnia** and other sleep disturbances are reported in as many as 36% of hospitalized patients, with the elderly inpatient population being disproportionately affected.[1] Older adults are already prone to sleep cycle disturbances because of changing physiology associated with age, and the inpatient setting seems to exacerbate these symptoms.[2] Proper sleep is essential to the healing process, and the increasing prevalence of **insomnia** has affected hospital outcomes, mortality, as well as patient satisfaction; even federal patient satisfaction surveys ask about the quietness of the hospital environment at night.[3,4] With the rising emphasis of creating a "healing environment," improving sleep quality has become a growing area of concern. Current commonly used pharmacologic sleep aids have questionable efficacy or dangerous side effect profiles, especially in older populations.[5] This widespread problem of **insomnia** has left a therapeutic gap in the elderly population necessitating safer alternatives and strategies.

### Aging and Sleep Physiology

A usual night's sleep has a predictable pattern and combination of the different sleep stages, which is referred to as "sleep architecture."[6] Normal sleep architecture consists of non–rapid eye movement (REM) and REM sleep alternating several times over the course of a night and varies with age. As individuals get older, the amount of deep sleep, stage N3, decreases; and although less N3 sleep leads to weaker sleep, the need for sleep never decreases.[2]

In addition to the physiologic changes that occur with age, the older adult has other obstacles that prevent them having a restful night of sleep. **Insomnia** can be distressing to the elderly patient, as demonstrated by a recent study in which elderly patients were asked to rate their overall self-perceived health. They were also asked about other factors such as **insomnia**, independence in activities of daily living, family support, falls, and frailty. **Insomnia** was the strongest predictor of poor self-perceived health in these patients, therefore addressing **insomnia** is crucial in elderly patients.[7] Rates of **insomnia** rise in prevalence as patients age and can be attributed to a primary process, not caused by other health conditions, or a secondary process, difficulty sleeping because of interference by a comorbid illness.[8] Secondary **insomnia** is commonly a consequence of medications or chronic disease. Many commonly prescribed classes of medications have effects on sleep including $\alpha$-blockers, $\beta$-blockers, corticosteroids, and selective serotonin reuptake inhibitors. $\beta$-Blockers, specifically, are known to cause decreased endogenous melatonin secretion, with melatonin supplementation shown to improve sleep quality in patients with hypertension.[9] Chronic illnesses such as obstructive sleep apnea, chronic obstructive pulmonary disease, and congestive heart failure are among the common long-standing medical conditions associated with poor sleep. Indeed, patients with these chronic conditions represent a significant portion of hospitalizations.

When evaluating **insomnia**, it is often the patient's perceived sleep quality that is of critical importance. Therefore, numerous patient-reported questionnaires have been developed to screen for **insomnia** and to assess treatment outcomes in **insomnia** research. The Pittsburgh Sleep Quality Index is a commonly used questionnaire to subjectively measure sleep in patients. The questionnaire assesses duration of sleep, perceived sleep efficiency, and number of sleep disturbances over a 1-month period.[10] Additionally, the Insomnia Severity Index is a 7-item questionnaire assessing the severity of **insomnia** and its impact on daytime functioning.[11] These two questionnaires, while helpful in the outpatient setting, are often not appropriate for hospitalized patients, as they require patients to reflect on their sleep over a time frame of at least 2 weeks. In the inpatient setting, sleep assessment instruments are not routinely used, despite the fact that **insomnia** is a common complaint among inpatients. There is a need for brief and practical sleep assessment tools for hospitalized patients.

# AREAS OF UNCERTAINTY

## Sleep in the Inpatient Setting

The inpatient setting further exacerbates sleep disturbances through a variety of unintended mechanisms.[1] As a new and unknown environment, many patients report more difficulty than usual with initiating and maintaining sleep. This unusual environment brings with it incessant interruptions in the form of intrusive monitoring, disruptive medication administrations, and bothersome blood draws. Because of fragmented and poor quality sleep, hospitalized patients are at risk of marked disruption of their circadian rhythm. Some of this disruption can be attributed to shifts in the patient's routine that impact the cyclic nature of the circadian rhythm, such as changes in medication times and meal times and sun exposure. With the presence of acute illness compounded by the multitude of excessive stimuli present in the inpatient setting, it is no surprise that patients, especially the elderly, frequently have difficulty getting a restful night's sleep while hospitalized. The recommended first-line treatment for **insomnia** revolves around behavioral approaches, but the inpatient setting is not always conducive to these modalities. Benzodiazepines and nonbenzodiazepines have been helpful in increasing total sleep and reducing time to sleep onset, but are coupled with the risk of abnormal sleep-related behaviors, increased falls, and potential for abuse. Newer agents and patient-friendly hospital policies may be the key to improving sleep quality for the hospitalized older adult. This chapter will aim to review commonly used sleep aids as well as introduce novel therapeutics and nonpharmacologic strategies that may be beneficial in the acute inpatient setting.

# NONPHARMACOLOGIC STRATEGIES

## Structural Changes

As the inpatient setting offers distinct challenges, policy and patient care changes may offer additional benefits where medications fail. It is likely that focused, short-term behavioral intervention can play a part to improve sleep quality in hospitalized geriatric inpatients. An example of its integration could be as an adjunct to a comprehensive nonpharmacologic inpatient bundle such as the Hospital Elder Life Program.[12] These programs screen elderly patients for delirium-inducing risk factors including cognitive impairment, visual/hearing difficulties, immobilization, and sleep deprivation. A trained interdisciplinary team with the assistance of volunteers employs interventions such as reality orientation, early mobilization, sleep enhancement programs, and avoiding psychoactive medications when possible. Although establishing wards or floor plans designed for the older adult are not necessary, doing so can help geriatric units facilitate better sleep quality and patient satisfaction (Table 12.1).[13]

Avoiding sleep interruptions by minimizing nonemergent lab draws or identifying patients who are low risk and can tolerate fewer vitals checks overnight has been shown to improve sleep quality.[14] Improving patient environment by decreasing excess light and judicious use of monitors and alarms are among potential areas that can be improved.[15] Another strategy for environment modification could include sound masking systems to help minimize unwanted auditory stimuli and facilitate sleep.

## Cognitive Behavioral Therapy

Cognitive behavioral therapy for **insomnia** (CBT-I) is a multimodal technique, which includes components such as sleep education, sleep hygiene, sleep restriction, relaxation

**TABLE 12.1 • Nonpharmacologic Strategies**

| Program | Intervention | Resources Needed |
|---|---|---|
| Hospital Elder Life Program (HELP) | Screen patients at risk for delirium. Use interdisciplinary teams for reality orientation, early mobilization, sleep enhancement, and medication optimization | Early identification<br>Trained volunteers |
| Geriatric units | Dedicated wards designed for elderly patients, utilizing open floor plans, clocks for time orientation, natural lighting, etc. | Significant floor plan redesign/structural changes<br>Less space-efficient |
| Sleep improvement bundles | Systems to improve sleep quality by minimizing overnight vitals and nonemergent blood draws in low-risk patients | Early identification<br>Less time-efficient |
| Environmental modifications | Creating more hospitable sleep environments with reduced lightning, minimize monitor alarms, ambient noise machines for sound masking, etc. | Structural changes<br>Equipment purchases |

training, and cognitive therapy. This multicomponent approach is beneficial given that multiple factors can contribute to a patient's **insomnia** and can be tailored to each patient.

Many professional organizations recommend that all adult patients receive CBT-I as an initial treatment for **insomnia**.[16,17] In older adults, moderate quality evidence showed that CBT-I improved subjective sleep scores on the Insomnia Severity Index and the Pittsburgh Sleep Quality Index. Low-quality to moderate-quality evidence showed that CBT-I improved sleep onset latency, wake after sleep onset, and sleep efficiency. Adverse events were not reported for CBT-I; however, the authors determined that given its noninvasive nature, harms are likely to be mild. CBT-I seems to have longer-lasting benefits with fewer adverse effects as compared to pharmacologic therapy. The American College of Physicians (ACP) recommends that if patients fail treatment with CBT-I, clinicians use a shared decision-making approach to decide whether or not to add pharmacologic therapy.

# PHARMACOLOGIC STRATEGIES

## Benzodiazepines

It is widely established that benzodiazepines should be avoided in the elderly population. The American Geriatrics Society in its Beers Criteria includes a strong recommendation to avoid benzodiazepines in the treatment of **insomnia**.[18] In addition, the ACP recommends that all patients receive cognitive behavioral therapy as the initial treatment for chronic **insomnia**.[16] However, despite these recommendations, benzodiazepines continue to be prescribed frequently to older adults.[19] A recent study showed that although benzodiazepines are still being frequently prescribed to patients over 65, less than 1% of patients are offered psychotherapy, even though cognitive behavioral therapy is effective and is appropriate as a first-line treatment for **insomnia** (Table 12.2).[20-22]

A meta-analysis conducted evaluated perceived barriers to minimizing inappropriate medications, including benzodiazepines.[23] Some barriers associated with prescribers are: unawareness of the adverse events, belief that the benefits outweigh the risks, and believing that stopping a long-term benzodiazepine prescription in an elderly user with limited life expectancy could do more harm than good. Among practitioners, the most frequently mentioned barrier was reluctance to question a colleague's prescribing decisions or reluctance to question a specialist prescriber. Factors external to the prescriber are the patient not accepting alternative therapies, limited time during clinic visits to review all medications, limited availability of nonpharmacologic options, and inadequate reimbursement and access to support services such as mental health workers. On the inpatient setting, a recent study from the *Journal of Hospital Medicine* showed that 15.9% of elderly patients were newly prescribed an inappropriate medication such as a benzodiazepine or zopiclone, and that the majority of these medications were prescribed for **insomnia** during overnight hours.[24] Many of these medications were prescribed by first year trainees, highlighting the need for increased education on sedative-hypnotics in the elderly.

An increasing amount of data has emerged that support the recommendations to avoid benzodiazepines in older adults. Among the adverse effects listed in the 2015

**TABLE 12.2 • Pharmacologic Strategies**

| Drug | Benefits | Side Effects |
| --- | --- | --- |
| **Benzodiazepines** | Increased subjective total sleep time | Cognitive deficits, falls, fractures, daytime sedation |
| **Nonbenzodiazepine receptor agonists** | Increased objective total sleep time<br>Decreased sleep onset latency | Delirium, somnolence, falls |
| **Ramelteon** | Increased total sleep time<br>Decreased sleep onset latency | Fatigue, somnolence, indigestion<br>Abdominal pain |
| **Doxepin** | Decreased sleep onset latency<br>Increased total sleep time<br>Decreased early morning awakenings<br>Improved sleep maintenance | Avoid doses ≥6 mg in the elderly because of increased anticholinergic effects, sedation, orthostatic hypotension |
| **Orexin receptor antagonist (Suvorexant)** | Increased subjective sleep time<br>Decreased objective waking after sleep | Sleep terrors<br>Next day drowsiness<br>Difficulty operating heavy machinery |

Beers Criteria are increased cognitive deficits, falls, fractures, dependence, and motor vehicle accidents.[18] Benzodiazepines are associated with falls through numerous mechanisms, including daytime sedation, cognitive decline, dizziness, ataxia, balance, and memory impairment.[25-27] A few studies have also indicated that even after benzodiazepines are discontinued, long-term users continue to have cognitive deficits, suggesting lasting and potentially irreversible cognitive deficits.[28,29] A meta-analysis of risks and benefits of sedative-hypnotics in older adults found that although patients did achieve significant improvement in sleep, the magnitude of the effect was small, with total sleep time increased by 34 minutes.[27] However, the cognitive and psychomotor effects associated with benzodiazepines led the authors to conclude that the benefits may not justify the increased risk in the elderly population.

## Nonbenzodiazepine Receptor Agonists

The nonbenzodiazepine receptor agonists (non-BzRAs) are also used for the treatment of **insomnia** and were designed to avoid the potential adverse effects associated with benzodiazepines. Prescriptions for non-BzRAs increased about 30-fold from 1994 to 2007, and they are now among the most commonly prescribed sleep medications worldwide.[30] The 2006 Medicare Part D restriction that excluded benzodiazepines from mandatory drug coverage has also increased the use of non-BzRAs, particularly in nursing homes and residential care facilities.[31]

The non-BzRAs were among the medications that were included in the 2015 update to the American Geriatrics Society Beers Criteria. Prior editions of the Beers Criteria considered non-BzRAs acceptable to use for **insomnia** in the elderly if used for less than 90 days.[18] However, the American Geriatric Society changed their recommendation following two trials showing increased adverse events in patients taking non-BzRAs. A retrospective study, reviewing public health surveillance data between 2009 and 2011, showed an increase in emergency department visits related to adverse drug reactions in patients taking zolpidem.[32] Zolpidem was implicated in 11.5% of emergency department visits related to all adult psychiatric medication adverse drug events, with the most common adverse events being delirium and somnolence. This effect was especially high in patients 65 years and older, where zolpidem was involved in 21.0% of visits to the emergency department for a psychiatric medication adverse drug event. Interestingly, zolpidem was implicated in more emergency department visits per 10 000 outpatient prescriptions than the benzodiazepines alprazolam, lorazepam, and clonazepam. This is consistent with prior studies that have demonstrated that zolpidem is associated with increased falls and fractures in the elderly, both in hospitalized patients and in the community.[33-35] These effects are likely related to the fact that similar to benzodiazepines, non-BzRAs can affect cognitive function, balance, attention, and memory, even in young, healthy individuals.[36,37]

The second study that the American Geriatrics Society cited as a reason to change the 2015 Beers Criteria showed an increase in hip fractures in nursing home residents who were prescribed a non-BzRA. A case-crossover study reviewed a large sample of US longstay nursing home residents and found that there was a 66% increase in hip fractures within 30 days of using a non-BzRA, with the risk being the greatest in the first 15 days.[38]

Studies of non-BzRAs have yet to demonstrate significant clinical benefits, with one meta-analysis showing non-BzRAs decreased sleep onset latency by 12 minutes[9-18] and increased total sleep time by 11.4 minutes as measured by polysomnography.[39] Similar to the benzodiazepines, the risk of adverse events may outweigh the small benefit of these drugs, particularly in older adults. However, the non-BzRAs remain Food and Drug Administration (FDA) approved for the treatment of **insomnia** in the elderly. They do recognize that older adults are particularly sensitive to sedative-hypnotic drugs and recommend decreasing the dose by half (5 mg at bedtime) to decrease the risks related to motor and cognitive performance.[40]

## Ramelteon

The well-established role of melatonin on the circadian rhythm led to the development of a melatonin agonist for the treatment of **insomnia**. The dietary supplement melatonin, which can be bought over the counter, is commonly used as a sleep aid. However, the efficacy of melatonin has been inconsistent across trials. Older studies from the 1990s showed that melatonin can improve sleep,[41,42] but more recent studies have not shown the same beneficial effects.[43,44] Ramelteon is the first selective melatonin agonist to be approved by the FDA. Ramelteon exhibits 6- and 4-fold higher binding affinity for melatonin receptors, MT1 and MT2, respectively, compared with melatonin.[44,45] Ramelteon has demonstrated efficacy in older adults with chronic **insomnia**, decreasing sleep latency and improving total sleep time but the magnitude was small (4.6 minutes and 7.3 minutes, respectively).[46,47] The most commonly reported adverse effects were abdominal pain, indigestion, somnolence, and fatigue. Ramelteon has not shown evidence of next-day drowsiness, dependence, withdrawal effect, cognitive deficit, or impaired middle-of-the-night balance, mobility, or memory.[46-48] It also demonstrated no significant difference from placebo in subjective total sleep time and number of awakenings during the night. These conflicting results demonstrate the need for larger long-term studies to be done to evaluate the efficacy of ramelteon. However, given the positive side-effect profile compared to the sedative-hypnotic sleep aids, it may be considered an early option for elderly patients who fail nonpharmacologic therapy for **insomnia**.[45]

## Novel Therapeutics

### *Orexin Receptor Antagonism*

The orexin system comprises a group of neuropeptides that were found to have a significant role in regulating arousal and sleep states.[49] The lateral hypothalamus projects thousands of neurons that produce orexin neuropeptides and modulate wakefulness throughout the brain. Two types of orexin neuropeptides are known, orexin-A and orexin-B, and these excitatory signaling molecules bind two different orexin G protein–coupled receptors, OX1 and OX2. Orexin-A has been found to have relatively equal binding affinity with both OX1 and OX2; orexin-B has a significantly high affinity for OX2.[50] The activation of the orexin system is implicated in centrally promoting wakefulness and increasing appetite. Suvorexant is a dual orexin receptor antagonist that was approved in 2014 as a novel therapeutic to treat **insomnia**. As the first medication in its class, suvorexant offers an entirely new pathway to promote better sleep. Suvorexant exerts its therapeutic effect through antagonism of both OX1 and OX2 receptors.[51] This novel medication prevents the binding of orexin neuropeptides and therefore dampens an unwanted wake drive that interferes with restful sleep.

In randomized clinical trials to test the efficacy of suvorexant, there was moderate-level evidence that the medication increases subjective sleep time and decreases objective waking after sleep. In the study of safety and tolerability, NCT01021813, a randomized, blinded, controlled trial, 781 patients with **insomnia** were treated with nightly suvorexant for 1 year and extended for 2 months for discontinuation monitoring.[52] Although primary outcomes revolved around adverse events, secondary efficacy outcomes showed that suvorexant had a statistically significant decrease in time to sleep onset, and that subjective total sleep was increased by 27.5 minutes in the intervention arm. In a randomized, controlled clinical trial, NCT00792298, dose-dependent suvorexant had statistically significant improvements in sleep efficiency, including on day 1 of administration, and demonstrated a decrease in waking after sleep onset by 21 to 37 minutes.[53]

Suvorexant appears to be well tolerated; NCT00792298 showed there were no significant major adverse drug events associated with suvorexant compared with placebo in the 254 participants randomized to varying doses or placebo. Although FDA approval came without major warnings, patients should be advised that some sleep disturbances have been reported such as nightmares and sleep terrors as well as next day sleepiness and difficulty operating heavy machinery.[54] Suvorexant is not recommended for patients with hepatic impairment and during pregnancy.

When looking specifically at elderly patients, suvorexant has also been shown to be effective and without major adverse events. In a recent pooled analysis of two phase III clinical trials looking only at patients older than 65, suvorexant demonstrated efficacy compared to placebo both in subjective and in objective sleep measures over a 3-month period.[55] Additionally, suvorexant was also well tolerated in elderly patients, with the most common adverse event being mild to moderate somnolence compared to placebo, however, with no increase in falls or motor vehicle accidents.

Further evaluation is needed to compare suvorexant with other commonly used sleep aids in terms of efficacy and safety. It would also be beneficial to reevaluate suvorexant's potential for abuse and dependency; suvorexant was classified as a Schedule IV medication by the Drug Enforcement Administration regulators because of its similar effects to zolpidem despite having a completely distinct mechanism of action.[56]

# CONCLUSIONS

In the geriatric population, commonly used sleep aids are associated with significant harms and adverse effects but, nonetheless, patients are frequently already dependent on these drugs as an outpatient. In the inpatient setting, it can be very difficult to discontinue long-standing medications despite careful risk/benefit discussions. Given the risks and harms in the above medications, pharmacotherapy should be avoided in favor of other strategies if possible for patients having new difficulty with sleep in the hospital.

Targeted inpatient environmental interventions such as fewer nighttime vitals monitoring when appropriate or noise reduction have already been demonstrated to reduce patient requests of pharmacologic sleeping aids.[12,14] It is doubtful that the harms of behavioral interventions can compare to the risks of pharmacologic therapy, and the improvement was seen in the same exact domains of measured outcomes. The limiting factor for these approaches in the inpatient setting is the lack of time and available resources.

When pharmacotherapy is indicated, it is important to consider that the present state of literature lacks direct comparison of different pharmacologic agents and therefore is inadequate to guide the choice of medications. For elderly, sleep aid–naive patients, we suggest starting with melatonin or selective melatonin receptor agonists given the minimal amount of adverse events and short onset for sleep improvement that suits the inpatient setting. For patients seeking long-term medication, **orexin receptor antagonists** such as suvorexant may be a more natural target for improving sleep quality with tolerable side effects.

# SUMMARY

Sleep disturbances are a source of significant challenge to the care of geriatric hospitalized patients. Commonly used medications to promote sleep are fraught with side effects, especially in the geriatric population. The management of this issue is very important to many patients. We reviewed current data on the effectiveness of current pharmacologic and nonpharmacologic strategies to improve **insomnia** in elderly patients.

Environmental adjustments to the inpatient setting have been shown to improve sleep with no adverse effects. Cognitive behavioral therapy has also been shown to improve objective and subjective sleep measures in older patients with similar efficacy to medications. Benzodiazepines are still popular medications despite evidence demonstrating adverse outcomes including falls, fractures, and cognitive decline. Nevertheless, they have been shown to have a generally small effect on total sleep time. Non-BzRAs have also been demonstrated to pose significant risks of harm to the elderly patient, including delirium and, again, falls and fractures as the price for a small increase in total sleep time. Ramelteon is also shown to have an even smaller effect on sleep time, however, with a more positive side-effect profile. Suvorexant is a new agent that works through a novel mechanism inhibiting the orexin activating system. It has been shown to have similar objective efficacy on sleep as other medications already mentioned and was approved by the FDA without major warnings. However, more study is required to determine if it will elude the risks of medications already available.

Given the lack of adverse consequences, a persuasive case can be made for a comprehensive behavioral approach to sleep promotion before pharmacologic agents are attempted. Studies comparing individual medications are unavailable and thus cannot guide therapy further.

## References

1. Isaia G, Corsinovi L, Bo M, et al. Insomnia among hospitalized elderly patients: prevalence, clinical characteristics and risk factors. *Arch Gerontol Geriatr*. 2011;52:133-137.
2. Espiritu JRD. Aging-related sleep changes. *Clin Geriatr Med*. 2008;24:1-14.
3. Manabe K, Matsui T, Yamaya M, et al. Sleep patterns and mortality among elderly patients in a geriatric hospital. *Gerontology*. 2000;46:318-322.
4. Montague K, Blietz C, Kachur M. Ensuring quieter hospital environments. *Am J Nurs*. 2009;109:65-67.
5. Kelly J. Insomnia treatment for the medically ill hospitalized patient. Ment Health Clin. 2014;4:82-90.
6. Iber C, Ancoli-Israel S, Chesson A, et al. *The AASM Manual for the Scoring of Sleep and Associated Events: Rules, Terminology and Technical Specifications*. Westchester, IL: American Academy of Sleep Medicine; 2007:1.
7. Silva J, Truzzi A, Schautsz F, et al. Impact of insomnia on self-perceived health in the elderly. *Arquivos de Neuro-Psiquiatria*. 2017;75(5):277-281.
8. Roth T. Insomnia: definition, prevalence, etiology, and consequences. *J Clin Sleep Med*. 2007;3:S7-S10.
9. Scheer FA, Morris CJ, Garcia JI, et al. Repeated melatonin supplementation improves sleep in hypertensive patients treated with beta-blockers: a randomized controlled trial. *Sleep*. 2012;35:1395-1402.
10. Buysse D, Reynolds C, Monk T, Berman SR, Kupfer DJ. The Pittsburgh Sleep Quality Index (PSQI): a new instrument for psychiatric research and practice. *Psychiatry Res*. 1989;28:193-213.
11. Bastien C, Vallières A, Morin C. Validation of the insomnia severity index as an outcome measure for insomnia research. *Sleep Med*. 2001;2:297-307.
12. Inouye S, Bogardus S, Charpentier PA, et al. A multicomponent intervention to prevent delirium in hospitalized older patients. *N Engl J Med*. 1999;340:669-676.
13. McDowell JA, Mion LC, Lydon TJ, et al. A nonpharmacologic sleep protocol for hospitalized older patients. *J Am Geriatr Soc*. 1998;46:700-705.
14. Yoder J, Yuen T, Churpek M, et al. A prospective study of nighttime vital sign monitoring frequency and risk of clinical deterioration. *JAMA Intern Med*. 2013;173:1554-1555.
15. Bartick M, Thai X, Schmidt T, et al. Decrease in as needed sedative use by limiting nighttime sleep disruptions from hospital staff. *J Hosp Med*. 2010;5:E20-E24.
16. Qaseem A, Kansagara D, Forciea MA, et al; Clinical Guidelines Committee of the American College of Physicians. Management of chronic insomnia disorder in adults: a clinical practice guideline from the American College of Physicians. *Ann Intern Med*. 2016;165:125-133.

17. Foley D, Ancoli-Israel S, Britz P, Walsh J. Sleep disturbances and chronic disease in older adults—results of the 2003 National Sleep Foundation *Sleep in America* Survey. *J Psychosom Res.* 2004;56:497-502.

18. American Geriatrics Society Beers Criteria Update Expert Panel. American geriatrics Society 2015 updated Beers criteria for potentially inappropriate medication use in older adults. *J Am Geriatr Soc.* 2015;63:2227-2246.

19. Olfson M, King M, Schonenbaum M. Benzodiazepine use in the United States. *JAMA Psychiatry.* 2015;72:136-142.

20. Maust DT, Kales HC, Wiechers IR, et al. No end in sight: benzodiazepine use in older adults in the United States. *J Am Geriatr Soc.* 2016;64:2546-2553.

21. Montgomery P, Dennis J. Cognitive-behavioral interventions for sleep problems in adults aged 60+. *Cochrane Database Syst Rev.* 2003:CD003161.

22. Spinewine A, Swine C, Dhillon S, et al. Appropriateness of use of medicines in elderly inpatients: qualitative study. *BMJ.* 2005;331:935.

23. Anderson K, Stowasser D, Freeman C, et al. Prescriber barriers and enablers to minimizing potentially inappropriate medications in adults: a systematic review and thematic synthesis. *BMJ Open.* 2014;4:e006544.

24. Pek, E, Remfry A, Pendrith C, et al. High prevalence of inappropriate benzodiazepine and sedative hypnotic prescriptions among hospitalized older adults. *J. Hosp. Med.* 2017;5:310-316.

25. Holbrook AM, Crowther R, Lotter A, et al. Meta-analysis of benzodiazepine use in the treatment of insomnia. *Can Med Assoc J.* 2000;162:225-233.

26. Cutson TM, Gray SL, Hughes MA, et al. Effect of a single dose of diazepam on balance measures in older people. *J Am Geriatr Soc.* 1997;45:435-440.

27. Glass J, Lanctot KL, Herrmann N, et al. Sedative hypnotics in older people with insomnia: meta-analysis of risks and benefits. *BMJ.* 2005;331:1169.

28. Barker MJ, Greenwood KM, Jackson M, et al. Persistence of cognitive effects after withdrawal from long-term benzodiazepine use: a meta-analysis. *Arch Clin Neuropsychol.* 2004;19:437-454.

29. Rummans TA, Davis LJ Jr, Morse RM, et al. Learning and memory impairment in older, detoxified, benzodiazepine dependent patients. *Mayo Clin Proc.* 1993;68:731-737.

30. Moloney ME, Konrad TR, Zimmer CR. The medicalization of sleeplessness: a public health concern. *Am J Public Health.* 2011;101:1429-1433.

31. Briesacher BA, Soumerai SB, Field TS, et al. Medicare Part D's exclusion of benzodiazepines and fracture risk in nursing homes. *Arch Intern Med.* 2010;170:693-698.

32. Hampton LM, Daubresse M, Chang HY, et al. Emergency department visits by adults for psychiatric medication adverse events. *JAMA Psychiatry.* 2014;71:1006-1014.

33. Kolla BP, Lovely JK, Mansukhani MP, et al. Zolpidem is independently associated with increased risk of inpatient falls. *J Hosp Med.* 2013;8:1-6.

34. Wang PS, Bohn RL, Glynn RJ, et al. Zolpidem use and hip fractures in older people. *J Am Geriatr Soc.* 2001;49:1685-1690.

35. Tom SE, Wickwire EM, Park Y, Albrecht JS. Nonbenzodiazepine sedative hypnotics and risk of fall-related injury. *Sleep.* 2016;39:1009-1014.

36. Frey DJ, Ortega JD, Wiseman C, et al. Influence of zolpidem and sleep inertia on balance and cognition during nighttime awakening: a randomized placebo-controlled trial. *J Am Geriatr Soc.* 2011;59:73-81.

37. Kleykamp BA, Griffiths RR, McCann UD, et al. Acute effects of zolpidem extended-release on cognitive performance and sleep in healthy males after repeated nightly use. *Exp Clin Psychopharmacol.* 2012;20:28-39.

38. Berry SD, Lee Y, Cai S, et al. Nonbenzodiazepine sleep medication use and hip fractures in nursing home residents. *JAMA Intern Med.* 2013;173:754-761.

39. Buscemi N, Vandermeer B, Friesen C, et al. The efficacy and safety of drug treatments for chronic insomnia in adults: a meta-analysis of RCTs. *J Gen Intern Med.* 2007;22:1335-1350.

40. Sanofi-Aventis. Ambien (zolpidem tartrate tablet) [prescribing information]. Bridgewater, NJ: Sanofi-Aventis; 2016.

41. Garfinkel D, Laudon M, Nof D, et al. Improvement of sleep quality in elderly people by controlled-release melatonin. *Lancet.* 1995;346:541-544.

42. Jean-Louis G, von Gizycki H, Zizi F. Melatonin effects on sleep, mood, and cognition in elderly with mild cognitive impairment. *J Pineal Res*. 1998;25:177-183.

43. Buscemi N, Vandermeer B, Hooton N, et al. The efficacy and safety of exogenous melatonin for primary sleep disorders: a meta-analysis. *J Gen Intern Med*. 2005;20:1151-1158.

44. Singer C, Tractenberg RE, Kaye J, et al; Alzheimer's Disease Cooperative Study. A multicenter, placebo-controlled trial of melatonin for sleep disturbance in Alzheimer's disease. *Sleep*. 2003; 26(7):893-901.

45. Schroeck JL, Ford J, Conway EL, et al. Review of safety and efficacy of sleep medicines in older adults. *Clin Ther*. 2016;38:2340-2372.

46. Mini LJ, Wang-Weigand S, Zhang J. Self-reported efficacy and tolerability of ramelteon 8 mg in older adults experiencing severe sleep-onset difficulty. *Am J Geriatr Pharmacother*. 2007;5:177-184.

47. Kuriyama A, Honda M, Hayashino Y. Ramelteon for the treatment of insomnia in adults: a systematic review and meta-analysis. *Sleep Med*. 2014;15:385-392.

48. Roth T, Seiden D, Sainati S, et al. Effects of ramelteon on patient-reported sleep latency in older adults with chronic insomnia. *Sleep Med*. 2006;7:312-318.

49. Ebrahim IO, Howard RS, Kopelman MD, et al. The hypocretin/orexin system. *J R Soc Med*. 2002; 95:227-230.

50. Langmead CJ, Jerman JC, Brough SJ, et al. Characterization of the binding of [3H]-SB-674042, a novel nonpeptide antagonist, to the human orexin-1 receptor. *Br J Pharmacol*. 2004;141:340-346.

51. Mieda M, Sakurai T. Orexin (hypocretin) receptor agonists and antagonists for treatment of sleep disorders: rationale for development and current status. *CNS Drugs*. 2013;27:83-90.

52. Michelson D, Snyder E, Paradis E, et al. Safety and efficacy of suvorexant during 1-year treatment of insomnia with subsequent abrupt treatment discontinuation: a phase 3 randomized, double-blind, placebo-controlled trial. *Lancet Neurol*. 2014;13:461-471.

53. Herring W, Snyder E, Budd K, et al. Orexin receptor antagonism for treatment of insomnia: a randomized clinical trial of suvorexant. *Neurology*. 2012;79:2265-2274.

54. Bennett T, Bray D, Neville MW. Suvorexant, a dual orexin receptor antagonist for the management of insomnia. *Pharm Ther*. 2014;39:264-266.

55. Herring WJ, Connor KM, Snyder E et al. Suvorexant in elderly patients with insomnia: pooled analyses of data from phase III randomized controlled clinical trials. *Am J Geriatr Psychiatry*. 2017;25(7): 791-802.

56. Drug Enforcement Administration, Department of Justice. Schedules of controlled substances: placement of suvorexant into Schedule IV. Final rule. *Fed Regist*. 2014;79:51243-51247.

# Therapeutic Advances in Sub-Specialty Geriatric Care

# CHAPTER 13

# New Innovations in Treatment and Monitoring of Heart Failure

Shikha Sheth, MD, Shankar Thampi, MD, Chinedu Madu, MD, Alicia Chionchio, MD, and Evangelos Loukas, DO

## BACKGROUND

Heart failure is a clinical syndrome with a substantial impact on modern society. Currently, more than 5 million Americans have heart failure and that number is predicted to exceed 8 million by 2030.[1] Heart failure exacerbation is the leading cause of hospitalizations in patients older than 65 years. In addition, heart failure is a major cause of hospital readmissions, with 25% of patients readmitted within 30 days and up to 50% within 6 months.[1] Heart failure hospitalizations are also strong predictors of mortality, with 10% at 1 month and nearly 25% at 1 year.[1] The resulting disease burden within society is profound, because financial costs of heart failure are currently estimated to be greater than US$30 billion per year and expected to increase.[1]

Key factors driving the prevalence of heart failure include the aging population; increasing prevalence of comorbid conditions that lead to heart failure such as coronary artery disease (CAD), hypertension, valvular heart disease, obesity, and diabetes; and advances in the treatment of myocardial infarction, which have led to improved survival.[1] Despite the therapeutic advances in the management of heart failure over the past three decades, there are still many challenges to developing effective therapies and prognosis remains poor, particularly with geriatric patients.[2] In response to this critical, global issue, there are many ongoing collaborative efforts, both pharmacologic and nonpharmacologic, to advance the therapeutic field of heart failure.

This review aims to assess established effective pharmacotherapies in the management and treatment of heart failure and analyze and summarize key clinical research trials, highlighting recent advances in medical therapy and management of heart failure, so that providers can incorporate the findings to optimize care for this challenging patient population.

# ESTABLISHED THERAPIES

## Angiotensin-Converting Enzyme Inhibitors and Angiotensin Receptor Blockers

One of the mainstays of treatment of **heart failure** (particularly with reduced ejection fraction [EF]) is the angiotensin-converting enzyme inhibitors (ACEIs). These drugs block the renin–angiotensin–aldosterone system (RAAS) by inhibiting the conversion of angiotensin I to its more active metabolite angiotensin II, thus preventing its downstream effects of increased systemic vascular resistance (SVR), sodium retention, and cardiac remodeling.[3] In patients with **heart failure** with reduced ejection fraction (HFrEF), ACEIs have been shown to be beneficial in all age groups, including those older than 60 years, in both improving quality of life and decreasing hospitalizations and mortality related to **heart failure**.[4] However, some more recent data suggest that in those older than 75 years, the relative benefit is smaller.[5] In addition, older patients are more prone to adverse complications, such as hypotension, kidney injury, and electrolyte disturbances, especially if interacting with other medications.[6] Hypotension is particularly problematic because of the risk of orthostatic hypotension, which may lead to falls and fractures, a major cause of morbidity and mortality in the elderly. In regard to renal dysfunction, although ACEIs are not advised in patients with acute kidney injury, they are generally considered safe in those with chronic kidney disease. No creatinine level or clearance is established as an absolute contraindication, although levels should be watched closely after the initiation of therapy.

Angiotensin receptor blockers (ARBs) have beneficial effects similar to those of ACEIs while avoiding the common side effect of cough by blocking angiotensin II directly at its receptor and thus allowing the metabolism of bradykinin by angiotensin-converting enzyme (ACE) and still inhibiting the RAAS. Although equivalence of ARBs to ACEIs has not yet been established, both classes of drugs have independently been shown to significantly decrease all-cause mortality, development of new arrhythmias, and hospitalizations due to **heart failure**, making ARBs a viable option in those unable to tolerate ACEIs.[7-10] The Evaluation of Losartan in the Elderly (ELITE) study, a randomized controlled trial comparing losartan with captopril using 722 ACEI-naive patients older than 65 years with New York Heart Association (NYHA) Class II–IV **heart failure** and EFs <40%, noted an apparent benefit in mortality with the ARB compared with the ACEI; however, the ELITE II follow-up trial that assessed a larger cohort of patients (3,152) within the same population (average age 71.5) was not able to replicate this finding.[7,8] In addition, most of the adverse risks of ACEIs are unfortunately still present with ARBs and, for older populations, substantial.

Multiple studies have attempted to assess the utility of both ACEIs and ARBs in patients with concern for diastolic dysfunction, with no clear significant benefit.[11-13] Data from studies geared toward the geriatric population, however, such as the Heart Outcomes Prevention Evaluation (HOPE) trial, which looked at patients older than 55 years with a significant cardiovascular risk, and the Losartan Intervention for Endpoint Reduction (LIFE) trial, which looked at patients aged 55 to 80 years with signs of concentric left ventricular hypertrophy, suggest some benefit likely by treating the most common underlying cause of diastolic **heart failure**: uncontrolled hypertension.[14,15]

## β-Blockers

Another common class of medications used for systolic **heart failure** management are β-blockers because of their negative inotropic and chronotropic effects. Although decreasing cardiac output with β-blockers can transiently worsen **heart failure** symptoms, especially in older patients, there is a well-established benefit on morbidity and mortality regardless of the age group, thus making them a standard of therapy.[16] However, because β-blockers are less well tolerated in the elderly because of side effects such as bradycardia, hypotension, and initial worsening of symptoms of **heart failure**, appropriate dosing can be a challenge.[17]

Although no large clinical trials have definitively proved the efficacy of β-blockers in HFpEF, preliminary data strongly suggest a beneficial effect likely because of its effects on hypertension, CAD, and atrial fibrillation, all common causes of HFpEF exacerbations.[18-20] Data gathered from the Swedish Heart Failure Registry, for example, looking at 19 083 patients with an average age of 76 years and known HFpEF were found to have a lower risk of all-cause mortality (but no reduction in **heart failure** hospitalization) through a propensity score–matched cohort study. However, the authors are quick to point out that further data from randomized clinical trials are needed to strongly support this conclusion.[19,20]

## Aldosterone Antagonists

In addition to ACEIs/ARBs, and β-blockers, the only other class of pharmaceuticals that has been shown to cause a significant reduction in overall mortality in patients with severe HFrEF (NYHA Class IV, LEFT VENTRICULAR [LV] EF <35%) are the aldosterone antagonists such as spironolactone, eplerenone, and amiloride.[21] These medications are diuretics that act on the RAAS as well by competitively binding with the aldosterone receptor in the distal renal tubules, increasing sodium and water excretion. The results from the Randomized Aldactone Evaluation Study (RALES), a double-blind trial comparing Aldactone with placebo in 1663 patients with NYHA Class III–IV HFrEF already on multidrug therapy, found a nearly 30% reduction in mortality with Aldactone.[21] These data can be extrapolated for the geriatric population, because the average age of the patients was 65 years (standard deviation [SD] 12).

The common side effects of this class of medicine include hypotension, kidney injury, and electrolyte abnormalities (particularly hyperkalemia), and are prevalent in the elderly; thus, reduced dosing may be necessary.[6,22]

## Digoxin

One of the oldest medications used for treating **heart failure**, digoxin is a compound isolated from the foxglove plant and has been a standard of therapy for **heart failure** and other cardiac illnesses for ages. The Digitalis Investigation Group (DIG), which looked at nearly 7000 patients with an average age of 63 and EF <45% in a double-blind study, however, found that although digoxin can create symptomatic improvement and reduce hospitalizations when used in conjunction with ACEIs, regardless of the age group, it did not have a significant effect in reducing cardiovascular morbidity and mortality compared with placebo.[23] Given its benefits at reducing chronic **heart failure** (CHF)-related hospitalizations, it is still considered a useful adjunctive treatment in severe HFrEF. In addition, although digoxin can have adverse and toxic effects such as gastrointestinal disturbance, vision changes, and abnormal heart rhythms, the DIG found that these effects were not age dependent.[24] However, because digoxin is renally cleared, it must be used judiciously in those with decreased kidney function, such as the elderly.[6,25] Digoxin toxicity is common among older patients because of their decreased filtration rate, as well as their decreased size, drug interactions, and comorbidities.[26] For this reason, recommendations from the latest Beers Criteria update are that digoxin should be avoided as a first-line agent in geriatric patients, with daily doses of no more than 0.125 mg if used.[6]

Of note, an ancillary to the DIG trial focusing on a subset of patients with HFpEF suggested that digoxin was still beneficial in preventing **heart failure**–related hospitalizations in this population; however, this relationship was not statistically significant.[26]

## Diuretics

Some of the most commonly used classes of medications in both HFrEF and HFpEF are the diuretics, all of which work to help patients manage their volume status. These include the thiazide diuretics (such as hydrochlorothiazide), which act at the distal tubules to inhibit sodium reabsorption causing increased sodium and water excretion, as well as the loop diuretics (such as furosemide), which act on the ascending loop of Henle as well as the proximal and distal renal tubules to affect the chloride-binding cotransport system leading to electrolyte and water excretion, and the aldosterone antagonists noted earlier. Although the aldosterone antagonists have been shown to have some effect on mortality, the other diuretics have not been shown to have any significant effect on outcomes and are mainly used for symptom control and to help patients maintain a state of euvolemia.[16] The most common side effects of these medications are related to overdiuresis and include hypotension, kidney injury, and electrolyte imbalances. In patients with diastolic dysfunction, overdiuresis may worsen **heart failure** by decreasing preload and thus cardiac output. Another factor to take into consideration is that although increased urination is the intended effect of the medication, it may also lead to incontinence and decreased quality of life from increased frequency, which in turn may lead to noncompliance. There are no major data assessing the effects of diuretics in patients with **heart failure** on the basis of age group.

## Vasodilators (Nitrates and Hydralazine)

For patients who are unable to tolerate treatment with ACEIs/ARBs, such as those with kidney disease or who are prone to electrolyte imbalances, a viable alternative is to use a combination vasodilator therapy with hydralazine and a nitrate. Hydralazine works to reduce SVR (afterload) by the direct vasodilatory effect on arterioles, whereas nitrates have a vasodilatory effect more primarily on the veins, thus decreasing preload. In combination, these medications have been proved to decrease cardiovascular mortality, however not to as significant an extent as ACEI/ARB therapy.[27] Before the development of ACEIs/ARBs, vasodilators were often used in patients with HFrEF because data suggested a survival benefit, especially in those with mild to moderate **heart failure**.[28] The Vasodilator Heart Failure Trial (V-HeFT), a double-blind, randomized study comparing hydralazine and isosorbide dinitrate with placebo in 642 men with dilated cardiomyopathy (or EF <45%), showed a significant benefit in survival with vasodilator therapy.[28] Unfortunately, although the average age of patients was 60 years, no subgroup analysis was performed on the data to quantify the effect on the basis of age range.

# AREAS OF UNCERTAINTY

Despite therapeutic advances in the field of **heart failure**, there are two noteworthy gaps within that need to be further defined. First, there has been limited research and effective pharmacotherapies identified for patients with **heart failure** with preserved EF, which constitute about half of all **heart failure** cases.[29,30] Second, most of the randomized controlled trials do not reflect accurately the types of patients physicians encounter daily—the elderly and those with several comorbidities.[29] A multicenter trial in the United States across 274 hospitals and 105 388 patients found that 52% of the patients admitted for acute decompensated **heart failure** were women, with a mean age across the group of 72 (SD 14).[31] Of these, 54% of the patients had HFrEF. Most trials assessing the reduction in hospitalization rates and all-cause mortality in patients with HFrEF fall significantly short of this age group and do not have appropriate representation of women, making it questionable to what extent the guidelines can be applied to the elderly patients. Consequently, the clinical reproducibility of the outcomes achieved in these studies becomes challenging, because physicians must leverage other competing chronic diseases in an effort to achieve the desired result.

The classification and diagnosis of **heart failure** with preserved EF is not straightforward, because EF can be normal or slightly reduced, and there may be no clinical symptoms of **heart failure**. Timely recognition and early intervention become very important, because patients may have evidence of underlying abnormalities in heart function even without symptoms of **heart failure**.[32] Clinical biomarkers, most notably brain natriuretic assays, are often used to help aid in the diagnosis; but diagnostic thresholds are variable, and other cardiac and noncardiac disease processes can influence the levels, making interpretation difficult at times. In older adults, these conditions commonly include renal dysfunction, sepsis, anemia, and advancing age.[1] The use of biomarkers to affect decisions on therapeutic regimens is still underdeveloped.[33]

**Heart failure** is a chronic syndrome manifested by episodes of acute exacerbation with a rehospitalization rate suggestive of multifactorial causes contributing to disease progression. A better understanding of these influences coupled with a need for a comprehensive, integrated, and multidisciplinary approach focused on optimizing care transitions, using available resources, and providing patient education is necessary to help address this complex syndrome.[32,34] The efficacy of various transitional care interventions in an effort to prevent **heart failure** readmissions and reduce mortality has been studied; however, the results have been equivocal. There have been some promising data with high-intensity home-visiting programs and multidisciplinary **heart failure** clinic interventions resulting in reductions in all-cause readmissions and mortality over 3 to 6 months.[35] The inherent issues with these interventions lie in their reproducibility because of the intensity of resources and costs required, coupled with the necessity to manage patient comorbidities, education, and socioeconomic factors. It seems that a combination of inpatient, transitional, and outpatient strategies that solidify and reinforce the continuum of integrated care for these patients could prove to be most efficacious in improving outcomes.

# NEW THERAPEUTICS

## Angiotensin Receptor Blocker with Neprilysin Inhibitor

A combination drug, **sacubitril/valsartan** (angiotensin receptor blocker with **neprilysin inhibitor** [ARNi]), has recently gained Class 1B recommendation for treatment of HFrEF.[36] ARNi combines a **neprilysin inhibitor**, sacubitril, with an ARB, valsartan. Neprilysin is a neutral endopeptidase, which degrades endogenous natriuretic peptides (NTs) and angiotensin II. Inhibition of neprilysin leads to a buildup of NTs, including brain-type natriuretic peptides (BNPs) and atrial and c-type NTs, as well as angiotensin II.[37] NTs are released in response to increased intracardiac pressures, atrial and ventricular wall stress, and increase in cytokines. These peptides act as potent vasodilators, reducing systemic blood pressure, and also act on the kidneys to decrease the intravascular volume, resulting in a decrease of both preload and afterload and a consequent decrease in cardiac stress.[38] However, neprilysin inhibition also leads to a buildup of angiotensin II and subsequent adverse effects through the RAAS pathway.

The first novel agent targeting the neprilysin inhibition pathway was candoxatril.[39] However, it was studied as a monotherapy without the addition of ACE or ARB. Although the result increased NTs, there was also an increase in angiotensin II that had a stronger net effect of increased SVR and decreased cardiac output. A second trial was conducted with omapatrilat, a drug that combined the effects of neprilysin inhibitor with ACEI (omapatrilat) to combat the increase of angiotensin II.[40] Although the drug showed noninferiority in the phase III trial, it was discontinued because of a 3-fold increase in angioedema secondary to the combination effect of both medications in inhibition of bradykinin metabolism.

The next trial used a combination of sacubitril and valsartan, which achieved successful inhibition of angiotensin II without increasing bradykinin.[41] The Prospective Comparison of ARNi with ACEI to Determine Impact on Global Mortality and Morbidity in Heart Failure (PARADIGM-HF) trial, a randomized controlled trial, established the efficacy of this drug against enalapril for patients with NYHA Class IIIV HFrEF, demonstrating a 20% reduction in primary end points including cardiovascular mortality and rehospitalization rate ($P < 0.001$) and a 16% reduction in all-cause mortality over the course of 27 months.[42,43] Secondary outcomes, including new-onset atrial fibrillation and decline in renal function, were similar between the two drugs. The incidence of symptomatic hypotension was higher in ARNi, whereas that of hyperkalemia and cough was higher in enalapril.

The concern for the PARADIGM-HF trial and the older studies assessing the efficacy of ACEIs and ARBs is that the average age of the studied population was 64 years (SD 11) in a sample size of 8442 patients, and only 20% of the patients were women.[42] This is similar to the population enrolled in previous studies assessing the efficacy of enalapril and the novel agent **ivabradine**.[10,44] In addition, although a little more diverse than the previous studies having 80% of white ethnicity, the PARADIGM-HF still has 66% of white patients despite being conducted across 47 nations and 1043 centers. The trial remains focused on the younger end of the spectrum of patients with **heart failure**. Therefore, it is not clear what the implications are for using this class of medications in patients who are older than 75 years.

Identification of the optimal patient population for ARNi as opposed to ACE or ARB remains unclear. New subanalysis of the PARADIGM-HF suggests that measurement of the N-terminal pro-BNP provides a valuable insight into this concern. Patients who have NT-pro-BNP ≤ 1000 have a 59% lower risk of the primary end point, regardless of which medication was used to maintain that level.[45] For patients with NT-pro-BNP > 1000, however, ARNi was nearly twice as effective as enalapril (31% vs. 17%) at achieving a goal of NT-pro-BNP ≤ 1000 at 1 month, and 15% more likely to maintain this reduction over 8 months than enalapril. On the basis of this study, measurement of NT-pro-BNP would be a valuable tool in the determination of which patients may benefit from ARNi—with those patients in advance **heart failure** and high levels of NT-pro-BNP having the maximum benefit of this novel agent.

## Ivabradine

A novel agent, **ivabradine**, is an inhibitor of the If channel at the sinoatrial node, which allows for selective reduction in heart rate without detrimentally affecting cardiac contractility.[46] It has a Class IIa B-evidence recommendation in regard to **heart failure**.[36] Instrumental in validating **ivabradine** was the Systolic Heart Failure Treatment with If Inhibitor Ivabradine Trial (SHIFT), a randomized, double-blind, placebo-controlled, parallel group study (6558 total patients, over 18-28 months).[44] This trial was directed at patients with symptomatic stable systolic **heart failure**. Inclusion criteria were a previous hospital admission in the past year, active medical management, and a heart rate with a sinus rhythm of 70 beats per minute or higher.[44] Using **ivabradine**, researchers noted a significant reduction in hospital admissions for worsening **heart failure** ($P < 0.0001$) and deaths due to **heart failure** ($P = 0.014$).[44]

In contrast to the SHIFT was the morbidity–mortality evaluation of the If inhibitor **ivabradine** in patients with coronary disease and left ventricular dysfunction or the BEAUTIFUL trial. This was a randomized, double-blind, placebo-controlled, parallel group study (10 917 total patients), which included patients 55 years or older, with stable CAD and systolic EF <40%.[47] The BEAUTIFUL trial did not show an improvement of the primary end point of the study (composite of admission for **heart failure** and cardiovascular death and admission for myocardial infarction).[47]

Of note, the use of **ivabradine** may be limited to patients in sinus rhythm and with **heart failure**. In the BEAUTIFUL trial, **ivabradine** seemed to reduce admission for myocardial infarction ($P = 0.001$) and revascularization ($P = 0.016$).[47] However, in the study assessing the morbidity–mortality benefits of the If inhibitor **ivabradine** in patients with CAD, which assessed patients without **heart failure**, there was no significant improvement in clinical outcomes with **ivabradine**.[48] **Ivabradine** may also be limited in patients with atrial fibrillation. It has an increased relative risk of atrial fibrillation, and it was an exclusion criterion for the SHIFT.[49,50] This is a potential limitation in the elderly, given the increasing prevalence of atrial fibrillation in that population.

Overall, **ivabradine** seems promising as a new agent for the elderly population, because it was well tolerated in both the SHIFT and BEAUTIFUL trials.[44,47] Each of these included the elderly population (the SHIFT had 11% of patients older or equal to 75 years, and the BEAUTIFUL had a median age of 64.8 years in the **ivabradine** group).[37,44] The main side effects included asymptomatic bradycardia and visual changes such as blurred vision and phosphenes. Subsequent subanalyses have also shown improvement in quality of life.[50,51]

## Nesiritide

Nesiritide is a recombinant human BNP that is shown to cause arterial and venous dilatation and suppression of RASS. Early clinical trials showed the efficacy of the drug in short-term treatment of **heart failure** exacerbation in the hospital setting, with a dose-dependent decrease in baseline pulmonary–capillary wedge pressure within 6 hours of the start of therapy and a decrease in SVR and systolic blood pressure.[52] **Nesiritide** was shown to improve dyspnea and fatigue more rapidly at 6 hours after infusion and at 24 hours after infusion than did the placebo drug. However, when compared with the use of inotropes such as dobutamine and milrinone, outcomes were similar across the drugs in decreasing the symptoms of acute **heart failure** exacerbation. Subsequent investigations have found that although **nesiritide** infusion in acute decompensated **heart failure** results in a rapid reduction of pulmonary–capillary wedge pressure compared with placebo or nitroglycerine, symptomatic relief of dyspnea or hospital readmission rates are not affected.[53] This led to further investigation of **nesiritide** in **heart failure** management, with the largest prospective randomized study evaluation in the Acute Study of Clinical Effectiveness of **Nesiritide** in Decompensated Heart Failure (ASCEND-HF) trial with 398 sites across four continents. This trial revealed similar outcomes, with nonsignificant effects on rehospitalization rates or on mortality.[54] The median age was 67 years (SD 9) in a sample size of 7141 patients, slightly higher than that in other study drugs in **heart failure**. Furthermore, the use of **nesiritide** was not shown to improve renal function in the patients with acute kidney injury or in patients with chronic kidney disease, but instead it has been associated with an increase in rates of hypotension.[36,55] There have not been significant trials assessing for its use in chronic **heart failure** management. Given the findings, **nesiritide** is not recommended in acute or chronic management of **heart failure** except in extreme circumstances with severe **heart failure** exacerbation symptoms refractory to other medications in intensive care settings.

# NONPHARMACOLOGIC TREATMENTS FOR CONGESTIVE HEART FAILURE IN THE ELDERLY

## Left Ventricular Assist Device

A ventricular assist device is a mechanical device that can assist the pumping mechanism of the heart. It can be inserted in either ventricle, although it is most commonly used in the left ventricle. The implanted pump takes blood from the apex of the left ventricle and propels it to the ascending aorta. The pump is connected to the percutaneous lead that connects to an external power source.[56] Left ventricular assist devices (LVADs) were originally developed for patients with end-stage **heart failure** as a bridge to a heart transplant. Recent studies have shown that long-term LVAD can provide a meaningful survival benefit and improved quality of life in patients who are not good candidates for a heart transplant.[57] In 2014, a single-center retrospective study involving 64 patients showed that patients older than 65 years who received an LVAD as either a bridge to transplantation or destination therapy showed improved survival compared with what their Seattle Heart Failure Model score would have predicted.[58] Although there are sparse data about outcomes of implementation in the very elderly, manufacturer data indicate that a device should be expected to function for 7 to 10 years. Primary risks of LVAD include increased risk of infection, bleeding, stroke, and pump malfunction primarily due to pump thrombosis.[59] Technological advances in LVAD are fast growing, with initial designs focused on pulsatile flow designs now being replaced with continuous flow devices. A newer pump model that employs magnetically levitated centrifugal continuous flow was recently shown to reduce the risk of pump thrombosis.[60,61] This pump employs intrinsic artificial pulse to reduce blood stasis within the pump and employ wider blood flow passages to decrease friction, resulting also in a decrease in stroke in addition to device thrombosis. As technology becomes more advanced to minimize device failure, use of these LVADS is increasingly geared toward patients in clinical need for circulatory support as a destination therapy and not just as a bridge toward transplant. There is still a need to establish criteria for risk stratification for LVAD implantation in elderly patients.

## Pulmonary Artery Pressure Monitoring Device

Pulmonary artery pressure monitoring devices have been developed as a way to predict worsening acute on chronic **heart failure** before the development of symptoms. An increase in pulmonary artery pressure is used as a proxy for volume overload. The CardioMEMS **heart failure** system is U.S. Food and Drug Administration approved for patients with NYHA Class III **heart failure** who have been hospitalized with **heart failure** in the previous year. Physicians can monitor the pressures remotely to help prevent hospitalizations. A multicenter randomized controlled trial involving 550 patients, known as the CHAMPION trial, showed that patients (average age 67 years) with Class III **heart failure** who have the hemodynamic monitoring device had a significant decrease in hospital admissions over a 6-month period.[62] Follow-up studies showed similar effects at 18 months as well.[63] In 2016, a randomized control trial looked specifically at 245 Medicare-eligible patients (65 years and older) and showed that pulmonary artery pressure monitoring leads to a 49% decrease in **heart failure**–related 30-day hospital readmissions and a 58% reduction in all-cause readmissions.[64] In this study, the average age of the patients was 73 years (66 years).

## Defibrillators

The implantable cardioverter–defibrillator (ICD) is indicated as primary prophylaxis for patients with NYHA Class II–III and an EF < 35%, based on results from the sudden cardiac death-HeFT, a randomized control trial involving 2521 patients (average age 60 years) that compared outcomes after ICD implantation versus amiodarone.[65] An ICD is also indicated as secondary prophylaxis in patients who have previously had life-threatening arrhythmias such as ventricular tachycardia. In the geriatric population, it is extremely important for there to be a goals-of-care discussion between a patient and their provider. A study has shown that approximately 10% of Medicare beneficiaries who receive an ICD have significant frailty or dementia. These patients have a higher 1-year mortality than do patients with similar comorbidities.[66] Overall, patients with less risk factors have been shown to have success similar to that of younger patients with ICDs.[67,68]

# STEM CELL–BASED TREATMENT

There are many etiologies of **heart failure** including myocardial infarction, hypertensive heart disease, as well as nonischemic cardiomyopathy secondary to immune dysregulation, among others. Bone marrow–derived human mesenchymal stem cells (hMSCs) are gaining attention as a possible source of new treatment strategy, with cell-based development of pro-regenerative effect for ventricular architecture. The working theory is that mesenchymal stem cells can enhance angiogenesis, mitigate inflammation, and reduce scarring and fibrosis via immune-modulation and cytoprotective cytokine release.[69] The POSEIDON-DCM trial (Percutaneous Stem Cell Injection Delivery Effects on Neomyogenesis in Dilated Cardiomyopathy) prospectively evaluated the effects of autologous versus allogenic hMSC injection treatments in patients with nonischemic dilated cardiomyopathy.[70] Allogenic hMSC treatment resulted in improved EF, 6-min walk test, and decreased adverse cardiac events. Although the trial was limited, with only 37 patients enrolled, the results are promising and encourage development of larger adequately powered trials to assess this treatment modality.

# CONCLUSIONS/GUIDELINES

**Heart failure** is a clinical syndrome that carries a significant amount of morbidity and mortality. Numerous treatment options are available from the well-established therapeutics (as summarized in Table 13.1) to the more novel agents (summarized in Table 13.2). In general, however, these modalities can be divided into two categories: those that have demonstrated improvements in survival and those that can be used for the management of symptoms. In a mortality benefit, medications such as ACEIs, β-blockers, and aldosterone antagonists have been well established to improve survival in patients with **heart failure** of all ages. With the data found in the PARADIGM-HF trial, ARNi joins the list of agents available for consideration in a mortality benefit. In addition, relief of debilitating symptoms and prevention of hospitalizations are crucial in improving quality of life for patients with **heart failure**. Loop diuretics are important in the control of volume status. Initiation of diuretics should be considered in all patients who develop symptoms of dyspnea, orthopnea, paroxysmal nocturnal dyspnea, and edema. However, even with these symptoms, providers should still be cautious of the risk of dehydration, orthostatic hypotension, and incontinence. **Ivabradine** is a novel agent that is still under consideration as a

**TABLE 13.1 • Established Therapeutics: Current Pharmacologic Options in Treatment of Heart Failure**

| Medication Class | Mechanism of Action | Adult Dosing in Heart Failure | Adverse Reactions |
|---|---|---|---|
| Angiotensin-converting enzyme inhibitor | Prevents the conversion of angiotensin I to angiotensin II<br>Net decrease in vasopressor activity | • Lisinopril—initial 5 mg orally daily; maximum 40 mg daily<br>• Enalapril—initial 2.5 mg orally bid; maximum 20 mg bid<br>• Captopril—initial 25 mg orally tid (can start lower in patients with normal/low blood pressure); maximum 450 mg daily<br>• Ramipril—initial 2.5 mg orally bid; maintenance 5 mg orally bid | • Cardiovascular—chest pain, hypotension, syncope<br>• Neurologic—dizziness, headache<br>• Metabolic-hyperkalemia<br>• Respiratory—cough<br>• Renal—acute renal failure<br>• Other—angioedema |
| Angiotensin II receptor blocker | Specifically intercepts the binding of angiotensin II to the angiotensin I receptor<br>Net decrease in vasopressor activity | • Losartan—initial 25-50 mg orally; daily maximum 150 mg daily<br>• Valsartan—initial 40 mg orally bid; maximum 320 mg orally daily | • Musculoskeletal—backache<br>• Neurologic—dizziness<br>• Renal—acute renal failure |
| β-blockers | Blocks β-adrenergic and in some cases also α-1 adrenergic activity<br>Net decrease in heart rate, cardiac remodeling | • Carvedilol—initial 3.125 mg orally daily; maximum dose patient <85 kg 25 mg bid; Maximum dose patient >85 kg 50 mg orally bid<br>Metoprolol succinate—initial 12.5-25 mg orally daily; maximum 200 mg daily | • Cardiovascular—bradycardia, hypotension<br>• Gastrointestinal—constipation, diarrhea, indigestion, nausea<br>• Neurologic—dizziness, fatigue, headache<br>• Psychiatric—depression<br>• Respiratory—dyspnea, wheezing<br>• Reproductive—erectile dysfunction |
| Aldosterone antagonist | Inhibits the effect of aldosterone by competing for the aldosterone-dependent sodium-potassium exchange site in the distal tubule cells in the kidneys<br>Net increase in water and sodium excretion, decrease in potassium excretion | Spironolactone—initial 25 mg orally daily, conditional: serum potassium <5 mEq/L, serum creatinine <2.5 mg/dL; maximum dose 50 mg once daily[a]<br>• Eplerenone—initial 25 mg orally daily; maximum dose 50 mg orally daily[a] | • Endocrine—gynecomastia<br>• Gastrointestinal—diarrhea, nausea<br>• Metabolic—hyperkalemia<br>• Reproductive—erectile dysfunction |

**TABLE 13.1 • Established Therapeutics: Current Pharmacologic Options in Treatment of Heart Failure (continued)**

| Medication Class | Mechanism of Action | Adult Dosing in Heart Failure | Adverse Reactions |
|---|---|---|---|
| Digoxin | Inhibits sodium–potassium ADENOSINE TRIPHOSPHATase Net increase in intracellular sodium and calcium concentration, resulting in increased contractility, decreased heart rate, smooth muscle relaxation, and vasoconstriction | • For gradual digitalization and/or maintenance dosing—3.4-5.1 µg/kg orally daily[a] | • Cardiovascular—bradycardia<br>• Gastrointestinal—nausea and vomiting<br>• Neurologic—dizziness, headache<br>• Psychiatric—mental disorder |
| Loop diuretics | Blocks the absorption of sodium and chloride in the loop of Henle (proximal and distal tubules), causing a profound increase in urine output | • Furosemide—initial 20-80 mg orally as single dose, may repeat in 6-8 h; titration may increase by 20-40 mg until desired response; may titrate up to 600 mg/d<br>• Torsemide—initial 10-20 mg orally daily; titrate to desired response, maximum dose 200 mg orally once daily<br>• Bumetanide—0.5-2 mg orally, up to q4h; maximum total dose 10 mg daily | • Metabolic—hyperuricemia, hypomagnesemia, hypokalemia<br>• Gastrointestinal—loss of appetite<br>• Renal—bladder spasm |
| Vasodilators—nitrates | Relaxes vascular smooth muscle, resulting in dilation of peripheral arteries and veins | • Isosorbide dinitrate—30-160 mg/d orally in divided doses; maximum 240 mg/d | • Cardiovascular—hypotension<br>• Neurologic—headache, light headedness |
| Vasodilators—hydralazine | Mechanism is mostly unknown. It appears to decrease blood pressure by exhibiting a peripheral-vasodilating effect through a direct relaxation of vascular smooth muscle. | 200-300 mg orally daily in two to three divided doses | • Cardiovascular—angina, edema, palpitations, tachycardia<br>• Gastrointestinal—diarrhea, loss of appetite, nausea/vomiting<br>• Neurologic—headache |

[a]Beers Criteria – use with caution in older adults.
Abbreviations: bid, twice a day; tid, thrice a day.
Opie LH, Gersh BJ. *Drugs for the Heart.* Rochester, MN: Elsevier; 2013.

**TABLE 13.2** • Therapeutic Advances: New Pharmacological Options in Treatment of Heart Failure

| Medication | Mechanism of Action | Adult Dosing in Heart Failure | Adverse Reactions |
|---|---|---|---|
| Angiotensin II receptor blocker + neprilysin inhibitor—valsartan/sacubitril | Valsartan—see ARB mechanism of action Sacubitril—inhibits neprilysin, thereby increasing levels of natriuretic peptides Net vasodilation and suppression of renin-angiotensin system | • If not previously taking ACE-I or ARB, sacubitril/valsartan 24 mg/26 mg orally bid • If switching from ACE-I or ARB, 49 mg/51 mg orally bid • Maintenance dose is 97 mg/103 mg bid. | • Cardiovascular—hypotension • Metabolic—hyperkalemia • Neurologic—dizziness • Renal—renal failure |
| Ivabradine | Reduces spontaneous pacemaker activity at the cardiac sinus by blocking the hyperpolarization-activated cyclic nucleotide-gated channel to selectively inhibit If current, thus reducing the heart rate. | • Initial 5 mg orally bid; dose increased as heart rate tolerates • Maximum dose 7.5 mg orally twice daily | • Cardiovascular—atrial fibrillation, bradycardia |
| Nesiritide | Recombinant form of brain natriuretic peptide, increases intracellular cyclic GUANOSINE MONOPHOSPHATE and smooth muscle relaxation by binding to the particulate guanylate cyclase receptor of vascular smooth muscle and endothelial cells Net vasodilation | • In acute heart failure, 2 µg/kg IV bolus followed by 0.01 µg/kg/min continuous IV infusion • For titration, may increase by 0.005 µg/kg/min no more frequently than every 3 h up to a maximum dose of 0.03 µg/kg/min | • Cardiovascular – hypotension • Gastrointestinal – nausea • Neurologic—dizziness, headache • Renal—increased serum creatinine |

Abbreviations: ACE-I, angiotensin-converting enzyme inhibitor; ARB, angiotensin receptor blocker; bid, twice a day; IV, intravenous.

Yancy CW, Jessup M, Bozkurt B, et al. 2017 ACC/AHA/HFSA focused update on new pharmacological therapy for heart failure: an update of the 2013 ACCF/AHA Guideline for the Management of Heart Failure: a report of the American College of Cardiology/American Heart Association Task Force on Clinical Practice Guidelines and the Heart Failure Society of America. *J Am Coll Cardiol.* 2017;70(6):776-803; Coons JC, Mcgraw M, Murali S. Pharmacotherapy for acute heart failure syndromes. *Am J Health Syst Pharm.* 2010;68:21-35.

second line for symptomatic management. Finally, devices such as the CardioMEMS have been shown to allow patients and their physicians to keep volume status under control and prevent hospitalizations. Implantable devices such as ICD and LVAD can improve mortality in advanced **heart failure**, but their implementation should be considered on an individual basis.

# SUMMARY

**Heart failure** is a clinical syndrome that carries a significant burden of morbidity and is associated with poor long-term prognosis. Treatment of **heart failure** is constantly evolving, with large amounts of research going into the development of new medications, in the hope of improving symptom management as well as reducing morbidity and mortality.

One of the major areas of uncertainty regarding recent advances in **heart failure** management is the applicability of data from existing trials to the geriatric population. The majority of current research focuses on patients in a younger age group with a median age around 60, and there is a lack of randomized control trials assessing efficacy in the geriatric population specifically.

This chapter describes the mechanism of action and evidence for the established medications recommended for mortality benefit, including angiotensin receptor inhibitors, β-blockers, and aldosterone antagonists, and now adds a new medication to the list, **sacubitril/valsartan**. In addition, the chapter describes the medications used for symptomatic improvement and decrease in hospitalization including digoxin, diuretics, and vasodilators, and adding **ivabradine** as a new medication. Studies and guidelines for **nesiritide** as well as nonpharmacologic options such as ventricular assist devices, pulmonary pressure monitoring devices, and implantable defibrillators are also included.

As the population of the United States continues to age, the number of patients with **heart failure** will continue to rise. Understanding the wide range of treatment options available to elderly patients is increasingly important for clinicians. Determining whether any of the new therapeutic options is appropriate for a patient will be a collaborative effort between a clinician and patient and will depend heavily on the patient's comorbidities, functional status, and goals of care.

## References

1. Yancy CW, Jessup M, Bozkurt B, et al. 2013 ACCF/AHA guideline for the management of heart failure. *J Am Coll Cardiol.* 2013;62:e147-e239.
2. Cowie MR, Anker SD, Cleland JGF, et al. Improving care for patients with acute heart failure: before, during and after hospitalization. *ESC Heart Fail.* 2014;1:110-145.
3. Richards AM. The renin-angiotensin-aldosterone system and the cardiac natriuretic peptides. *Heart.* 1996;76:36-44.
4. Garg R, Yusuf S; for the Collaborative Group on ACE Inhibitor Trials. Overview of randomized trials of angiotensin-converting enzyme inhibitors on mortality and morbidity in patients with heart failure. *JAMA.* 1995;273:1450-1456.
5. Flather MD, Yusuf S, Køber L, et al. Long-term ACE inhibitor therapy in patients with heart failure or left ventricular dysfunction: a systematic overview of data from individual patients. *Lancet.* 2000;355:1575-1581.
6. American Geriatrics Society 2015 Beers Criteria Update Expert Panel. American Geriatrics Society 2015 updated Beers criteria for potentially inappropriate medication use in older adults. *J Am Geriatr Soc.* 2015;63:2227-2246.

7. Pitt B, Segal R, Martinez FA, et al. Randomised trial of losartan versus captopril in patients over 65 with heart failure (Evaluation of Losartan in the Elderly Study, ELITE). *Lancet.* 1997;349:747-752.

8. Pitt B, Poole-Wilson PA, Segal R, et al. Effect of losartan compared with captopril on mortality in patients with symptomatic heart failure: randomized trial: the Losartan Heart Failure Survival Study ELITE II. *Lancet.* 2000;355:1582-1587.

9. CONSENSUS Trial Study Group. Effects of enalapril on mortality in severe congestive heart failure: results of the Cooperative North Scandinavian Enalapril Survival Study (CONSENSUS). *N Engl J Med.* 1987;316:1429-1435.

10. SOLVD Investigators. Effect of enalapril on survival in patients with reduced left ventricular ejection fractions and congestive heart failure. *N Engl J Med.* 1991;325:293-302.

11. Cleland JG, Tendera M, Adamus J, et al. The perindopril in elderly people with chronic heart failure (PEP-CHF) study. *Eur Heart J.* 2006;27:2338-2345.

12. Yusuf S, Pfeffer MA, Swedberg K, et al. Effects of candesartan in patients with chronic heart failure and preserved left-ventricular ejection fraction: the CHARM-Preserved Trial. *Lancet.* 2003;362:777-781.

13. Massie BM, Carson PE, McMurray JJ, et al. Irbesartan in patients with heart failure and preserved ejection fraction. *N Engl J Med.* 2008;359:2456-2467.

14. Yusuf S, Sleight P, Pogue J, et al. Effects of an angiotensin-converting-enzyme inhibitor, ramipril, on cardiovascular events in high-risk patients. *N Engl J Med.* 2000;342:145-153.

15. Dahlöf B, Devereux RB, Kjeldsen SE, et al. Cardiovascular morbidity and mortality in the Losartan Intervention for Endpoint reduction in hypertension study (LIFE): a randomized trial against atenolol. *Lancet.* 2002;359:995-1003.

16. Rich MW. Drug therapy of heart failure in the elderly. *Am J Geriatr Cardiol.* 2003;12:235-242.

17. Schumann S, Hickner J. When not to use beta-blockers in seniors with hypertension. *J Fam Pract.* 2008;57:18-21.

18. Aronow WS, Ahn C, Kronzon I. Effect of propranolol versus no propranolol on total mortality plus nonfatal myocardial infarction in older patients with prior myocardial infarction, congestive heart failure, and left ventricular ejection fraction $\geq$40% treated with diuretics plus angiotensin-converting enzyme inhibitors. *Am J Cardiol.* 1997;80:207-209.

19. Lund L, Benson L, Dahlstrom U, et al. Association between use of $\beta$-blockers and outcomes in patients with heart failure and preserved ejection fraction. *JAMA.* 2014;312:2008-2018.

20. Cheng S, Pfeffer MA. Searching for treatments of heart failure with preserved ejection fraction. *JAMA.* 2014;312:1977-1978.

21. Pitt B, Zannad F, Remme WJ, et al; for the Randomized Aldactone Evaluation Study Investigators. The effect of spironolactone on morbidity and mortality in patients with severe heart failure. *N Engl J Med.* 1999;341:709-717.

22. Juurlink DN, Mamdani MM, Lee DS, et al. Rates of hyperkalemia after publication of the randomized Aldactone Evaluation Study. *N Engl J Med.* 2004;351:543-551.

23. Digitalis Investigation Group. The effect of digoxin on mortality and morbidity in patients with heart failure. *N Engl J Med.* 1997;336:525-533.

24. Rich MW, McSherry F, Williford WO, et al. Effect of age on mortality, hospitalizations, and response to digoxin in patients with heart failure: the DIG Study. *J Am Coll Cardiol.* 2001;38:806-813.

25. Ware JA, Snow E, Luchi JM, et al. Effect of digoxin on ejection fraction in elderly patients with congestive heart failure. *J Am Geriatr Soc.* 1984;32:631-635.

26. Currie GM, Wheat JM, Hosen K. Pharmacokinetic considerations for digoxin in older people. *Open Cardiovasc Med J.* 2011;5:130-135.

27. Cohn JN, Johnson G, Ziesche S, et al. A comparison of enalapril with hydralazine-isosorbide dinitrate in the treatment of chronic congestive heart failure. *N Engl J Med.* 1991; 325:303-310.

28. Cohn JN, Archibald DG, Ziesche S, et al. Effect of vasodilator therapy on mortality in chronic congestive heart failure. Results of a Veterans Administration Cooperative Study. *N Engl J Med.* 1986;314:1547-1452.

29. Jessup M, Brozena S. Heart failure. *N Engl J Med.* 2003;348:2007-2018.

30. Sacks C, Jarcho J, Curfman G. Paradigm shifts in heart failure therapy—a timeline. *N Engl J Med.* 2014;371:989-991.

31. Adams KF, Fonarow GC, Emerman CL, et al. Characteristics and outcomes of patients hospitalized for heart failure in the United States: rationale, design and preliminary observations from the first 100,000 cases in the Acute Decompensated Heart Failure National Registry (ADHERE). *Am Heart J.* 2005;149:209-216.

32. Ponikowski P, Voors A, Anker, SD, et al. 2016 ESC Guidelines for the diagnosis and treatment of acute and chronic heart failure. *Eur Heart J.* 2016;37:2129-2200.

33. Ahmad T, Fiuzat M, Pencina M, et al. Charting a roadmap for heart failure biomarker studies. *J Am Coll Cardiol HF.* 2014;2:477-487.

34. Roger V. Epidemiology of heart failure. *Circ Res.* 2013;113:646-659.

35. Feltner C, Jones C, Cene C, et al. Transitional care interventions to prevent readmissions for persons with heart failure. *Ann Intern Med.* 2014;160:774-784.

36. Yancy CW, Jessup M, Bozkurt B, et al. 2017 ACC/AHA/HFSA focused update on new pharmacological therapy for heart failure: an update of the 2013 ACCF/AHA Guideline for the Management of Heart Failure: a report of the American College of Cardiology/American Heart Association Task Force on Clinical Practice Guidelines and the Heart Failure Society of America. *J Am Coll Cardiol.* 2017;70(6):776-803.

37. Potter LR, Abbey-Hosch S, Dickey DM. Natriuretic peptides, their receptors, and cyclic guanosine monophosphate-dependent signaling functions. *Endocr Rev.* 2006;27:47-72.

38. Levin ER, Gardner DG, Samson WK. Natriuretic peptides. *N Engl J Med.* 1998;339:321-328.

39. McDowell G, Nicholls DP. The therapeutic potential of candoxatril, a neutral endopeptidase inhibitor, in humans. *Cardiovasc Drug Rev.* 2000;18:259-270.

40. Packer M, Califf RM, Konstam MA, et al. Comparison of omapatrilat and enalapril in patients with chronic heart failure: the Omapatrilat Versus Enalapril Randomized Trial of Utility in Reducing Events (OVERTURE). *Circulation.* 2002;106:920-926.

41. Gu J, Noe A, Chandra P, et al. Pharmacokinetics and pharmacodynamics of LCZ696, a novel dual-acting Angiotensin Receptor-Neprilysin Inhibitor (ARNi). *J Clinc Pharmacol.* 2010;50:401-414.

42. McMurray JJ, Packer M, Desai AS, et al. Dual angiotensin receptor and neprilysin inhibition as an alternative to angiotensin-converting enzyme inhibition in patients with chronic systolic heart failure: rationale for and design of the Prospective comparison of ARNI with ACEI to Determine Impact on Global Mortality and morbidity in Heart Failure trial (PARADIGM-HF). *Eur J Heart Fail.* 2013;15:1062-1073.

43. McMurray JJ, Packer M, Desai AS, et al; PARADIGM-HF Committees and Investigators. Angiotensin-neprilysin inhibition versus enalapril in heart failure. *N Engl J Med.* 2014;371:993-1004.

44. Swedberg K, Komajda M, Böhm M, et al; SHIFT Trial investigators. Ivabradine and outcomes in chronic heart failure (SHIFT): a randomized placebo controlled study. *Lancet.* 2010;376(9744):875-885.

45. Zile MR, Claggett BL, Prescott MF, et al. Prognostic implications of changes in n-terminal pro-b-type natriuretic peptide in patients with heart failure. *J Am Col Card.* 2016;68:2425-2436.

46. DiFrancesco D, Camm JA. Heart rate lowering by specific and selective I(f) current inhibition with ivabradine: a new therapeutic perspective in cardiovascular disease. *Drugs.* 2004;64:1757-1765.

47. Fox K, Ford I, Steg PG, et al. Ivabradine for patients with stable coronary artery disease and left-ventricular systolic dysfunction (BEAUTIFUL): a randomized, double-blind, placebo-controlled trial. *Lancet.* 2008;372:807-816.

48. Fox K, Ford I, Steg PG, et al; SIGNIFY Investigators. Ivabradine in stable coronary artery disease without clinical heart failure. *N Engl J Med.* 2014;371:1091-1099.

49. Martin RI, Pogoryelova O, Koref MS, et al. Atrial fibrillation associated with ivabradine treatment: meta-analysis of randomized controlled trials. *Heart.* 2014;100:1506-1510.

50. Werdan K, Ebelt H, Nuding S, et al. Ivabradine in combination with beta-blocker improves symptoms and quality of life in patients with stable angina pectoris: results from the ADDITIONS study. *Clin Res Cardiol.* 2012;101:365-373.

51. Ekman I, Chassany O, Komajda M, et al. Heart rate reduction with ivabradine and health related quality of life in patients with chronic heart failure: results from the SHIFT study. *Eur Heart J.* 2011;32:2395-2404.

52. Colucci WS, Eikayam U, Horton DP, et al. Intravenous nesiritide, a natriuretic peptide, in the treatment of decompensated congestive heart failure. *N Engl J Med*. 2000;343:246-253.

53. Publication Committee for the VMAC Investigators. Intravenous nesiritide vs nitroglycerine for treatment of decompensated congestive heart failure a randomized controlled trial. *JAMA*. 2002;287:1531-1540.

54. O'Connor CM, Starling RC, Hernandez AF, et al. Effect of nesiritide in patients with acute decompensated heart failure. *N Engl J Med*. 2011;365:32-43.

55. Wang DJ, Dowling TC, Meadows D, et al. Nesiritide does not improve renal function in patients with chronic heart failure and worsening serum creatinine. *Circulation*. 2004;110:1620-1625.

56. Slaughter MS, Rogers JG, Milano CA, et al. Advanced heart failure treated with continuous-flow left ventricular assist device. *N Engl J Med*. 2009;361:2241-2251.

57. Rose EA, Gelijns AC, Moskowitz AJ, et al. Long-term use of a left ventricular assist device for end-stage heart failure. *N Engl J Med*. 2001;345:1435-1443.

58. Rosenbaum AN, John R, Liao KK, et al. Survival in elderly patients supported with continuous flow left ventricular assist device as bridge to transplantation or destination therapy. *J Card Fail*. 2014;20:161-167.

59. Capoccia M. Mechanical circulatory support for advanced heart failure. Are we about to witness a new "Gold Standard?" *J Cardiovasc Dev Dis*. 2016;3(4):35.

60. Mehra MR, Naka Y, Uriel N, et al. A fully magnetically levitated circulatory pump for advanced heart failure. *N Engl J Med*. 2017;376(5):440-450.

61. Urien N, Colombo PC, Clevelend JC, et al. Hemocompatibility-related outcomes in the MOMENTUM 3 trial at 6 months: a randomized controlled study of a fully magnetically levitated pump in advanced heart failure. *Circulation*. 2017;135(21):2003-2012.

62. Abraham WT, Adamson PB, Bourge RC, et al. Wireless pulmonary artery hemodynamic monitoring in chronic heart failure: a randomized controlled trial. *Lancet*. 2011;377:658-666.

63. Abraham WT, Stevenson LW, Bourge RC, et al. Sustained efficacy of pulmonary artery pressure to guide adjustment of chronic heart failure therapy: complete follow-up results from the CHAMPION randomized trial. *Lancet*. 2016;387:453-461.

64. Adamson PB, Abraham WT, Stevenson LW, et al. Pulmonary artery pressure–Guided heart failure management reduces 30-day readmissions. *Circ Heart Fail*. 2016;9;e002600.

65. Bardy GH, Lee KL, Mark DB, et al. Amiodarone or an implantable cardioverter–defibrillator for congestive heart failure. *N Engl J Med*. 2005;352:225-237.

66. Green AR, Leff B, Wang Y, et al. Geriatric conditions in patients undergoing defibrillator implantation for prevention of sudden cardiac death. *Circ Cardiovasc Qual Outcomes*. 2015;9:23-30.

67. Rees JBV, Borleffs CJW, Thijssen J, et al. Prophylactic implantable cardioverter-defibrillator treatment in the elderly: therapy, adverse events, and survival gain. *Europace*. 2011;14:66-73.

68. Barra S, Providencia R, Paiva L, et al. Implantable cardioverter-defibrillators in the elderly: rationale and specific age-related considerations. *Europace*. 2014;17:174-186.

69. Pandey AC, Lancaster JJ, Harris DT, Goldman S, Juneman E. Cellular therapeutics for heart failure: focus on mesenchymal stem cells. *Stem Cells Int*. 2017;2017:9640108.

70. Hare JM, DiFede DL, Rieger AC, et al. Randomized comparison of allogeneic versus autologous mesenchymal stem cells for nonischemic dilated cardiomyopathy: POSEIDON-DCM trial. *J Am Coll Cardiol*. 2017;69(5):526-537.

# Therapeutic Approaches to Secondary Fracture Prevention in High-Risk Populations: Current Recommendations and Advances

Huei-Wen Lim, MD, Melissa Chamblain, MD, Benny Wong, MD, and Siddharth Raghavan, MD

## BACKGROUND

**Osteoporosis** is the most common bone disease in humans, affecting approximately 10 million Americans as per data from the National Health and Nutrition Examination Survey (NHANES III).[1] Another 43 million individuals are at risk for fracture because of low bone mass, with 1.5 million fractures being attributed to **osteoporosis** annually in the United States.[2] In their lifetimes, 30% to 50% of women and 15% to 30% of men will suffer from a fragility fracture accounting for 432 000 hospital admissions, 2.5 million medical office visits, and an annual healthcare expenditure of approximately US$15 billion.[2,3] Because a history of fracture is a strong risk factor for future fractures, appropriate outpatient follow-up and effective interventions to improve **osteoporosis** care are needed in this at-risk patient population.

In 1999, the National Osteoporosis Foundation (NOF) first published a guide for the management of **osteoporosis** and postfracture care.[4] Since then, it has become increasingly evident that many patients are not being diagnosed with **osteoporosis** after fragility fractures and are not receiving any of the U.S. Food and Drug Administration (FDA)–approved, effective therapies. After this initial guide, the Joint Commission in 2008 and Physician Quality Reporting System (PQRS) for the Centers for Medicare and Medicaid Services (CMS) in 2014 further developed evidence-based, consensus-driven performance measures after low-trauma or fragility fractures.[5,6]

Performance measures guiding postfracture care include the following:

1. Bone mineral density (BMD) or equivalent testing (eg, Fracture Risk Assessment Tool [FRAX] score) in postmenopausal women and men aged 50 years and older to diagnose and determine the degree of **osteoporosis** within 3 months of recognition of fracture.

2. Initiation of FDA-approved pharmacotherapy for **osteoporosis** in postmenopausal women and men aged 50 and older within 3 months of recognition of fracture.

Despite the availability of therapy, low rates of treatment after fragility fractures have been detected. A cross-sectional study ($N = 60$) in Connecticut depicted that only 13% of women above the age of 65 with nontraumatic hip fractures received adequate treatment for **osteoporosis**, whereas 40% received no treatment and 47% received partial treatment depending on the NOF guidelines.[7] The National Committee for Quality Assistance estimated that in 2015, 23% of women above the age of 65 who had **osteoporosis** and related fractures were not offered a BMD test or treatment in the 6 months after a fracture.[4,8] The underdiagnosis of **osteoporosis** after fragility fractures has resulted in increased risk of secondary fractures, higher costs, and increased morbidity and mortality. We aim to demonstrate the importance of **secondary fracture prevention** after initial fragility fracture by systematically reviewing current and novel therapeutic agents for **osteoporosis**.

# AREAS OF UNCERTAINTY

**Osteoporosis** is defined on the basis of T-scores generated by DEXA (dual-energy X-ray absorptiometry) scans assessing BMD at the femoral neck and lumbar spine. T-scores represent standard deviations from the mean value expected in young healthy adults. A score of 22.5 or more defines **osteoporosis**. An estimated fracture risk can be obtained with a FRAX score. FRAX is a computer-based algorithm that can estimate a 10-year probability of a major fracture (hip, spine, humerus, or wrist fracture) or a hip fracture. Treatment is recommended when the risk of a major osteoporotic fracture is ≥20% or the risk of a hip fracture is ≥3%. A cross-sectional review of screening tools demonstrated that the FRAX alone may be as effective as DEXA or DEXA combined with FRAX, especially in the younger age population.[9] Despite the effectiveness of screening tools, they are not readily used in the community.

In patients with a hip or spine fracture, the T-score is not as important as the fracture itself in predicting future risk of fracture. Fragility fractures (ie, low-trauma fracture occurring spontaneously or from a fall no higher than standing height) in someone older than 45 years should raise suspicion of **osteoporosis**. Vertebral fractures may present as backache, height loss, spinal deformity, or incidental radiologic findings. Although most fractures present clinically, two-thirds may be asymptomatic.[10] Untreated **osteoporosis** leads to an even higher risk of future fragility fractures. Studies have shown that sustaining a wrist fracture increases the risk of further fractures by 2-fold.[11,12] Previous nonhip fractures have been identified in around half of the women admitted with hip fractures.[12,13]

The underdiagnosis of **osteoporosis** after fragility fractures may be attributed to a variety of factors including loss of follow-up, lack of patient awareness of the diagnosis, and neglecting to identify the disease after minor trauma fractures. Interventions aimed at coordinating the care between hospitals and outpatient clinics have the potential to decrease the rates of patients lost to follow-up.

Fracture liaison services (FLSs) are coordinator-based services that use clinical nurses as case managers to enhance communication between the patient, the inpatient provider, and the primary care provider. FLSS have been proved to be the most effective nonpharmacologic intervention method in **secondary fracture prevention**.[14] In the most intensive service model that includes the identification, assessment, and treatment of selected patients, the risk of future fractures and mortality associated with fragility fractures was significantly reduced (hazard ratio [HR] 0.18-0.67 over 2-4 years and HR 0.65 over 2 years, respectively). Adherence to treatment (65%-88% at 1 year) and cost-effective care were also centerpieces of such an FLS model.[12] In a randomized controlled study ($N = 220$) in Alberta, Canada, assessing the use of a case manager to improve **osteoporosis** treatment after a hip fracture in the elderly, the intervention group was almost five times as likely to receive bisphosphonate therapy than the control group (22%) (odds ratio = 4.7; 95% confidence interval [CI], 2.4-8.9; $P < 0.001$).[15]

Successful **secondary fracture prevention** measures can be limited by patient-related factors such as medical nonadherence. Nonetheless, the evidence clearly supports that secondary fractures can be significantly prevented by appropriate management. However, the decision to treat the geriatric population with decreased functional status and/or multiple comorbidities oftentimes remains debatable. In a study composed of U.S. Medicare beneficiaries from 1999 to 2008 with a fragility fracture occurring in 2000 or 2001, the risk of death after a 5-year period almost exceeded the risk of a subsequent fracture.[17] Subgroup analyses were performed depending on the type of fracture, age, and demographics. The risk difference was noted to be higher in men and African Americans of both sexes compared with that in women. In the extreme subgroup analysis, individuals aged 85 and older with dementia who experienced a hip fracture were found to have a 7-fold greater risk of death (81%) than subsequent fractures (12%).[16] It is unclear if some underwent surgical fixation of the hip. Surgical fixation of a hip fracture significantly reduces complications and risk of death and perhaps could have significantly modified the results of this study.

It is important to consider reduced life expectancy when considering treatment in patients with a high mortality index. Thus, a patient should be expected to live for at least 6 months to justify the use of therapeutic agents. Irrespective of age and comorbidities, the risk of a subsequent fracture at the same site or another site remains substantially high despite the similarly high risk of death. Moreover, the NOF recommends treatment for all persons with a hip or vertebral fracture regardless of BMD or 10-year fracture risk. The clinician should assess the potential benefits versus risks of therapy in each patient and the effectiveness of any given treatment in reducing further fragility fractures.

Initiation of treatment in the hospital may be paramount to improve **osteoporosis** management. However, intravenous (IV) bisphosphonate infusion given within 2 weeks of an acute hip fracture may not be beneficial to prevent secondary fracture.[17] Animal studies suggest that zoledronic acid is deposited at the site of the acute fracture if given within 2 weeks, leaving the rest of the body unprotected. Alternatively, some models suggest that oral bisphosphonates can be initiated in the hospital and later switched to IV treatment at a follow-up visit.[17]

## FDA-Approved Drugs for Osteoporosis

Current FDA-approved pharmacologic treatment for the prevention of future fractures include bisphosphonates, receptor activator of nuclear factor kappa-B (RANK) ligand inhibitor (denosumab), hormonal receptor therapy, calcitonin, and selective estrogen replacement modulators (SERMs) such as raloxifene and parathyroid hormone (teriparatide).

Their efficacy has been mostly studied in postmenopausal women with **osteoporosis**, who have had fragility fractures and/or **osteoporosis** identified on DXA. There is limited data on the efficacy of these FDA-approved drugs in men 50 years and older and in steroid-induced **osteoporosis**.

# THERAPEUTIC ADVANCES

## Bisphosphonates

Bisphosphonates have long been considered first-line therapy for secondary prevention of vertebral fragility fractures in older patients because of their efficacy, relative cost, and the availability of long-term safety data. Randomized controlled trials (RCTs) of postmenopausal women with **osteoporosis** with existing fractures demonstrate a relative risk reduction (RRR) compared with placebo for alendronate of 45% (relative risk [RR] 0.55, 95% CI, 0.43-0.69),[18] 39% for daily risedronate (RR = 0.61, 95% CI, 0.50-0.76),[19] 48% to 49% for oral ibandronate ($P = 0.012$ for 2.5 mg and $P = 0.014$ for 20 mg),[20] and 70% for IV zoledronic acid (RR = 0.30, 95% CI, 0.24-0.38).[21] Bisphosphonates also reduce nonvertebral fractures by 23% for alendronate (RR = 0.77, 95% CI, 0.64-0.92),[18] 20% for risedronate (RR = 0.80, 95% CI, 0.72-0.90),[19] and 25% for IV zoledronic acid (RR = 0.75, 95% CI, 0.64-0.87)[21] compared with placebo. For hip fractures, RRR for alendronate, risedronate, and IV zoledronic acid compared with placebo were 53% (RR = 0.47, 95% CI, 0.26-0.85),[18] 26% (RR = 0.74, 95% CI, 0.59-0.94),[19] and 41% (RR = 0.59, 95% CI, 0.42-0.83),[21] respectively. A randomized trial ($N = 2027$) evaluated women with low femoral neck BMD with at least one vertebral fracture from population-based listings in 11 metropolitan areas in the United States and found that women in the alendronate group had less new morphometric vertebral fractures (8% vs 15%, RR = 0.53, 95% CI, 0.41-0.68) and less clinically apparent vertebral fractures (2.3% vs 5.0%, RR = 0.45, 95% CI, 0.27-0.72) compared with the placebo group.[22] In another meta-analysis of four randomized studies, two of which recruited women with low BMD and one to four clinically significant vertebral fractures, high-dose ibandronate (150 mg once a month and 3 mg quarterly IV injection) was associated with a significant reduction in nonvertebral fragility fractures (RRR = 0.34, $P$ = 0.032).[23] The efficacy and safety profile of bisphosphonates in treatment for preventing secondary fragility fractures has been well studied in numerous other trials.[24-26]

Current bisphosphonates indicated for the treatment of **osteoporosis** include alendronate, risedronate, ibandronate, and zoledronic acid and may be given orally on a daily, weekly, or monthly basis or IV every 3 months or once yearly.[4,27,28]

Oral bisphosphonates should not be used in patients with esophageal disorder or an inability to follow the dosing requirements (Table 14.1).[4,27,28] Esophageal ulceration

**TABLE 14.1  •  Overview of Medications for Treatment of Osteoporosis and Prevention of Secondary Fragility Fractures**

| Drug | Vertebral Fracture | Nonvertebral Fracture | Hip Fracture | Bone Mineral Density Increase | Dosing | Route | Adverse Events |
|---|---|---|---|---|---|---|---|
| Biphosphonate Alendronate | Yes | Yes | Yes | Yes | 10 mg once daily or 70 mg once weekly | Oral | Dyspepsia, abdominal pain, musculoskeletal pain |
| Ibandronate | Yes | Yes | | Yes | Oral: 2.5 mg once daily or 150 mg once a month IV: 3 mg every 3 mo | Oral, IV | Dyspepsia, back pain, musculoskeletal pain, headache, abdominal pain |
| Risedronate | Yes | Yes | Yes | | Immediate release: 5 mg once daily or 35 mg once weekly or 150 mg once a month Delayed release: 35 mg once weekly | Oral | Rash, abdominal pain, dyspepsia, diarrhea, arthralgia |

*(continued)*

**TABLE 14.1 • Overview of Medications for Treatment of Osteoporosis and Prevention of Secondary Fragility Fractures (*continued*)**

| Drug | Vertebral Fracture | Nonvertebral Fracture | Hip Fracture | Bone Mineral Density Increase | Dosing | Route | Adverse Events |
|---|---|---|---|---|---|---|---|
| Zoledronic acid | Yes | Yes | Yes | Yes | 5 mg once a year | IV | Acute reaction (flulike symptoms, fever, myalgia) may occur within 3 d of infusion; hypotension, fatigue, eye inflammation, nausea, vomiting, abdominal pain |
| Monoclonal antibody Denosumab | Yes | Yes | Yes | Yes | 60 mg every 6 mo | SC | Dermatitis, rash, mild bone/muscle pain, urinary tract infections |
| Hormonal therapy Estrogen only, progestin only, combination estrogen/progestin | Yes | Yes | Yes | Yes | Continuous daily or cyclical | Oral, transdermal | Coronary heart disease, VTE, stroke |
| Selective estrogen replacement modulators Raloxifene | Yes | | | Yes | 60 mg once daily | Oral | VTE, arthralgia, leg cramps, flu syndrome, peripheral edema, hot flashes |
| Calcitonin | Yes | | | Yes | 200 IU in 1 nostril daily alternating each day or 100 IU every day; Injectable formulations available | | Rhinitis, nasal irritation, dizziness, nasal dryness, injection site reactions, nausea, vomiting, abdominal cramping, flushing |
| Parathyroid hormone analog Teriparatide | Yes | Yes | | Yes | 20 mg once daily | Subcutaneous | Transient hypercalcemia, nausea, rhinitis, arthralgia, pain |

Abbreviations: IV, intravenous; VTE, venous thromboembolism.

has been reported in multiple trials for oral bisphosphonates, although this has not been found in IV forms of the medication.[18,19,27,28] An acute-phase reaction (myalgia, fever, flulike symptoms) has been reported in both oral and IV formulations.[4,27,28] In an international, multicenter, randomized, double-blind study ($N$ = 3862) of once-yearly zoledronic acid for treatment of postmenopausal **osteoporosis**, 16.1% of the studied population experience pyrexia, 9.5% had myalgia, and 7.8% had flulike symptoms ($P < 0.001$).[21] Several articles also demonstrated an association between bisphosphonate and atypical femur fractures secondary to oversuppression of bone turnover.[4,28-30] A recent cohort study in California ($N$ = 1 835 116) suggested the incidence of atypical fracture to be 1.78 out of 100 000 persons per year (95% CI, 1.5-2.0) with exposure to bisphosphonates from 0.1 to 0.9 years. The incidence increased to 113.1 of 100 000 persons per year (95% CI, 69.3-156.8) with exposure to a bisphosphonate from 8 to 9.9 years.[30] Other reported adverse effects include osteonecrosis of the jaw, although it is much more common with high-dose IV bisphosphonate use in patients with malignancy than in patients receiving low doses of oral and IV bisphosphonate.[4,27,28,31] Both oral and IV bisphosphonates should be avoided in patients with chronic kidney disease (estimated glomerular filtration rate, 30 mL/min), which is of particular concern in the elderly population with fragility fracture.[4,27] Receptor activator of nuclear factor-κB ligand inhibitor (RANKL): denosumab.

Denosumab is a fully humanized monoclonal antibody that inhibits maturation of osteoclasts by binding to and inhibiting RANKL, thus inhibiting bone resorption.[28] It is approved by the FDA for the treatment of **osteoporosis** in postmenopausal women at high risk for fracture. In a 3-year, international, randomized, phase III study named Fracture Reduction Evaluation of Denosumab in Osteoporosis Every 6 Months (FREEDOM trial) ($N$ = 7688) conducted in women who had a BMD T-score of 22.5 to 24.0, approximately 23% of the population had at least one clinically significant vertebral fracture at the time of entry into the study. Compared with placebo, denosumab significantly decreases the risk of new vertebral fracture by 68% (HR = 0.32, 95% CI, 0.26-0.41), hip fracture by 40% (HR = 0.60, 95% CI, 0.37-0.97), and nonvertebral fracture by 20% (HR = 0.80, 95% CI, 0.67-0.95) without an increased risk of cancer, major cardiovascular events, hypocalcemia, or delayed fracture healing.[32] After 5 years of follow-up in the extension of the FREEDOM trial and in several other trials, denosumab has been shown to improve BMD and reduce bone turnover.[33,34] A phase III, multicenter, double-blind study ($N$ = 1189) conducted comparing denosumab to alendronate has shown that BMD gains were significantly higher with denosumab (12-month treatment difference: 0.6%, femoral neck; 1.0%, trochanter; 1.1%, lumbar spine; 0.6%, one-third radius; $P \leq 0.0002$ all sites), with greater reductions in biochemical markers of bone turnover (C-telopeptide and serum procollagen type 1 N-terminal propeptide) in the denosumab group compared with alendronate (89% vs 61% at month 1, 89% vs 66% at month 3, 77% vs 73% at month 6, $P < 0.0001$).[35] To date, several other studies have shown the efficacy of denosumab for the treatment of **osteoporosis**.[36,37] However, denosumab has not been shown to be superior to other **osteoporosis** drugs in reducing fractures because there are currently no head-to-head trials comparing efficacy.

Denosumab is dosed subcutaneously every 6 months and does not require dose adjustments for chronic kidney disease. Calcium level should be checked within 10 days of receiving denosumab in patients with chronic kidney disease or other conditions that may predispose them to hypocalcemia.[4,38]

Denosumab is generally well tolerated, but its use has been associated with severe skin reactions and cellulitis in the FREEDOM trial.[4,32] There is no evidence of increased overall risk of malignancies, major cardiovascular events, or delayed fracture healing.[32] Most common side effects reported were musculoskeletal pain, cystitis, and hypercholesterolemia.[38] Denosumab has been rarely associated with osteonecrosis of the jaw and atypical fractures.[4,38-40] In the extension of the FREEDOM trial, eight occurrences of osteonecrosis of the jaw and two occurrences of atypical fracture were confirmed; but incidence did not increase over time.[34]

## Hormone Therapy

Although the FDA approves estrogen/hormone replacement therapy (HRT) for prevention and not treatment of **osteoporosis**, data have shown that it is also effective in women with established **osteoporosis** and vertebral fractures.[4,28] In a double-blind, randomized clinical trial ($N = 75$) conducted in patients with more than one vertebral fracture due to **osteoporosis** in an outpatient clinic, there was a steady increase in BMD at the spine (5.3 vs 0.2, $P = 0.007$) and proximal femur (7.6 vs 2.1, $P = 0.03$) in the estrogen group compared with that in placebo, and reduction in vertebral fracture rate (RR = 0.39, 95% CI, 0.16-0.95).[41] In another 4-year prospective randomized study conducted ($N = 72$) in postmenopausal women with established **osteoporosis** defined as having at least one radiographically demonstrable atraumatic thoracic vertebral crush fracture and spine BMD T-score of 22.0 or below in England, HRT significantly increases BMD in the lumbar spine by 7.0% ($P < 0.001$) and in the hip by 4.8% ($P < 0.01$) after 4 years compared with that in the control group who received calcium and vitamin D. When combined with etidronate, the increases were 10.4% ($P < 0.001$) and 7.0% ($P < 0.001$) in the vertebrae and femora, respectively.[42] In addition, several meta-analyses and RCTs have illustrated the efficacy of hormonal therapy in the reduction of nonvertebral and vertebral fracture risk.[43,44]

HRT may be given orally or transdermally and includes estrogen only, progestin only, and a combination of estrogen and progestin. It may be given as a continuous or cyclical regimen. Discontinuation of treatment may result in rapid bone loss, hence alternative treatment such as bisphosphonate should be started to maintain BMD.[4]

Data from Women's Health Initiative reports increased incidence of breast cancer,[45,46] coronary heart disease, stroke,[46-48] and venous thromboembolism[47,49] in postmenopausal women treated with conjugated estrogens plus medroxyprogesterone acetate, or in the case of conjugated estrogens alone, an increased risk of stroke and venous thromboembolism.[50] The data demonstrated that there was no increased risk of cardiovascular disease if treatment was started within 10 years of menopause.[51]

Given the paucity of studies on other doses and combinations of HRT, risk profile should be assumed to be comparable.[4] Currently, guidelines recommend the use of HRT in the lowest effective doses consistent with treatment goals for the shortest duration to minimize the risk of adverse events.[28]

## Selective Estrogen Receptor Modulators: Raloxifene

Another promising therapy is SERMs such as raloxifene, which has been approved for the treatment of **osteoporosis** and secondary prevention of fragility fractures. It has a beneficial effect on BMD shown by the Multiple Outcomes of Raloxifene Evaluation (MORE) trial, a multicenter, randomized, placebo-controlled trial ($N = 7705$).[52] During the MORE trial, 60 mg/d of raloxifene was given for 3 years and vertebral fracture risk was reduced by 55% in women with a femoral neck or lumbar spine BMD T-score of 22.5 or below and by 30% in women with low T-scores and an existing vertebral fracture ($P < 0.001$). Persistent vertebral fracture risk was 50% and 38% in these two groups, respectively.[53] A separate analysis revealed that at 1 year, raloxifene decreased the risk of new clinical vertebral fracture by 68% (95% CI, 20-87) compared with placebo in the overall study population and by 66% (95% CI, 23-89) in women with existing fractures.[54]

Raloxifene is administered 60 mg/d as an oral tablet. One of the major concerns with raloxifene is its theoretical risk of major cardiovascular events because it selectively binds and activates estrogenic pathways. This acts as an estrogen agonist on bone to increase BMD. However, the Raloxifene Use for the Heart (RUTH) trial ($N = 10\,101$), an international, randomized, placebo-controlled trial suggests that there is no significant difference in the incidence of death from coronary causes, nonfatal myocardial infarction, or hospitalization from an acute coronary syndrome (HR = 0.95, 95% CI, 0.84-1.07).[55] The MORE trial demonstrates a significant increase in venous thromboembolic events (RR = 2.1, 95% CI, 1.2-3.8), but no difference in coronary events (533 vs 553, HR = 0.95, 95% CI, 0.84-1.07) or cerebrovascular events (249 vs 224, HR = 1.10, 95% CI, 0.92-1.32) when raloxifene is compared with placebo.[52] Women with higher cardiovascular risk such as established coronary heart disease, peripheral arterial disease, advanced age, diabetes mellitus, cigarette use, hypertension, and hyperlipidemia did not have a greater risk of adverse effects when compared with women with no cardiovascular risk.[55]

## Calcitonin

Calcitonin can be used for the treatment of **osteoporosis** and secondary prevention of fragility fractures when alternative therapies are not suitable.[4,28] In a 5-year, double-blind, randomized, placebo-controlled study ($N = 1255$) conducted in centers in the United States and United Kingdom, which stratified postmenopausal women with lumbar spine T-score less than 22 and at least one vertebral fracture to either placebo or intranasal calcitonin daily for 5 years, 200 IU/d calcitonin nasal spray was associated with a decreased risk of secondary vertebral fracture by 33% compared with placebo (RR = 0.67, 95% CI, 0.47-0.97). None of the doses used in the study had a reduction in nonvertebral or hip fractures.[56] A randomized study performed in Spain evaluated 72 postmenopausal osteoporotic women having more than one atraumatic vertebral crush fracture and found that at 24 months, the calcitonin group showed a 60% reduction in the number of new fractures compared with a 45% increase in the group receiving calcium only ($P < 0.001$).[57] Other studies yielded positive results for the secondary prevention of fragility fractures in **osteoporosis**.[58-60] Calcitonin may also provide an analgesic effect in patients with acute painful vertebral fractures.[61]

Calcitonin can be administered daily using single intranasal spray or subcutaneous/intramuscular administration by injection.[4,28]

Long-term use of calcitonin has been shown to increase the risk of cancer.[4] The European Medicine Agency reported that calcitonin increases the risk of malignancy by 0.7% for oral and 2.4% for nasal formulations compared with placebo.[62] Given the risk of malignancy and the availability of more efficacious medications to prevent recurrent fragility fractures, the European Medicine Agency advised against the routine use of calcitonin to prevent secondary fragility fractures. An FDA advisory panel also conducted a meta-analysis of 21 RCTs and concluded that there was an increased risk of malignancy of 4.2% in the salmon calcitonin–treated group compared with 2.9% in the placebo group.[4,63] Although a direct causal relationship between calcitonin-containing products and malignancy cannot be established from the meta-analyses, given the availability of more effective drugs in the treatment of **osteoporosis** and fragility fractures, the benefits of calcitonin do not outweigh its risk for malignancy.[63]

## Parathyroid Hormone Analogs: Teriparatide

Teriparatide is a parathyroid hormone (PTH) analog that is used in the treatment of **osteoporosis** in patients to reduce the risk of osteoporotic fractures. PTH acts on osteoblasts to indirectly stimulate osteoclastic breakdown of bone through the RANK–RANK ligand interaction. A once-daily injection of teriparatide will activate osteoblasts more than osteoclasts, stimulating osteoblastic bone formation to increase trabecular bone density and connectivity. Several RCTs have demonstrated a significant increase in BMD in the spine by 8.14% (95% CI, 6.72-9.55; 8 trials, $N = 2206$) and total hip BMD by 2.48% (95% CI, 1.67-3.29; 7 trials, $N = 1303$).[64] Likewise, the incidence of new vertebral fractures was reduced by 65% (95% CI, 0.22-0.55) and new nonvertebral fractures by 53% (95% CI, 0.25-0.88).[65-67] Specifically, for secondary prevention of fractures, a randomized, placebo-controlled trial ($N = 1637$) evaluated postmenopausal women with previous vertebral fractures in 17 countries and found that teriparatide decreases the risk of new vertebral (20-µg dose: RR = 0.35, 95% CI, 0.22-0.55; 40-mg dose: RR = 0.31, 95% CI, 0.19-0.50) and nonvertebral fractures (20-mg dose: RR = 0.47, 95% CI, 0.25-0.88; 40-µg dose: RR = 0.46, 95% CI, 0.25-0.86) with an increase in BMD ($P < 0.01$).[67] There are several studies that suggest that teriparatide can augment BMD when used in conjunction with other therapies. RCTs comparing teriparatide and HRT to HRT alone have a pooled weighted mean difference of 10.98% (lumbar spine: 95% CI, 10.81-11.16) and 3.65% (total hip: 95% CI, 3.53-3.76), indicating that teriparatide in combination with HRT was superior to HRT therapy alone in restoring BMD.[68,69]

Teriparatide is administered 20 μg subcutaneously into the thigh or abdominal wall daily for the treatment of **osteoporosis**. High-dose teriparatide treatment has caused osteosarcomas in rat models at doses from 3 to 60 times the 20 μg per day dose, although this finding has not been replicated in human trials.[70] Other adverse effects include muscle cramps, nausea, dizziness, and, infrequently, hypercalcemia. When PTH therapy was abruptly discontinued, substantial bone loss resulted within the first-year postuse.[71] However, RCTs suggest that administering alendronate post-PTH therapy can maintain or even improve BMD.[72,73]

## Emerging Therapies

### Parathyroid Hormone Receptor Ligands

Abaloparatide is an investigational PTH-related protein analog drug developed for the treatment of **osteoporosis**. As does its counterpart teriparatide, abaloparatide binds more selectively to the RG conformation of the PTH receptor type 1, resulting in transient responses, stimulating bone formation with less bone resorption and less hypercalcemic effects seen with PTH.[74] In a phase III, double-blind, RCT ($N = 2463$) determining the efficacy and safety of abaloparatide in postmenopausal women with **osteoporosis** and existing fractures at 28 sites in 10 countries, new morphometric vertebral fractures occurred in 0.58% of patients receiving abaloparatide compared with 4.22% of those in the placebo group (RR 0.14, 95% CI, 0.05-0.39). BMD increases were also greater with abaloparatide than with placebo (all $P < 0.001$) (Table 14.2).[75]

**TABLE 14.2 • Emerging Therapies for Osteoporosis**

| Drug | Mechanism of Action | Dosing | Route | Adverse Events |
|---|---|---|---|---|
| PTH receptor ligands Abaloparatide | Binds more selectively to the RG conformation of PTH receptor type 1 → results in transient response → stimulates bone formation, less bone resorption | 80 mg once a day | SC | Hypercalciuria, dizziness, nausea, headache, palpitations, fatigue |
| Monoclonal antisclerostin antibody Romosozumab | Binds and inhibits sclerostin (protein with antianabolic effect) → increases bone formation | Variable doses | SC | Reported SC injection site reaction, osteonecrosis of the jaw in trials |
| Cathepsin K inhibitors Odanacatib | Inhibit cathepsin (protease that aids in osteoclast-mediated bone resorption) → inhibits bone resorption | Variable doses | Oral | Reported atypical femoral-shaft fractures in trials |

Abbreviations: PTH, parathyroid hormone; SC, subcutaneous.

## Monoclonal Antisclerostin Antibody

Sclerostin is a protein produced by osteocytes that has antianabolic effects on bone formation. Romosozumab, an investigative monoclonal antisclerostin antibody, has been shown to improve BMD in postmenopausal women. In an international, randomized, placebo-controlled trial ($N = 7180$) designed to assess radiographic vertebral fracture outcomes, the incidence of vertebral fracture was lower in the romosozumab group at 12 months compared with placebo (0.5 vs 1.8%, RR = 0.27, 95% CI, 0.16-0.47).[76] A recently published RCT ($N = 4093$) showed that romosozumab treatment for 12 months followed by alendronate resulted in a significantly lower risk of fracture than alendronate alone in postmenopausal women with **osteoporosis** and a fragility fracture.[77] Additional trials comparing romosozumab to other osteoporotic drugs have also yielded positive outcomes.[78,79] There are currently no trials in the literature assessing the efficacy of secondary prevention of fragility fractures because osteoporotic patients with existing fractures were excluded from the studies.

## Cathepsin K Inhibitors

Cathepsin is a protease expressed by osteoclasts that aids in osteoclast-mediated bone resorption. It causes degradation of the triple helical collagen, primarily in type 1 collagen.[80] In a multicenter, randomized, placebo-controlled trial ($N = 857$), lumbar spine and total hip BMD increased 5.5% and 3.2%, respectively, with 50-mg dose of odanacatib (cathepsin K inhibitor) and biochemical markers of bone turnover also exhibited dose-related changes. There were no dose-related adverse events relative to placebo.[81] Other studies have shown efficacy of cathepsin K inhibitor with great results.[82,83] However, in 2016, the development of odanacatib was discontinued after analysis discovered an increased risk of stroke.[84] There are currently no trials in the literature assessing the efficacy of secondary prevention of fragility fractures because osteoporotic patients with existing fractures were excluded from the studies.

# SUMMARY

Osteoporotic fragility fracture is a burgeoning health epidemic that is associated with high rates of disability, morbidity, and mortality. On the basis of the NHANES data, approximately 10 million Americans are affected by this disease.

Successful **secondary fracture prevention** measures are often limited by the underdiagnosis of **osteoporosis** after fragility fractures because of lack of patient and physician awareness of the disease, lack of follow-up, and medical nonadherence.

Current guidelines recommend the use of bisphosphonate as the first-line therapy for **secondary fracture prevention**. Compared with placebo, RCTs have demonstrated a significant reduction in vertebral and nonvertebral fractures using alendronate, risedronate, ibandronate, and zoledronic acid. All but ibandronate showed a significant reduction in hip fractures as well (all trials with $P < 0.05$). Denosumab is an option in patients with impaired renal function or who are unresponsive to other therapies. It significantly decreases the risk of new vertebral fracture (hazard ratio [HR] = 0.32, 95% confidence interval [CI], 0.26-0.41), hip fracture (HR = 0.60, 95% CI, 0.37-0.97), and nonvertebral fracture (HR = 0.80; 95% CI, 0.67-0.95) without an increase in adverse events. Hormonal therapy has been shown to be effective, but should be used in the lowest effective dose to minimize the risk of coronary heart disease, stroke, and venous thromboembolism. SERMs, calcitonin, and PTH are other alternatives described in this chapter. In addition to current therapies, emerging therapies under investigation such as abaloparatide, a **parathyroid receptor ligand**, and romosozumab, a **monoclonal antisclerostin antibody** both showed a reduction in new morphometric vertebral fractures compared with placebo (0.58% vs 4.22%, relative risk = 0.14, 95% CI, 0.05-0.39, and 0.5 vs 1.8%, relative risk = 0.27, 95% CI, 0.16-0.47, respectively). In this chapter, we summarize advances in current therapeutic agents used for **secondary fracture prevention** and provide insight into potential therapies that hold promise in the future of **osteoporosis**.

Secondary prevention of fragility fractures through care coordination and initiation of various pharmacologic agents is crucial in the elderly population. Careful risk assessment and stratification should be performed before the initiation of pharmacologic treatment to optimize disease management.

## References

1. National Health and Nutrition Examination Survey. Osteoporosis. https://www.cdc.gov/nchs/data/nhanes/databriefs/osteoporosis.pdf. Accessed February 2, 2017.

2. Tosi LL, Dell RM. Challenging orthopaedics to reduce osteoporotic hip fractures. *Am Acad Orthop Surg.* 2009.

3. Lyet JP. Fragility fractures in the osteoporotic patient: special challenges. *J Lancaster Gen Hosp.* 2006;1:91-95.

4. Cosman F, de Beur SJ, LeBoff MS, et al. Clinician's guide to prevention and treatment of osteoporosis. *Osteoporos Int.* 2014;25:2359-2381.

5. The Joint Commission. Improving and measuring osteoporosis management. https://www.jointcommission.org/assets/1/18/OsteoMono_REVFinal_31208.pdf. Accessed February 2, 2017.

6. Centers for Medicare & Medicaid Services. 2014 Physician Quality Reporting System (PQRS) measure specifications manual for claims and registry reporting of individual measures. https://www.cms.gov/apps/ama/license.asp?file=/PQRS/downloads/2014_PQRS_IndClaimsRegistry_Measure-Specs_SupportingDocs_12132013.zip. Accessed February 2, 2017.

7. Bellantonio S, Fortinsky R, Prestwood K. How well are community-living women treated for osteoporosis after hip fracture? *J Am Geriatr Soc.* 2001;49:1197-1204.

8. National Committee for Quality Assurance. HEDIS & performance measurement. Proposed changes to existing measure for HEDIS 2015: osteoporosis management in women who had a fracture (OMW). 2015.

9. Gadam RK, Schlauch K, Izuora KE. FRAX prediction without BMD for assessment of osteoporotic fracture risk. *Endocr Pract.* 2013;19:780-784.

10. Cooper C, Atkinson EJ, O'Fallon WM, et al. Incidence of clinically diagnosed vertebral fractures: a population-based study in Rochester, Minnesota, 1985–1989. *J Bone Miner Res.* 1992;7:221-227.

11. Klotzbuecher CM, Ross PD, Landsman PB, et al. Patients with prior fractures have an increased risk of future fractures: a summary of the literature and statistical synthesis. *J Bone Miner Res.* 2000;15:721-739.

12. Walters S, Khan T, Ong T, et al. Fracture liaison services: improving outcomes for patients with osteoporosis. *Clin Interv Aging.* 2017;12:117-127.

13. Port L, Center J, Briffa NK, et al. Osteoporotic fracture: missed opportunity for intervention. *Osteoporos Int.* 2003;14:780-784.

14. Eisman JA, Bogoch ER, Dell R, et al. Making the first fracture the last fracture: ASBMR task force report on secondary fracture prevention. *J Bone Miner Res.* 2012;27:2039-2046.

15. Majumdar SR, Beaupre LA, Harley CH, et al. Use of a case manager to improve osteoporosis treatment after hip fracture: results of a randomized controlled trial. *Arch Intern Med.* 2007;167:2110-2115.

16. Curtis JR, Arora T, Matthews RS, et al. Is withholding osteoporosis medication after fracture sometimes rational? A comparison of the risk for second fracture versus death. *J Am Med Dir Assoc.* 2010;11:584-591.

17. Gosch M, Kammerlander C, Roth T, et al. Surgeons save bones: an algorithm for orthopedic surgeons managing secondary fracture prevention. *Arch Orthop Trauma Surg.* 2013;133:1101-1108.

18. Wells GA, Cranney A, Peterson J, et al. Alendronate for the primary and secondary prevention of osteoporotic fractures in postmenopausal women. *Cochrane Database Syst Rev.* 2008:CD001155.

19. Wells G, Cranney A, Peterson J, et al. Risedronate for the primary and secondary prevention of osteoporotic fractures in postmenopausal women. *Cochrane Database Syst Rev.* 2008:CD004523.

20. Chesnut CH III, Skag A, Christiansen C, et al. Effects of oral ibandronate administered daily or intermittently on fracture risk in postmenopausal osteoporosis. *J Bone Miner Res.* 2004;19:1241-1249.

21. Black DM, Delmas PD, Eastell R, et al. Once-yearly zoledronic acid for treatment of postmenopausal osteoporosis. *N Engl J Med.* 2007;356:1809-1822.

22. Black DM, Cummings SR, Karpf DB, et al; Fracture Intervention Trial Research Group. Randomised trial of effect of alendronate on risk of fracture in women with existing vertebral fractures. *Lancet.* 1996;348:1535-1541.

23. Harris ST, Blumentals WA, Miller PD. Ibandronate and the risk of non-vertebral and clinical fractures in women with postmenopausal osteoporosis: results of a meta-analysis of phase III studies. *Curr Med Res Opin.* 2008;24:237-245.

24. Harris ST, Watts NB, Genant HK, et al; Vertebral Efficacy with Risedronate Therapy (VERT) Study Group. Effects of risedronate treatment on vertebral and nonvertebral fractures in women with postmenopausal osteoporosis: a randomized controlled trial. *JAMA.* 1999;282:1344-1352.

25. Black DM, Thompson DE, Bauer DC, et al; FIT research group. Fracture risk reduction with alendronate in women with osteoporosis: the fracture intervention trial. *J Clin Endocrinol Metab.* 2000;85:4118-4124.

26. Reginster J, Minne HW, Sorensen OH, et al; Vertebral Efficacy with Risedronate Therapy (VERT) Study Group. Randomized trial of the effects of risedronate on vertebral fractures in women with established postmenopausal osteoporosis. *Osteoporos Int.* 2000;11:83-91.

27. Bobba RS, Beattie K, Parkinson B, et al. Tolerability of different dosing regimens of bisphosphonates for the treatment of osteoporosis and malignant bone disease. *Drug Saf.* 2006;29:1133-1152.

28. Management of osteoporosis in postmenopausal women: 2010 position statement of the North American Menopause Society. *Menopause.* 2010;17:25-54; quiz 55-56.

29. Schneider JP. Bisphosphonates and low-impact femoral fractures: current evidence on alendronate-fracture risk. *Geriatrics.* 2009;64:18-23.

30. Dell RM, Adams AL, Greene DF, et al. Incidence of atypical nontraumatic diaphyseal fractures of the femur. *J Bone Miner Res.* 2012;27:2544-2550.

31. Khosla S, Burr D, Cauley J, et al. Bisphosphonate-associated osteonecrosis of the jaw: report of a task force of the American Society for Bone and Mineral Research. *J Bone Miner Res.* 2007;22:1479-1491.

32. Cummings SR, San Martin J, McClung MR, et al. Denosumab for prevention of fractures in postmenopausal women with osteoporosis. *N Engl J Med.* 2009;361:756-765.

33. Miller PD, Wagman RB, Peacock M, et al. Effect of denosumab on bone mineral density and biochemical markers of bone turnover: six-year results of a phase 2 clinical trial. *J Clin Endocrinol Metab.* 2011;96:394-402.

34. Papapoulos S, Lippuner K, Roux C, et al. The effect of 8 or 5 years of denosumab treatment in postmenopausal women with osteoporosis: results from the FREEDOM extension study. *Osteoporos Int.* 2015;26:2773-2783.

35. Brown JP, Prince RL, Deal C, et al. Comparison of the effect of denosumab and alendronate on BMD and biochemical markers of bone turnover in postmenopausal women with low bone mass: a randomized, blinded, phase 3 trial. *J Bone Miner Res*. 2009;24:153-161.

36. Miller PD, Bolognese MA, Lewiecki EM, et al. Effect of denosumab on bone density and turnover in postmenopausal women with low bone mass after longterm continued, discontinued, and restarting of therapy: a randomized blinded phase 2 clinical trial. *Bone*. 2008;43:222-229.

37. Miller PD. Denosumab: anti-RANKL antibody. *Curr Osteoporos Rep*. 2009;7:18-22.

38. Amgen Inc. Prolia prescribing information. http://pi.amgen.com/ ~ /media/amgen/repositorysites/pi-amgen-com/prolia/prolia_pi.ashx. Accessed February 2, 2017.

39. Rachner TD, Platzbecker U, Felsenberg D, et al. Osteonecrosis of the jaw after osteoporosis therapy with denosumab following long-term bisphosphonate therapy. *Mayo Clin Proc*. 2013;88:418-419.

40. Cating-Cabral MT, Clarke BL. Denosumab and atypical femur fractures. *Maturitas*. 2013;76:1-2.

41. Lufkin EG, Wahner HW, O'Fallon WM, et al. Treatment of postmenopausal osteoporosis with transdermal estrogen. *Ann Intern Med*. 1992;117:1-9.

42. Wimalawansa SJ. A four-year randomized controlled trial of hormone replacement and bisphosphonate, alone or in combination, in women with postmenopausal osteoporosis. *Am J Med*. 1998;104:219-226.

43. Wells G, Tugwell P, Shea B, et al. Meta-analyses of therapies for postmenopausal osteoporosis. V. Meta-analysis of the efficacy of hormone replacement therapy in treating and preventing osteoporosis in postmenopausal women. *Endocr Rev*. 2002;23:529-539.

44. Lindsay R, Tohme JF. Estrogen treatment of patients with established postmenopausal osteoporosis. *Obstet Gynecol*. 1990;76:290-295.

45. Chlebowski RT, Hendrix SL, Langer RD, et al. Influence of estrogen plus progestin on breast cancer and mammography in healthy postmenopausal women: the Women's Health Initiative Randomized Trial. *JAMA*. 2003;289:3243-3253.

46. Wassertheil-Smoller S, Hendrix SL, Limacher M, et al. Effect of estrogen plus progestin on stroke in postmenopausal women: the Women's Health Initiative: a randomized trial. *JAMA*. 2003;289:2673-2684.

47. Rossouw JE, Anderson GL, Prentice RL, et al. Risks and benefits of estrogen plus progestin in healthy postmenopausal women: principal results from the Women's Health Initiative randomized controlled trial. *JAMA*. 2002;288:321-333.

48. Manson JE, Hsia J, Johnson KC, et al. Estrogen plus progestin and the risk of coronary heart disease. *N Engl J Med*. 2003;349:523-534.

49. Cushman M, Kuller LH, Prentice R, et al. Estrogen plus progestin and risk of venous thrombosis. *JAMA*. 2004;292:1573-1580.

50. Anderson GL, Limacher M, Assaf AR, et al. Effects of conjugated equine estrogen in postmenopausal women with hysterectomy: the Women's Health Initiative randomized controlled trial. *JAMA*. 2004;291:1701-1712.

51. Manson JE, Allison MA, Rossouw JE, et al. Estrogen therapy and coronary-artery calcification. *N Engl J Med*. 2007;356:2591-2602.

52. Ettinger B, Black DM, Mitlak BH, et al; Multiple Outcomes of Raloxifene Evaluation (MORE) Investigators. Reduction of vertebral fracture risk in postmenopausal women with osteoporosis treated with raloxifene: results from a 3-year randomized clinical trial. *JAMA*. 1999;282:637-645.

53. Messalli EM, Scaffa C. Long-term safety and efficacy of raloxifene in the prevention and treatment of postmenopausal osteoporosis: an update. *Int J Womens Health*. 2009;1:11-20.

54. Maricic M, Adachi JD, Sarkar S, et al. Early effects of raloxifene on clinical vertebral fractures at 12 months in postmenopausal women with osteoporosis. *Arch Intern Med*. 2002;162:1140-1143.

55. Barrett-Connor E, Mosca L, Collins P, et al. Effects of raloxifene on cardiovascular events and breast cancer in postmenopausal women. *N Engl J Med*. 2006;355:125-137.

56. Chesnut CH III, Silverman S, Andriano K, et al; PROOF Study Group. A randomized trial of nasal spray salmon calcitonin in postmenopausal women with established osteoporosis: the prevent recurrence of osteoporotic fractures study. *Am J Med*. 2000;109:267-276.

57. Rico H, Revilla M, Hernandez ER, et al. Total and regional bone mineral content and fracture rate in postmenopausal osteoporosis treated with salmon calcitonin: a prospective study. *Calcif Tissue Int*. 1995;56:181-185.

58. Civitelli R, Gonnelli S, Zacchei F, et al. Bone turnover in postmenopausal osteoporosis. Effect of calcitonin treatment. *J Clin Invest.* 1988;82:1268-1274.

59. Gruber HE, Ivey JL, Baylink DJ, et al. Long-term calcitonin therapy in postmenopausal osteoporosis. *Metabolism.* 1984;33:295-303.

60. Mazzuoli GF, Passeri M, Gennari C, et al. Effects of salmon calcitonin in postmenopausal osteoporosis: a controlled double-blind clinical study. *Calcif Tissue Int.* 1986;38:3-8.

61. Knopp-Sihota JA, Newburn-Cook CV, Homik J, et al. Calcitonin for treating acute and chronic pain of recent and remote osteoporotic vertebral compression fractures: a systematic review and meta-analysis. *Osteoporos Int.* 2012;23:17-38.

62. European Medicines Agency. European Medicines Agency recommends limiting long-term use of calcitonin medicines. http://www.ema.europa.eu/docs/en_GB/document_library/Press_release/2012/07/WC500130122.pdf. Accessed February 2, 2017.

63. U.S. Food & Drug Administration. Background document for meeting of advisory committee for reproductive health drugs and drug safety and risk management advisory committee. https://www.fda.gov/Drugs/Drugsafety/postmarketdrugsafetyinformationforpatientsandproviders/ucm388641.htm. Accessed February 2, 2017.

64. Han SL, Wan SL. Effect of teriparatide on bone mineral density and fracture in postmenopausal osteoporosis: meta-analysis of randomised controlled trials. *Int J Clin Pract.* 2012;66:199-209.

65. Dempster DW, Cosman F, Kurland ES, et al. Effects of daily treatment with parathyroid hormone on bone microarchitecture and turnover in patients with osteoporosis: a paired biopsy study. *J Bone Miner Res.* 2001;16:1846-1853.

66. Lindsay R, Nieves J, Formica C, et al. Randomised controlled study of effect of parathyroid hormone on vertebral-bone mass and fracture incidence among postmenopausal women on oestrogen with osteoporosis. *Lancet.* 1997;350:550-555.

67. Neer RM, Arnaud CD, Zanchetta JR, et al. Effect of parathyroid hormone (1–34) on fractures and bone mineral density in postmenopausal women with osteoporosis. *N Engl J Med.* 2001;344:1434-1441.

68. Cosman F, Nieves J, Woelfert L, et al. Parathyroid hormone added to established hormone therapy: effects on vertebral fracture and maintenance of bone mass after parathyroid hormone withdrawal. *J Bone Miner Res.* 2001;16:925-931.

69. Ste-Marie LG, Schwartz SL, Hossain A, et al. Effect of teriparatide [rhPTH(1–34)] on BMD when given to postmenopausal women receiving hormone replacement therapy. *J Bone Miner Res.* 2006;21:283-291.

70. Andrews EB, Gilsenan AW, Midkiff K, et al. The US postmarketing surveillance study of adult osteosarcoma and teriparatide: study design and findings from the first 7 years. *J Bone Miner Res.* 2012;27:2429-2437.

71. Black DM, Bilezikian JP, Ensrud KE, et al. One year of alendronate after one year of parathyroid hormone (1–84) for osteoporosis. *N Engl J Med.* 2005;353:555-565.

72. Cosman F, Nieves J, Zion M, et al. Daily and cyclic parathyroid hormone in women receiving alendronate. *N Engl J Med.* 2005;353:566-575.

73. Finkelstein JS, Wyland JJ, Lee H, et al. Effects of teriparatide, alendronate, or both in women with postmenopausal osteoporosis. *J Clin Endocrinol Metab.* 2010;95:1838-1845.

74. Hattersley G, Dean T, Corbin BA, et al. Binding selectivity of abaloparatide for PTH-type-1-receptor conformations and effects on downstream signaling. *Endocrinology.* 2016;157:141-149.

75. Miller PD, Hattersley G, Riis BJ, et al. Effect of abaloparatide vs placebo on new vertebral fractures in postmenopausal women with osteoporosis: a randomized clinical trial. *JAMA.* 2016;316:722-733.

76. Cosman F, Crittenden DB, Adachi JD, et al. Romosozumab treatment in postmenopausal women with osteoporosis. *N Engl J Med.* 2016;375:1532-1543.

77. Saag KG, Petersen J, Brandi ML, et al. Romosozumab or alendronate for fracture prevention in women with osteoporosis. *N Engl J Med.* 2017;377(15):1417-1427.

78. McClung MR, Grauer A, Boonen S, et al. Romosozumab in postmenopausal women with low bone mineral density. *N Engl J Med.* 2014;370:412-420.

79. Genant HK, Engelke K, Bolognese MA, et al. Effects of romosozumab compared with teriparatide on bone density and mass at the spine and hip in postmenopausal women with low bone mass. *J Bone Miner Res*. 2017;32:181-187.

80. Vasiljeva O, Reinheckel T, Peters C, et al. Emerging roles of cysteine cathepsins in disease and their potential as drug targets. *Curr Pharm Des*. 2007;13:387-403.

81. Bone HG, McClung MR, Roux C, et al. Odanacatib, a cathepsin-K inhibitor for osteoporosis: a two-year study in postmenopausal women with low bone density. *J Bone Miner Res*. 2010;25:937-947.

82. Eastell R, Nagase S, Ohyama M, et al. Safety and efficacy of the cathepsin K inhibitor ONO-5334 in postmenopausal osteoporosis: the OCEAN study. *J Bone Miner Res*. 2011;26:1303-1312.

83. Langdahl B, Binkley N, Bone H, et al. Odanacatib in the treatment of postmenopausal women with low bone mineral density: five years of continued therapy in a phase 2 study. *J Bone Miner Res*. 2012;27:2251-2258.

84. Mullard A. Merck & Co. drops osteoporosis drug odanacatib. *Nat Rev Drug Discov*. 2016;15:669.

# CHAPTER 15

# Therapeutic Advances in the Management of Older Adults in the Intensive Care Unit: A Focus on Pain, Sedation, and Delirium

Samantha Moore, PharmD

## BACKGROUND

Adults older than the age of 65 are the fastest growing segment of the U.S. population, with the most rapidly growing subgroup being those older than the age of 80.[1] By the year 2030, it is estimated that the population of **elderly** adults (age > 65 years) will increase to more than 72 million, or 19% of the U.S. population.[2] **Elderly** adults currently account for approximately half of all **intensive care unit** (ICU) admissions and 60% of ICU days.[3,4] These numbers are only expected to increase in the upcoming years as the population ages.

Despite the increasing proportion of **elderly** patients in the ICU, the overall rates of survival from critical illness continue to improve. This is likely a result of improved medical technologies and advancements in the management of illnesses such as acute respiratory distress syndrome and sepsis.[5-7] With the increased use of critical care services, the growth of the **elderly** population, and improvements in medical management, there has been an increasing number of ICU survivors. In fact, every year more than a million patients in the United States survive a critical illness.[8] As a result, there has been increased recognition and understanding of the significant long-term disabilities ICU survivors commonly struggle with.[9,10] Specifically, they often have a multitude of physical, cognitive, and mental health problems that affect their ability to perform activities of daily living and have a major impact on their quality of life[11-20] (Table 15.1). They may experience symptoms of depression and anxiety, posttraumatic stress disorder, chronic pain, new or significantly worsened cognitive impairments,

**TABLE 15.1 • Long-term Complications of Critical Illness**

| Complications | Consequences | Nonmodifiable Risk Factors | Potentially Modifiable Risk Factors | Recommended Interventions |
|---|---|---|---|---|
| **Physical** | | | | |
| • ICU-acquired weakness<br>• Muscle atrophy<br>• Critical illness polyneuropathy and myopathy | Prolonged mechanical ventilation, increased ICU and hospital LOS, neuromuscular weakness, fatigue, mobility impairments, dependence in ADLs and IADLs, institutionalization, reduced QOL | Increased age, baseline frailty and functional state, severity of illness, systemic inflammatory response syndrome, multiorgan dysfunction | Duration of mechanical ventilation, corticosteroids, neuromuscular blocking agents, hyperglycemia, immobility/bed rest, uncontrolled pain | Early mobility and participation with PT and OT, minimize bed-rest, minimize sedation to reduce time on ventilator and allow for participation in care, monitor for and treat pain |
| **Cognitive** | | | | |
| • Reduced attention, memory, executive function, visual-spatial activities | Overall reduction in global cognition, functional impairment, inability to return to work or reduced work productivity, reduced QOL | Increased age, baseline cognitive impairment, severity of illness | ICU delirium, deep sedation, sedatives (especially BZDs), immobility, hyper- and hypoglycemia, hypotension, hypoxia | Minimize or lighten sedation, avoid BZDs, monitor for delirium and reduce risk factors (through early mobility, lightening sedation) |
| **Psychiatric** | | | | |
| • Anxiety<br>• Depression<br>• PTSD | Distressing flashbacks, memory lapses, nightmares, reduced QOL | History of psychiatric disorder, severity of illness, multiorgan dysfunction | Deep sedation, sedatives (especially BZDs), agitation, sleep deprivation, uncontrolled pain | Minimize or lighten sedation, avoid BZDs, monitor for and treat pain, optimize sleep-wake cycle |

Abbreviations: ADL, activity of daily living; BZD, benzodiazepine; IADL, instrumental activity of daily living; ICU, intensive care unit; LOS, length of stay; OT, occupational therapy; PT, physical therapy; PTSD, posttraumatic stress disorder; QOL, quality of life.

profound skeletal muscle atrophy, and muscle weakness.[11-17,21-24] These disabilities may be collectively referred to as post–intensive care syndrome, which can be long-lasting and extend for years after a patient is discharged from the ICU.[18]

There are many factors that influence patient outcomes after critical illness, including baseline comorbidities, premorbid cognitive and functional status, admission diagnosis, and severity of illness.[19,25-27] **Elderly** patients frequently have multiple comorbidities, baseline cognitive, and/or functional impairments, as well as age-related physiologic changes.[27-29] As a result, it is more difficult for **elderly** patients to "bounce back" from their critical illness and they are particularly vulnerable to developing long-term disabilities.[13,14,21,25-28,30-32]

Given the impairments many **elderly** patients have post–critical illness, it is essential that critical care providers focus on interventions that not only improve acute survival but also improve the chances of returning to a reasonable quality of life, free from significant cognitive, functional, and psychological impairments.[10,18] In the words of Angus et al,[9] "The goals of critical care must extend beyond patient survival." Although many of the disabilities observed in post–intensive care syndrome are a consequence of the critical illness itself and are nonmodifiable, there are also many iatrogenic and modifiable risk factors.[18,27,33] For example, the choice of sedative and the depth of sedation may influence the ability to participate in physical therapy, the risk of developing **delirium**, the duration of mechanical ventilation, and **ICU** length of stay, all of which have been shown to have a negative impact on long-term outcomes.[24,34-45] Similarly, patients with inadequate pain control have difficulty participating in physical therapy and weaning from mechanical ventilation and are at increased risk of **ICU delirium** and developing chronic pain.[22,46-48] Finally, the development of **ICU delirium** has been associated with a longer duration of mechanical ventilation, increased risk of long-term cognitive impairment, and worse functional recovery.[15,49-53]

In an effort to improve acute patient care and minimize the development of post-ICU disabilities, there has been a focus on reducing iatrogenic risks patients are exposed to while in the **ICU**. Recently, the Society of Critical Care Medicine published an updated set of evidence-based recommendations titled the "Clinical Practice Guidelines for the Prevention and Management of Pain, Agitation/Sedation, Delirium, Immobility, and Sleep Disruption in Adult Patients in the **ICU**".[54] In addition, in 2015 the Institute for Healthcare Improvement sponsored the "Rethinking Critical Care" initiative, which focuses on patient comfort and safety in the **ICU** because it relates to pain, sedation, **delirium**, and early mobility. Finally, the ABCDEF bundle, which is described in detail elsewhere, incorporates recommendations from these guidelines. It focuses on reducing **delirium**, minimizing sedation, getting patients out of bed and moving, optimizing pain management, and providing patient-centered care with active family involvement.[33,48,55-58] The bundle and its individual components have demonstrated success in improving both short-term and long-term outcomes in critically ill patients.[30,42,43,59-61] However, there is limited data regarding the optimal pharmacologic management of analgesia, sedation, and **delirium** in **elderly ICU** patients specifically. This is significant given the alterations in pharmacokinetics and pharmacodynamics in **elderly** patients and the importance of these components of the bundle in improving patient outcomes.[62,63] Although more research is needed on this topic, this chapter summarizes the literature and provides recommendations on the pharmacologic management of pain, sedation, and **delirium** in **elderly** patients in the **ICU**.

At baseline, **elderly** patients have significant physiologic changes that result in altered **medication** pharmacokinetics and pharmacodynamics.[29,62,63] Specifically, the **elderly** often have impaired gastric absorption of **medications**, which may be further worsened by bowel wall edema and impaired gastric perfusion during critical ill-ness.[64-66] Older patients also have increased fat tissue, resulting in increased volume of distribution and subsequently increased half-life of lipophilic **medications**.[62,67] In regard to drug metabolism, hepatic function declines with age and primarily affects phase 1 or cytochrome P450 enzyme metabolism; this may be further impaired by poor hepatic blood flow during critical illness.[65,66,68] In addition, there is a steady decline in renal function with age, resulting in reduced renal elimination of **med-ications**.[69,70] This can be further complicated by acute kidney injury, which often occurs during the course of critical illness.[65,66] The pharmacodynamic changes that occur with aging are variable, but typically result in increased sensitivity to **medica-tions**; this is particularly true with centrally acting **medications** such as opioids and sedatives.[62,63]

# PAIN

Patients in the ICU have many sources of pain, including invasive devices, surgery, and bedside procedures.[47,71] Uncontrolled pain in **elderly** critically ill patients can have many adverse consequences including prolonged immobility, increased inci-dence of **ICU delirium**, and the development of chronic pain.[22,46,47] In addition, if pain is not recognized as such, it may be mistaken for agitation and inappropriately treated with sedatives.[72,73] The first component of pain management is frequent mon-itoring. Patients who are able to self-report their pain should do so, whereas validated scales such as the Critical-care Pain Observation Tool or Behavioral Pain Scale can be used in patients who are unable to self-report.[54,74,75] Monitoring for pain allows for early detection, effective treatment, and prevents the unnecessary use of analgesics and the inappropriate use of sedatives.[72] In addition, monitoring for pain has been shown to reduce the duration of mechanical ventilation and the ICU length of stay.[72]

Intravenous (IV) opioids, such as morphine, hydromorphone, and fentanyl, are the first-line treatment for pain in the ICU.[54,71] All opioids are equally effective at equi-analgesic doses; however, in **elderly** critically ill patients, morphine should generally be avoided because it is metabolized to an active metabolite that can accumulate in renal dysfunction and cause unpredictable and prolonged duration of effect.[76,77] Over-all, **elderly** patients are more sensitive to the therapeutic and adverse effects of opioids, and, as a result, initial doses should be reduced by 25% to 50%.[78] Whenever possible, **elderly** critically ill patients should receive opioids as intermittent bolus doses instead of continuous infusions as the former may reduce the risk of opioid accumulation and oversedation.

Multimodal analgesia may also be used to optimize pain control while reducing opi-oid requirements.[54,79] Acetaminophen is commonly used and has been shown to im-prove pain scores, reduce opioid use, and reduce opioid side effects.[80-82] Nonsteroidal anti-inflammatory drugs are also occasionally used as a part of multimodal analgesia. However, given the risk of acute renal dysfunction, gastric ulcers and bleeding, and cardiovascular events associated with their use, it is generally safest to avoid these **medications** in older critically ill patients.[54,71,83] If patients experience neuropathic pain while in the ICU, gabapentin may safely be used in most critically ill older adults.[54] However, because gabapentin clearance is almost completely dependent on renal elimination, it is recommended that older critically ill patients receive lower starting doses than do younger or healthier patients.[84]

# SEDATION

In addition to analgesia, critically ill patients often need sedation to remain calm and comfortable and to prevent agitation and removal of invasive medical devices. However, studies have demonstrated the numerous adverse outcomes associated with maintaining patients on deep levels of sedation.[41-45,85] Deeply sedated patients are unable to participate in their care and will remain immobile for prolonged periods of time.[24,86] In addition, they will have prolonged mechanical ventilation, prolonged hospital and ICU length of stay, and are more likely to suffer from long-term cognitive dysfunction.[41-45] To optimize sedation management, patients must first be assessed with a validated sedation scale that assesses level of consciousness, such as the Richmond Agitation-Sedation Scale.[54,87]

Commonly used sedatives in the ICU are benzodiazepines (midazolam and lorazepam), propofol, and dexmedetomidine. In general, benzodiazepines should be reserved as a last-line sedative for critically ill **elderly** patients. Several studies have demonstrated the increased risk of **delirium** with benzodiazepines as compared to nonbenzodiazepine sedatives.[34,35,39] In addition, benzodiazepines are lipophilic and tend to accumulate with prolonged use, particularly in the **elderly**, resulting in delayed emergence from sedation.[77,86,88,89] For most patients, propofol is preferred over benzodiazepines, although its use may be limited by dose-dependent hypotension.[39,40,90] A recent multicenter, retrospective, propensity-matched cohort study compared outcomes in more than 3000 mechanically ventilated patients who received propofol as compared to lorazepam or midazolam for ICU sedation. Patients who received propofol had earlier discontinuation of mechanical ventilation, reduced ICU and hospital length of stay, and reduced ICU mortality.[39] Lastly, dexmedetomidine is a unique sedative because it does not produce deep levels of sedation, which enables patients to interact with providers and family members and be active participants in their care.[54,91] In addition, dexmedetomidine does not cause respiratory depression and may be used in patients who are not receiving respiratory support.[91] However, the use of dexmedetomidine is limited by hemodynamic instability, particularly bradycardia.[92] When compared to benzodiazepines, sedation with dexmedetomidine has been associated with a lower prevalence of **delirium** and a shorter duration of mechanical ventilation.[34,35,93] Several studies have also suggested a lower risk of delirium with dexmedetomidine as compared to propofol.[38,94] As a result, the prior version of the SCCM Guidelines from 2013 recommended dexmedetomidine be considered as a first-line sedative in patients at high risk of developing ICU delirium.[48] However, this recommendation has been removed from the latest version of the SCCM Guidelines.[54] Instead, the 2018 guidelines state that both dexmedetomidine and propofol are appropriate first-line sedatives in mechanically ventilated critically ill patients. Despite this, in **elderly** patients at a very high risk of developing delirium, it may still be reasonable to consider dexmedetomidine as the first-line sedative in eligible high risk **elderly** patients.

# DELIRIUM

**Delirium** is a form of acute brain dysfunction that commonly occurs in critical illness and is characterized by acute changes and fluctuations in mental status with inattention, disorganized thinking, and altered levels of consciousness.[95] **Delirium** can be categorized as hyperactive (patient is restless, agitated, and combative), hypoactive (patient is apathetic, lethargic, and withdrawn), or mixed (patient fluctuates between the two).[96,97] Risk factors for **delirium** include benzodiazepines, physical restraints, immobilization, increased age, severity of illness, and preexisting cognitive dysfunction.[30,36,37,46,98-100] Both the development and the duration of **ICU delirium** are associated with prolonged duration of mechanical ventilation, prolonged **ICU** and hospital length of stay, long-term cognitive impairments, reduced quality of life after **ICU** discharge, and increased mortality.[15,46,49-51,53] In addition, in patients with preexisting dementia, the development of **delirium** can result in accelerated cognitive decline after hospital discharge.[101,102] The first step in **delirium** management is the detection of **delirium** through a validated monitoring tool. The two recommended tools include the Confusion Assessment Method for the **ICU** or the Intensive Care Delirium Screening Checklist, which are described elsewhere.[48,103,104]

Currently, nonpharmacologic interventions are recommended first line for the prevention and treatment of **ICU delirium**.[54] This includes removal of deliriogenic **medications**, such as benzodiazepines, antihistamines, anticholinergics, and corticosteroids, providing vision and hearing aids when necessary, frequent reorientation, optimizing the sleep–wake cycle, physical therapy and early mobility, and reinitiation of any psychiatric home **medications**.[30,54,105-107] In regard to the pharmacologic management, there are currently no approved **medications** for the treatment of **ICU delirium**. However, typical and atypical antipsychotics are commonly prescribed off-label for this condition.[108-109] Despite the frequency of use, published studies have not consistently demonstrated a benefit of antipsychotics in reducing the duration of **ICU delirium**, or, more importantly, in reducing the associated acute and long-term sequela.[110-112] In addition, antipsychotics are associated with serious adverse effects, including sedation, dizziness, extrapyramidal symptoms, and QT interval prolongation.[113-115] The use of atypical antipsychotics in **elderly** patients with dementia has also been associated with increased risk of stroke and death.[113,116,117]

Given the uncertain benefit of antipsychotics for this condition and the concern for **medication** adverse effects, particularly in the **elderly**, it is recommended that antipsychotics not be routinely used for the treatment of **ICU delirium**. This recommendation is supported by the SCCM 2018 guidelines as the authors recommend against the routine use of antipsychotics for the treatment of **ICU delirium**.[54] However, the guidelines also stipulate that in certain clinical scenarios short courses of haloperidol atypical antipsychotics may be beneficial. For example, **elderly** patients with hyperactive **delirium** may require some form of pharmacologic therapy to reduce agitation symptoms and prevent self- and caregiver-harm. Patients may also benefit from symptom control with antipsychotics if their **delirium** is associated with anxiety or hallucinations, which can be distressing. However, if an antipsychotic is initiated for **ICU delirium**, the need for continued use must be reassessed daily.[115]

Although the role of antipsychotics in the treatment of **ICU delirium** remains uncertain, there has also been interest in the use of antipsychotics for the prophylaxis of **ICU delirium**, particularly in high-risk populations such as the **elderly**. One study that evaluated this was a double-blind, randomized control trial of haloperidol for **ICU delirium** prophylaxis (Table 15.2).[118] A total of 457 adults 65 years and older, admitted to the **ICU** after noncardiac surgery, received either haloperidol 0.5 mg IV bolus followed by haloperidol 0.1 mg/h IV infusion or placebo for 12 hours. Patients who received haloperidol had reduced incidence of **delirium** in the first 7 days after surgery and a longer time to the onset of **delirium**. There was also a slight reduction in the **ICU** length of stay in the haloperidol group, but there was no difference in the hospital length of stay after surgery.

**TABLE 15.2 • Studies Evaluating Antipsychotics for ICU Delirium Prophylaxis**

| Study | Study Design | Population | Intervention | Outcomes |
|---|---|---|---|---|
| Wang et al[118] | RCT, double-blind, two-center | ICU patients, ≥65 y admitted after noncardiac surgery (n = 457) | Haloperidol 0.5 mg IV bolus, then 0.1 mg/h infusion or placebo for 12 h beginning at ICU admission; delirium screening with CAM-ICU once daily<br><br>Analgesia via epidural or PCA; if mechanically ventilated, sedation with propofol or midazolam infusion for a goal RASS −2 to +1 | Delirium incidence in 7 d after surgery, %<br>• haloperidol 15.3 vs placebo 23.2 (P = 0.031)<br>Time to onset of delirium, mean, d<br>• haloperidol 6.2 vs placebo 5.7 (P = 0.021)<br>Delirium-free days, mean, d<br>• haloperidol 6.8 vs placebo 6.7 (P = 0.027)<br>ICU LOS, median, h<br>• haloperidol 21.3 vs placebo 23 (P = 0.024)<br>Hospital LOS after surgery, median, d<br>• haloperidol 11 vs placebo 11 (P = 0.255) |

*(continued)*

**TABLE 15.2** • Studies Evaluating Antipsychotics for ICU Delirium Prophylaxis (*continued*)

| Study | Study Design | Population | Intervention | Outcomes |
|-------|-------------|-----------|--------------|----------|
| Hakim et al[119] | RCT, double-blind, single-center | Cardiothoracic surgical ICU patients, ≥65 y, nonintubated, with SSD after on-pump cardiac surgery (n = 101) | Risperidone 0.5 mg po q12h or placebo, continued until 24 h after resolution of SSD or until development of delirium. After development of delirium, open-label risperidone titrated to symptom control given to both groups. Delirium screening with ICDSC every 8 h<br><br>Analgesia with morphine infusion, acetaminophen IV, and ketorolac IV | Incidence of delirium, %<br>• risperidone 15.7 vs placebo 38 (P = 0.011)<br>Incidence of psychiatrist confirmed delirium, %<br>• risperidone 13.7 vs placebo 34 (P = 0.031)<br>ICU LOS, median, d<br>• risperidone 2 vs placebo 3 (P = 0.517)<br>Hospital LOS, median, d<br>• risperidone 6 vs placebo 6 (P = 0.056)<br>In patients who progressed to delirium, no difference between groups in duration of delirium, ICU or hospital LOS, highest risperidone dose, or highest score on ICDSC |
| Al-Qadheeb et al[120] | RCT, double-blind, single-center | Medical and surgical ICU patients, 18-84 y, mechanically ventilated, with SSD during first 4 d in ICU (n = 68) | Haloperidol 1 mg IV q6h or placebo, continued until patient developed clinical delirium, ICU discharge, 10 d of therapy, or adverse effect requiring discontinuation; delirium screening with ICDSC every 12 h<br><br>Analgesia and sedation was at the discretion of the bedside clinician | Incidence of delirium during study drug administration, %<br>• haloperidol 35.3 vs placebo 23.5 (P = 0.287)<br>Incidence of delirium during ICU admission, %<br>• haloperidol 35.3 vs placebo 26.5 (P = 0.43)<br>Time per study day spent agitated, median, h<br>• haloperidol 0 vs placebo 2 (P = 0.008)<br>Duration mechanical ventilation, median, d<br>• haloperidol 4.5 vs placebo 5 (P = 0.79)<br>ICU LOS, median, d<br>• haloperidol 6.5 vs placebo 7 (P = 0.66) |

ICDSC score— 0: not delirious, 1–3: subsyndromal delirium, ≥4: delirium; RASS score— −5: unarousable, −4: deep sedation, −3: moderate sedation, −2: light sedation, −1: drowsy, 0: alert and calm, +1: restless, +2: agitated, +3: very agitated, +4: combative.

Abbreviations: CAM-ICU, Confusion Assessment Method for the Intensive Care Unit; ICDSC, Intensive Care Delirium Screening Checklist; ICU, intensive care unit; IV, intravenous; LOS, length of stay; PCA, patient-controlled analgesia; po, orally; RASS, Richmond Agitation-Sedation Scale; RCT, randomized control trial; SSD, subsyndromal delirium.

Another double-blind, randomized control trial evaluated the use of risperidone for ICU **delirium** prophylaxis in patients who tested positive for subsyndromal **delirium** using the Intensive Care Delirium Screening Checklist (Table 15.2).[119] Unlike the Confusion Assessment Method for the ICU, the Intensive Care Delirium Screening Checklist allows for patients to be diagnosed with subsyndromal **delirium**, which indicates that a patient is at high risk of progressing to clinical **delirium**.[101,103] Other inclusion criteria included age 65 years or older, admitted to the ICU after on-pump cardiac bypass surgery, and extubated. A total of 101 patients were included and received either oral risperidone 0.5 mg every 12 hours or placebo, continued until 24 hours after resolution of subsyndromal **delirium** or until development of **delirium**. If patients in either group progressed to **delirium**, they were given open-label risperidone with up-titration for symptom control. Overall, fewer patients in the risperidone group transitioned to **delirium**. However, in patients who developed **delirium**, there was no difference in outcomes whether risperidone was initiated in the earlier, subsyndromal stages of **delirium** (risperidone group) or in the later stages of clinical **delirium** (placebo group).

Similarly, a recently published double-blind, randomized control trial also evaluated the use of antipsychotic prophylaxis to prevent the conversion from subsyndromal **delirium** to **delirium** (Table 15.2).[120] A total of 68 mechanically ventilated patients, aged 18 to 84 years, and diagnosed with subsyndromal **delirium** were randomized to receive either haloperidol 1 mg IV every 6 hours or placebo. The study drugs were given until the development of **delirium**, ICU discharge, 10 days of therapy had elapsed, or an adverse event that required discontinuation of the study drug occurred. There was no significant difference in the conversion to **delirium** during administration of the study drug or during ICU admission. However, patients who received haloperidol spent significantly less hours per day agitated. There was no difference between groups in the duration of mechanical ventilation or ICU length of stay.

Overall, there is inadequate evidence to recommend the use of antipsychotics for ICU **delirium** prophylaxis in critically ill older patients. The first two studies suggest a potential role of antipsychotic prophylaxis in postoperative **elderly** patients.[118,119] However, these patients had a low severity of illness and were discharged from the ICU in less than 24 hours. As a result, these findings cannot be applied to the general **elderly** critically ill population. In addition, although the last study was conducted in patients in the ICU with a higher severity of illness, it was not restricted to **elderly** patients, and excluded patients older than 85 years, again limiting the applicability to the **elderly** critically ill population.[120] Given the adverse effects associated with antipsychotics and the limited data to support their use for this indication, antipsychotic prophylaxis for ICU **delirium** in **elderly** critically ill patients is not recommended.

In addition to antipsychotics, there has been interest in the use of dexmedetomidine for prophylaxis and treatment of ICU **delirium**. As previously mentioned, studies have demonstrated reduced rates of **delirium** in patients who received dexmedetomidine for ICU sedation as compared to benzodiazepines or propofol.[34,35,38,94] However, it is unknown if this is due to a true anti-**delirium** effect of dexmedetomidine or is the result of dexmedetomidine being less deliriogenic than propofol and benzodiazepines. Several recently published studies have attempted to better elucidate the role of dexmedetomidine in the management of **ICU delirium**.

One study that evaluated dexmedetomidine for **delirium** prophylaxis was a double-blind, randomized control trial that included 700 patients aged 65 years and older who were admitted to the **ICU** after elective noncardiac surgery (Table 15.3).[121] Patients were randomized to a low dose dexmedetomidine infusion at 0.1 μg/kg/h or placebo, which began shortly after **ICU** admission on the day of surgery and continued until 08:00 AM the following day. Dexmedetomidine reduced the incidence of **delirium** and reduced the time to extubation. Although patients in the dexmedetomidine group also had a slight reduction in **ICU** length of stay, there was no difference in length of hospital stay or 30-day mortality.

Dexmedetomidine was also evaluated as a treatment for refractory **ICU delirium** in a nonrandomized control trial (Table 15.3).[122] A total of 132 nonintubated adult patients in the **ICU** with hyperactive **delirium** initially received escalating doses of haloperidol up to a total maximum daily dose of 30 mg. Forty-six (35%) patients did not achieve symptom control at the maximum daily dose and were switched to dexmedetomidine 0.2 to 0.7 μg/kg/h infusion. The 86 patients who responded to haloperidol subsequently received a haloperidol 1 mg/h infusion. Patients who failed haloperidol therapy and were switched to dexmedetomidine spent more time at goal sedation, had less oversedation, and a shorter **ICU** length of stay as compared to patients who received haloperidol. This study had several limitations, including the lack of randomization, lack of blinding, and, for the purposes of this review, was not specific to **elderly ICU** patients. Despite these limitations, the study does suggest a potential benefit of dexmedetomidine in treating the agitation associated with hyperactive **delirium**.

The benefit of dexmedetomidine for the treatment of hyperactive **delirium** was further supported in a recent double-blind, placebo-controlled trial (Table 15.3).[123] The study included 74 patients who were medically stable for extubation, but they required ongoing sedation and mechanical ventilation for severe agitation and **delirium**. Patients were randomized to receive a dexmedetomidine infusion, initiated at 0.5 μg/kg/h and titrated between 0 and 1.5 μg/kg/h, or placebo. Patients in the dexmedetomidine group had increased ventilator-free hours, had a shorter time to extubation, and a shorter time to the resolution of **delirium**. In addition, patients who received dexmedetomidine spent less time delirious in the **ICU** and were less likely to receive antipsychotics.

Overall, the literature suggests that there may be a role for dexmedetomidine in the management of **ICU delirium**.[121-123] One trial demonstrated reduced incidence of **delirium** when prophylactic dexmedetomidine was given to **elderly** patients.[121] However, this study included patients with low severity of illness who were briefly admitted

**TABLE 15.3** • Studies Evaluating Dexmedetomidine for ICU Delirium

| Study | Study Design | Population | Intervention | Outcomes |
|---|---|---|---|---|
| Su et al[121] | RCT, double-blind, two-center | ICU patients, ≥65 y, admitted after elective noncardiac surgery (n = 700) | DEX 0.1 μg/kg/h infusion or placebo beginning shortly after ICU admission on the day of surgery and continued until 8 AM on postoperative day 1 for ICU delirium prophylaxis. Delirium screening with CAM-ICU twice daily, starting ~24 h after surgery<br><br>Analgesia with epidural or PCA ± morphine IV or NSAIDs IV; if mechanically ventilated, sedation with propofol or midazolam bolus or infusion for a goal RASS of −2 to +1 | Incidence of delirium, %<br>• DEX 9.1 vs placebo 22.6 (P < 0.0001)<br>Time to onset of delirium, median, d<br>• DEX 6.5 vs placebo 5.8 (P < 0.0001)<br>Time to extubation, median, h<br>• DEX 4.6 vs placebo 6.9 (P = 0.031)<br>ICU LOS, median, h<br>• DEX 20.9 vs placebo 21.5 (P = 0.027)<br>Hospital LOS after surgery, median, d<br>• DEX 10 vs placebo 11 (P = 0.24)<br>All-cause 30-day mortality, %<br>• DEX 0.3 vs placebo 1.1 (P = 0.21) |
| Carrasco et al[122] | Nonrandomized controlled trial (quasi-experimental), single-center | Medical-surgical ICU patients, 18-95 y, nonintubated, with hyperactive delirium (n = 132) | Haloperidol 2.5-5 mg IV q10-30 min until RASS −2 to 0 or at max daily dose of 30 mg. Patients who reached 30 mg without response were nonresponders (n = 46) and switched to DEX 0.2-0.7 μg/kg/h infusion. Haloperidol responders (n = 86) received a haloperidol 0.5-1 mg/h infusion. The goal for both infusions was a RASS of 0. Delirium screening with ICDSC every 4 h and agitation screening with RASS every 1 h or less<br><br>Analgesia with acetaminophen IV q8h ± other analgesics as deemed necessary by nursing | Percentage of time RASS −2 to 0, %<br>• DEX 92.7 vs haloperidol 59.3 (P = 0.0001)<br>Percentage of time ICDSC < 4, %<br>• DEX 52 vs haloperidol 29.5 (P = 0.005)<br>Incidence excessive sedation (RASS −5 to −3), %<br>• DEX 0 vs haloperidol 11.6 (P = 0.01)<br>ICU LOS, mean, d<br>• DEX 3.1 vs haloperidol 6.4 (P < 0.0001)<br>ICU mortality, %<br>• DEX 0 vs haloperidol 2.3 (P = 0.69)<br>Hospital mortality, %<br>• DEX 8.6 vs haloperidol 8.1 (P = 0.09) |

*(continued)*

**TABLE 15.3** • Studies Evaluating Dexmedetomidine for ICU Delirium (*continued*)

| Study | Study Design | Population | Intervention | Outcomes |
|---|---|---|---|---|
| Reade et al.[123] | RCT, double-blind, multi-center | Medical-surgical ICU patients, ≥18 y, mechanically ventilated, with hyperactive delirium. Patients had a level of agitation that prevented sedative weaning and extubation (n = 74) | DEX infusion initiated at 0.5 µg/kg/h (range: 0-1.5 µg/kg/h) or placebo, titrated to RASS of 0 or physician goal. After 48 h of study drug, providers could stop the study drug and prescribe open-label DEX. If patient was receiving study drug at 7 d, it was considered a treatment failure and study drug was discontinued. Delirium screening with CAM-ICU every 8 h<br><br>Analgesia and additional sedation at discretion of treating physician | Time ventilator-free in 7 d after randomization, median, h<br>• DEX 144.8 vs placebo 127.5 (P = 0.01)<br>Time to RASS −2 to +1, IQR, h<br>• DEX 1 vs placebo 1 (P = 0.9)<br>Time to extubation, median, h<br>• DEX 21.9 vs placebo 44.3 (P < 0.001)<br>Time to first resolution of delirium, median, h<br>• DEX 23.3 vs placebo 40 (P = 0.01)<br>Time in ICU delirium, median, h<br>• DEX 36 vs placebo 62 (P = 0.009)<br>Received any antipsychotic on any day, %<br>• DEX 36.8 vs placebo 65.6 (P = 0.01)<br>No difference in ICU or hospital LOS |

ICDSC score— 0: not delirious, 1–3: subsyndromal delirium, ≥4: delirium; RASS score— −5: unarousable, −4: deep sedation, −3: moderate sedation, −2: light sedation, −1: drowsy, 0: alert and calm, +1: restless, +2: agitated, +3: very agitated, +4: combative.

Abbreviations: CAM-ICU, Confusion Assessment Method for the Intensive Care Unit; DEX, dexmedetomidine; ICDSC, Intensive Care Delirium Screening Checklist; ICU, intensive care unit; IV, intravenous; LOS, length of stay; NSAIDs, nonsteroidal anti-inflammatory drugs; PCA, patient-controlled analgesia; RASS, Richmond Agitation-Sedation Scale; RCT, randomized control trial.

to the ICU after an elective surgery. Therefore, the results may not be applicable to most **elderly** critically ill patients. Additionally, the 2018 SCCM guidelines suggest dexmedetomidine not be used as **ICU delirium** prophylaxis.[54] Although the two studies that evaluated dexmedetomidine for the treatment of hyperactive **delirium** were not restricted to **elderly** patients, dexmedetomidine seems to have a benefit in this specific subtype of **ICU delirium**.[122,123] Given the lack of other treatment options for this condition, it is reasonable to extrapolate these results to **elderly** critically ill patients with hyperactive **ICU delirium** and consider using dexmedetomidine before initiating antipsychotics. While the SCCM guidelines do not specifically mention dexmedetomidine for the treatment of **ICU delirium** in the **elderly**, they do suggest using dexmedetomidine for **delirium** in mechanically ventilated adults where agitation is preventing the patient from being extubated.[54] Ideally, future studies will assess the use of dexmedetomidine for the treatment of **ICU delirium** in the **elderly** population and assess if there is any role of dexmedetomidine in the management of hypoactive **delirium**.

# CONCLUSIONS

As the population is living longer and more **elderly** patients are admitted to the ICU, there is an increased need to understand how to optimize outcomes for this population.[1-4] Although overall survival from critical illness has improved, many of these **elderly** survivors leave the ICU with long-lasting cognitive, physical, and psychiatric impairments, or post–intensive care syndrome.[13,14,18,25-28] It is now known that short-term survival cannot be the only goal of critical care.[9,10,18,56] These disabilities have a devastating impact on patients; **elderly ICU** survivors often cannot return to work or to their homes, are newly dependent on others for their activities of daily living, and have a significantly reduced quality of life.[13,14,18,25-28,31] It is the responsibility of critical care providers to optimize a patient's chance of a quality recovery by reducing known iatrogenic risk factors, such as untreated pain, sedation, and **delirium**. However, this is often more challenging in **elderly** patients as a result of their physiologic changes and altered pharmacokinetics and pharmacodynamics.[29,62,63] Also, despite the significant amount of research regarding **ICU delirium**, how to best prevent and treat this condition is unknown. One therapy with promising benefits is the use of dexmedetomidine. Ideally, further studies will further describe the role of dexmedetomidine for **ICU delirium** in **elderly** patients and evaluate its impact on long-term outcomes.

# SUMMARY

Older adults currently account for over half of all ICU admissions. Although advances in critical care medicine have led to improved survival, critical illness is still associated with high short-term and long-term morbidity and mortality.

**Elderly** survivors of critical illness often have long-lasting physical, cognitive, and psychological disabilities. Several iatrogenic risk factors for post–critical illness impairments have been identified, including **delirium**, deep sedation, and inadequate analgesia. Multicomponent interventions or bundles, which target many of these risk factors, have been shown to improve patient outcomes. However, there is limited literature that addresses the optimal pharmacologic management of analgesia and sedation in **elderly** critically ill patients who are known to have altered pharmacokinetics and pharmacodynamics. There are also uncertainties regarding the treatment and prophylaxis of **delirium** in this patient population.

Various interventions can improve the pharmacologic management of pain, agitation, and **delirium** and subsequently improve outcomes in critically ill **elderly** patients. Pain should be managed with multimodal therapy and opioids used judiciously. Benzodiazepines should be avoided, and sedatives should be titrated to a light level of sedation. Only patients with hyperactive **delirium** should receive treatment with antipsychotics, and there is likely no role for antipsychotics in **delirium** prophylaxis. New literature suggests that dexmedetomidine may be effective in the prevention and treatment of ICU **delirium**.

**Elderly** patients are more sensitive to centrally acting **medications** and often require lower doses than do younger patients because of alterations in pharmacokinetics. A newer **medication**, dexmedetomidine, has demonstrated some benefit over other sedatives and may have a role in the management of **delirium**. Overall, more research is needed on the pharmacologic management of pain, sedation, and **delirium** in the **elderly** critically ill population.

## References

1. United Nations. Department of Economic and Social Affairs, Population Division. *World Population Ageing.* New York, NY: United Nations; 2013. Report Number: ST/ESA/SER.A/348.

2. Ortman JM, Velkoff VA, Hogan H. *An Aging Nation: The Older Population in the United States.* Washington, DC: US Census Bureau; 2014. Current Population Reports, P25-1140. https://www.census.gov/prod/2014pubs/p25-1140.pdf. Accessed June 15, 2017.

3. Angus DC, Shorr AF, White A, et al. Critical care delivery in the United States: distribution of services and compliance with Leapfrog recommendations. *Crit Care Med.* 2006;34:1016-1024.

4. Angus DC, Kelley MA, Schmitz RJ, et al. Caring for the critically ill patient. Current and projected workforce requirements for care of the critically ill and patients with pulmonary disease: can we meet the requirements of an aging population? *JAMA.* 2000;284:2762-2770.

5. Zambon M, Vincent JL. Mortality rates for patients with acute lung injury/ARDS have decreased over time. *Chest.* 2008;133:1120-1127.

6. Gaieski DF, Edwards JM, Kallan MJ, et al. Benchmarking the incidence and mortality of severe sepsis in the United States. *Crit Care Med.* 2013;41:1167-1174.

7. Stevenson EK, Rubenstein AR, Radin GT, et al. Two decades of mortality trends among patients with severe sepsis: a comparative meta-analysis. *Crit Care Med.* 2014;42:625-631.

8. Wunsch H, Guerra C, Barnato AE, et al. Three-year outcomes for Medicare beneficiaries who survive intensive care. *JAMA.* 2010;303:849-856.

9. Angus DC, Carlet J; 2002 Brussels Roundtable Participants. Surviving intensive care: a report from the 2002 Brussels Roundtable. *Intensive Care Med.* 2003;29:368-377.

10. Iwashyna TJ. Survivorship will be the defining challenge of critical care in the 21st century. *Ann Intern Med.* 2010;153:204-205.

11. Herridge MS, Cheung AM, Tansey CM. One-year outcomes in survivors of the acute respiratory distress syndrome. *N Engl J Med.* 2003;348:683-693.

12. Schelling G, Stoll C, Haller M, et al. Health-related quality of life and posttraumatic stress disorder in survivors of the acute respiratory distress syndrome. *Crit Care Med.* 1998;26:651-659.

13. Unroe M, Kahn JM, Carson SS, et al. One-year trajectories of care and resource utilization for recipients of prolonged mechanical ventilation: a cohort study. *Ann Intern Med.* 2010;153:167-175.

14. Jackson JC, Pandharipande PP, Girard TD, et al. Depression, posttraumatic stress disorder, and functional disability in survivors of critical illness: results from the BRAIN ICU investigation: a longitudinal cohort study. *Lancet Respir Med.* 2014;2:369-379.

15. Pandharipande PP, Girard TD, Jackson JC, et al. Long-term cognitive impairments after critical illness. *N Engl J Med.* 2013;369:1306-1316.

16. Timmers TK, Verhofstad MH, Moons KH, et al. Long-term quality of life after surgical intensive care admission. *Arch Surg.* 2011;146:412-418.

17. Weinert CR, Gross CR, Kangas JR, et al. Health-related quality of life after acute lung injury. *Am J Respir Crit Care Med.* 1997;156:1120-1128.

18. Needham DM, Davidson J, Cohen H, et al. Improving long-term outcomes after discharge from the intensive care unit: report from a stakeholders' conference. *Crit Care Med.* 2012;40:502-509.

19. Jackson JC, Mitchell N, Hopkins RO. Cognitive functioning, mental health, and quality of life in ICU survivors: an overview. *Crit Care Clin.* 2009;25:615-628.

20. Desai SV, Law TJ, Needham DM. Long-term complications of critical care. *Crit Care Med.* 2011;39:371-379.

21. Battle CE, Lovett S, Hutchings H. Chronic pain in survivors of critical illness: a retrospective analysis of incidence and risk factors. *Crit Care.* 2013;17:R101.

22. Kyranou M, Puntillo K. The transition from acute to chronic pain: might intensive care unit patients be at risk? *Ann Intensive Care.* 2012;2:36.

23. De Jonghe B, Lacherade JC, Sharshar T, et al. Intensive care unit-acquired weakness: risk factors and prevention. *Crit Care Med.* 2009;37:S309-S315.

24. Needham DM. Mobilizing patients in the intensive care unit: improving neuromuscular weakness and physical function. *JAMA.* 2008;300:1685-1690.

25. Heyland DK, Garland A, Bagshaw SM, et al. Recovery after critical illness in patients aged 80 years or older: a multi-center prospective observational cohort study. *Intensive Care Med.* 2015;41:1911-1920.

26. Dowdy DW, Eid MP, Sedrakyan A, et al. Quality of life in adult survivors of critical illness: a systematic review of the literature. *Intensive Care Med.* 2005;31:611-620.

27. Brummel NE, Balas MC, Morandi A, et al. Understanding and reducing disability in older adults following critical illness. *Crit Care Med.* 2015;43:1265-1275.

28. Malone ML. How to improve care for older patients in the intensive care unit. In: Boehm L, Ely EW, Mion L, eds. *Acute Care for Elders: A Model of Interdisciplinary Care.* New York, NY: Springer Science and Business Media; 2014.

29. Pisani MA. Considerations in caring for the critically ill older patient. *J Intensive Care Med.* 2009;24:83-95.

30. Schweickert WD, Pohlman MC, Pohlman AS, et al. Early physical and occupational therapy in mechanically ventilated, critically ill patients: a randomised controlled trial. *Lancet.* 2009;373:1874-1882.

31. Chelluri L, Im KA, Belle SH, et al. Long-term mortality and quality of life after prolonged mechanical ventilation. *Crit Care Med.* 2004;32:61-69.

32. Mira JC, Cuschieri J, Ozrazgat-Baslanti T, et al. The epidemiology of chronic critical illness after severe traumatic injury at two level-one trauma centers. *Crit Care Med.* 2017;45:1989-1996.

33. Vasilevskis EE, Ely EW, Speroff T, et al. Reducing iatrogenic risks: ICU-acquired delirium and weakness–crossing the quality chasm. *Chest.* 2010;138:1224-1233.

34. Riker RR, Shehabi Y, Bokesch PM, et al. Dexmedetomidine vs midazolam for sedation of critically ill patients: a randomized trial. *JAMA.* 2009;301:489-499.

35. Pandharipande PP, Pun BT, Herr DL, et al. Effect of sedation with dexmedetomidine vs lorazepam on acute brain dysfunction in mechanically ventilated patients: the MENDS randomized controlled trial. *JAMA.* 2007;298:2644-2653.

36. Pandharipande P, Shintani A, Peterson J, et al. Lorazepam is an independent risk factor for transitioning to delirium in intensive care unit patients. *Anesthesiology.* 2006;104:21–26.

37. Pandharipande P, Cotton BA, Shintani A, et al. Prevalence and risk factors for development of delirium in surgical and trauma intensive care unit patients. *J Trauma.* 2008;65:34-41.

38. Liu X, Xie G, Zhang K, et al. Dexmedetomidine vs propofol sedation reduces delirium in patients after cardiac surgery: a meta-analysis with trial sequential analysis of randomized controlled trials. *J Crit Care.* 2017;38:190-196.

39. Lonardo NW, Mone MC, Nirula R, et al. Propofol is associated with favorable outcomes compared to benzodiazepines in ventilated intensive care unit patients. *Am J Respir Crit Care Med.* 2014;189:1383-1394.

40. Carson SS, Kress JP, Rodgers JE, et al. A randomized trial of intermittent lorazepam versus propofol with daily interruption in mechanically ventilated patients. *Crit Care Med.* 2006;34:1326-1332.

41. Balzer F, Weib B, Kumpf O, et al. Early deep sedation is associated with decreased in-hospital and two-year follow-up survival. *Crit Care.* 2015;19:197.

42. Kress JP, Pohlman AS, O'Connor MF, et al. Daily interruption of sedative infusions in critically ill patients undergoing mechanical ventilation. *N Engl J Med.* 2000;342:1471-1477.

43. Treggiari MM, Romand JA, Yanez ND, et al. Randomized trial of light versus deep sedation on mental health after critical illness. *Crit Care Med.* 2009;37:2527-2534.

44. Shehabi Y, Bellomo R, Reade MC, et al. Early intensive care sedation predicts long-term mortality in ventilated critically ill patients. *Am J Respir Crit Care Med.* 2012;186:724-731.

45. Tanaka LM, Azevedo LC, Park M, et al. Early sedation and clinical outcomes of mechanically ventilated patients: a prospective multicenter cohort study. *Crit Care.* 2014;18:R156.

46. Ouimet S, Kavanagh BP, Gottfried SB, et al. Incidence, risk factors and consequences of ICU delirium. *Intensive Care Med.* 2007;33:66-73.

47. Diallo B, Kautz DD. Better pain management for elders in the intensive care unit. *Dimens Crit Care Nurs.* 2014;33:316-319.

48. Barr J, Fraser GL, Puntillo K, et al. Clinical practice guidelines for the management of pain, agitation, and delirium in adult patients in the intensive care unit. *Crit Care Med.* 2013;41:263-306.

49. Lin SM, Huang CD, Liu CY, et al. Risk factors for the development of early-onset delirium and the subsequent clinical outcome in mechanically ventilated patients. *J Crit Care.* 2008;23:372-379.

50. Lat I, McMillian W, Taylor S, et al. The impact of delirium on clinical outcomes in mechanically ventilated surgical and trauma patients. *Crit Care Med.* 2009;37:1898-1905.

51. Girard TD, Jackson JC, Pandharipande PP, et al. Delirium as a predictor of long-term cognitive impairment in survivors of critical illness. *Crit Care Med.* 2010;38:1513-1520.

52. Brummel NE, Jackson JC, Pandharipande PP, et al. Delirium in the ICU and subsequent long-term disability among survivors of mechanical ventilation. *Crit Care Med.* 2014;42:369-377.

53. Abelha FJ, Luis C, Veiga D, et al. Outcome and quality of life in patients with postoperative delirium during an ICU stay following major surgery. *Crit Care.* 2013;17:R257.

54. Devlin JW, Skrobik Y, Gélinas C, et al. Clinical practice guidelines for the prevention and management of pain, agitation/sedation, delirium, immobility, and sleep disruption in adult patients in the ICU. *Crit Care Med.* 2018;46(9):825-873.

55. Morandi A, Brummel NE, Ely EW. Sedation, delirium and mechanical ventilation: the "ABCDE" approach. *Curr Opin Crit Care.* 2011;17:43-49.

56. Ely EW. The ABCDEF bundle: science and philosophy of how ICU liberation serves patients and families. *Crit Care Med.* 2017;45:321-330.

57. Marra A, Ely EW, Pandharipande PP, et al. The ABCDEF bundle in critical care. *Crit Care Clin.* 2017;33:225-243.

58. ICU Liberation website. ICU Liberation: ABCDEF Bundles. http://www.iculiberation.org/SiteCollectionDocuments/Bundles-ICU-Liberation-ABCDEF.pdf. Accessed June 30, 2017.

59. Girard TD, Kress JP, Fuchs BD, et al. Efficacy and safety of a paired sedation and ventilator weaning protocol for mechanically ventilated patients in intensive care (Awakening and Breathing Controlled trial): a randomized controlled trial. *Lancet.* 2008;371:126-134.

60. Balas MC, Vasilevskis EE, Olsen KM, et al. Effectiveness and safety of the awakening and breathing coordination, delirium monitoring/management, and early exercise/mobility bundle. *Crit Care Med.* 2014;42:1024-1036.

61. Barnes-Daly MA, Phillips G, Ely EW. Improving hospital survival and reducing brain dysfunction at seven California community hospitals: implementing PAD guidelines via the ABCDEF bundle in 6064 patients. *Crit Care Med.* 2017;45:171-178.

62. Mangoni AA, Jackson SH. Age-related changes in pharmacokinetics and pharmacodynamics: basic principles and practical applications. *Br J Clin Pharmacol.* 2004;57:6-14.

63. Bowie MW, Slattum PW. Pharmacodynamics in older adults: a review. *Am J Geriatr Pharmacother.* 2007;5:263-303.

64. Bender AD. Effect of age on intestinal absorption: implications for drug absorption in the elderly. *J Am Geriatr Soc.* 1968;16:1331-1339.

65. Bodenham A, Shelly MP, Park GR. The altered pharmacokinetics and pharmacodynamics of drugs commonly used in critically ill patients. *Clin Pharmacokinet*. 1988;14:347-373.

66. Smith BS, Yogaratnam D, Levasseur-Franklin KE, et al. Introduction to drug pharmacokinetics in the critically ill patient. *Chest*. 2012;141:1327-1336.

67. Fulop T Jr, Worum I, Csongor J, Fóris G, Leövey A. Body composition in elderly people: determination of body composition by multiisotope method and the elimination kinetics of these isotopes in healthy elderly subjects. *Gerontology*. 1985;31:6-14.

68. Schmucker DL. Liver function and phase 1 metabolism in the elderly: a paradox. *Drugs Aging*. 2001;18:837-851.

69. Weinstein JR, Anderson S. The aging kidney: physiological changes. *Adv Chronic Kidney Dis*. 2010;17:302-307.

70. Rowe JW, Andres R, Tobin JD, et al. The effect of age on creatinine clearance in men: a cross-sectional and longitudinal study. *J Gerontol*. 1976;31:155-163.

71. Erstad BL, Puntillo K, Gilbert HC, et al. Pain management principles in the critically ill. *Chest*. 2009;135:1075-1086.

72. Payen JF, Bosson JL, Chanques G, et al. Pain assessment is associated with decreased duration of mechanical ventilation in the intensive care unit: a post hoc analysis of the DOLOREA study. *Anesthesiology*. 2009;111:1308-1316.

73. Liu D, Lyu J, Zhao H, et al. The influence of analgesic-based sedation protocols on delirium and outcomes in critically ill patients: a randomized controlled trial. *PloS One*. 2017;12:e0184310.

74. Gelinas C, Fillion L, Puntillo KA, et al. Validation of the critical-care pain observation tool in adult patients. *Am J Crit Care*. 2006;15:420-427.

75. Payen JF, Bru O, Bosson JL, et al. Assessing pain in critically ill sedated patients by using a behavioral pain scale. *Crit Care Med*. 2001;29:2258-2263.

76. Trescot AM, Datta S, Lee M, et al. Opioid pharmacology. *Pain Physician*. 2008;11:S133-S153.

77. Devlin JW, Roberts RJ. Pharmacology of commonly used analgesics and sedatives in the ICU: benzodiazepines, propofol, and opioids. *Anesthesiology Clin*. 2011;29:567-585.

78. Chau DL, Walker V, Pai L, et al. Opiates and elderly: use and side effects. *Clin Interv Aging*. 2008;3:273-278.

79. Joshi GP. Multimodal analgesia techniques and postoperative rehabilitation. *Anesthesiol Clin North Am*. 2005;23:185-202.

80. Mamoun NF, Lin P, Zimmerman NM, et al. Intravenous acetaminophen analgesia after cardiac surgery: a randomized, blinded, controlled superiority trial. *J Thorac Cardiovasc Surg*. 2016;152: 881-889.

81. Jelacic S, Bollag L, Bowdle A, et al. Intravenous acetaminophen as an adjunct analgesic in cardiac surgery reduces opioid consumption but not opioid-related adverse effects: a randomized controlled trial. *J Cardiothorac Vasc Anesth*. 2016;30:997-1004.

82. Memis D, Inal MT, Kavalci G, et al. Intravenous paracetamol reduced the use of opioids, extubation time, and opioid-related adverse effects after major surgery in intensive care unit. *J Crit Care*. 2010;25:458-462.

83. O'Day R, Graham GG. Non-steroidal anti-inflammatory drugs (NSAIDs). *BMJ*. 2013;346:f3195.

84. Neurontin (Gabapentin) [package Insert]. New York, NY: Pfizer; 2015.

85. Schweickert WD, Gehlbach BK, Pohlman AS, et al. Daily interruption of sedative infusions and complications of critical illness in mechanically ventilated patients. *Crit Care Med*. 2004;32:1272-1276.

86. Devlin JW. The pharmacology of oversedation in mechanically ventilated adults. *Curr Opin Crit Care*. 2008;14:403-407.

87. Sessler CN, Gosnell MS, Grap MJ, et al. The Richmond agitation-sedation scale: validity and reliability in adult intensive care unit patients. *Am J Respir Crit Care Med*. 2002;166:1338-1344.

88. Bauer TM, Ritz R, Haberthür C, et al. Prolonged sedation due to accumulation of conjugated metabolites of midazolam. *Lancet*. 1995;346:145-147.

89. Greenblatt DJ, Abernethy DR, Locniskar A, et al. Effect of age, gender, and obesity on midazolam kinetics. *Anesthesiology*. 1984;61:27-35.

90. Diprivan (Propofol) [package Insert]. Lake Zurich, IL: Fresenius Kabi; 2014.

91. Gerlach AT, Dasta JF. Dexmedetomidine: an updated review. *Ann Pharmacother*. 2007;41:245-254.

92. Djaiani G, Silverton N, Fedorko L, et al. Dexmedetomidine versus propofol sedation reduces delirium after cardiac surgery: a randomized controlled trial. *Anesthesiology*. 2016;124:362-368.

93. Jakob S, Ruokonen E, Grounds R, et al. Dexmedetomidine vs midazolam or propofol for sedation during prolonged mechanical ventilation: two randomized controlled trials. *JAMA*. 2012;307(11):1151-1160.

94. Precedex (Dexmedetomidine) [package Insert]. Lake Forest, IL: Hospira; 2016.

95. American Psychiatric Association. *Diagnostic and Statistical Manual of Mental Disorders*. 5th ed. Arlington, VA: American Psychiatric Publishing; 2013.

96. Peterson JF, Pun BT, Dittus RS, et al. Delirium and its motoric subtypes: a study of 614 critically ill patients. *J Am Geriatr Soc*. 2006;54:479-484.

97. Liptzin B, Levkoff SE. An empirical study of delirium subtypes. *Br J Psychiatry*. 1992;161:843-845.

98. Van Rompaey B, Elseviers MM, Schuurmans MJ, et al. Risk factors for delirium in intensive care patients: a prospective cohort study. *Crit Care*. 2009;13:R77.

99. Pisani MA, Murphy TE, Van Ness PH, et al. Characteristics associated with delirium in older patients in a medical intensive care unit. *Arch Intern Med*. 2007;167:1629-1634.

100. Hopkins RO, Suchyta MR, Farrer TJ, et al. Improving post-intensive care unit neuropsychiatric outcomes: understanding cognitive effects of physical activity. *Am J Respir Crit Care Med*. 2012;186:1220-1228.

101. Gross AL, Jones RN, Habtemariam BA, et al. Delirium and long-term cognitive trajectory among persons with dementia. *Arch Intern Med*. 2012;172:1324-1331.

102. Fong TG, Jones RN, Shi P, et al. Delirium accelerates cognitive decline in Alzheimer disease. *Neurology*. 2009;72:1570-1575.

103. Bergeron N, Dubois MJ, Dumont M, et al. Intensive care delirium screening checklist: evaluation of a new screening tool. *Intensive Care Med*. 2001;27:859-864.

104. Ely EW, Inouye SK, Bernard GR, et al. Delirium in mechanically ventilated patients: validity and reliability of the confusion assessment method for the intensive care unit (CAM-ICU). *JAMA*. 2001;286:2703-2710.

105. Brummel NE, Girard TD. Preventing delirium in the intensive care unit. *Crit Care Clin*. 2013;29:51-65.

106. Jackson P, Khan A. Delirium in critically ill patients. *Crit Care Clin*. 2015;31:589-603.

107. Hsieh SJ, Ely EW, Gong MN. Can intensive care unit delirium be prevented and reduced? Lessons learned and future directions. *Ann Am Thorac Soc*. 2013;10:648-656.

108. Tomichek JE, Stollings JL, Pandharipande PP, et al. Antipsychotic prescribing patterns during and after critical illness: a prospective cohort study. *Crit Care*. 2016;20:378.

109. Patel RP, Gambrell M, Speroff T, et al. Delirium and sedation in the intensive care unit: survey of behaviors and attitudes of 1384 healthcare professionals. *Crit Care Med*. 2009;37:825-832.

110. Page VJ, Ely EW, Gates S, et al. Effect of intravenous haloperidol on the duration of delirium and coma in critically ill patients (Hope-ICU): a randomised, double-blind, placebo-controlled trial. *Lancet Respir Med*. 2013;1:515-523.

111. Girard TD, Pandharipande PP, Carson SS, et al. Feasibility, efficacy, and safety of antipsychotics for intensive care unit delirium: the MIND randomized, placebo controlled trial. *Crit Care Med*. 2010;38:428-437.

112. Devlin JW, Skrobik Y, Riker RR, et al. Impact of quetiapine on resolution of individual delirium symptoms in critically ill patients with delirium: a post-hoc analysis of a double-blind, randomized, placebo-controlled study. *Crit Care*. 2011;15:R215.

113. Maher AR, Maglione M, Bagley S, et al. Efficacy and comparative effectiveness of atypical antipsychotic medications for off-label uses in adults. *JAMA*. 2011;306:1359-1369.

114. Muench J, Hamer AM. Adverse effects of antipsychotic medications. *Am Fam Physician*. 2010;81:617-622.

115. Inouye SK, Marcantonio ER, Metzger ED. Doing damage in delirium: the hazards of antipsychotic treatment in elderly persons. *Lancet Psychiatry*. 2014;1:312-315.

116. Schneider LS, Dagerman KS, Insel P. Risk of death with atypical antipsychotic drug treatment for dementia: meta-analysis of randomized placebo-controlled trials. *JAMA*. 2005;294:1934-1943.

117. Shin JY, Choi NK, Jung SY, et al. Risk of ischemic stroke with the use of risperidone, quetiapine and olanzapine in elderly patients: a population-based, case-crossover study. *J Psychopharmacol*. 2013;27:638-644.

118. Wang W, Li HL, Wang DX, et al. Haloperidol prophylaxis decreases delirium incidence in elderly patients after noncardiac surgery: a randomized controlled trial. *Crit Care Med.* 2012;40:731-739.

119. Hakim SM, Othman AI, Naoum DO. Early treatment with risperidone for subsyndromal delirium after on-pump cardiac surgery in the elderly: a randomized trial. *Anesthesiology.* 2012;116:987-997.

120. Al-Qadheeb NS, Skrobik Y, Schumaker G, et al. Preventing ICU subsyndromal delirium conversion to delirium with low-dose IV haloperidol: a double-blind, placebo controlled pilot study. *Crit Care Med.* 2016;44:583-591.

121. Su X, Meng ZT, Wu XH, et al. Dexmedetomidine for prevention of delirium in elderly patients after noncardiac surgery: a randomised, double-blind, placebo controlled trial. *Lancet.* 2016;388:1893-1902.

122. Carrasco G, Baeza N, Cabre L, et al. Dexmedetomidine for the treatment of hyperactive delirium refractory to haloperidol in nonintubated ICU patients: a nonrandomized controlled trial. *Crit Care Med.* 2016;44:1295-1306.

123. Reade MC, Eastwood GM, Bellomo R, et al. Effect of dexmedetomidine added to standard care on ventilator-free time in patients with agitated delirium: a randomized clinical trial. *JAMA.* 2016;315:1460-1468.

# Overview of the Diagnosis, Evaluation, and Novel Treatment Strategies for Ophthalmic Emergencies in the Hospitalized Geriatric Patient

# CHAPTER 16

Laura Palazzolo, MD and Matthew Gorski, MD

## BACKGROUND

The following review aims to familiarize the hospitalist with common **ophthalmic emergencies** that may present in the hospitalized **geriatric** patient. It highlights key features of the ophthalmic examination and early identification and treatment of **ophthalmic emergencies**, including transient monocular loss of vision with risk of future ischemic complications, **central retinal artery occlusion (CRAO)**, **giant-cell arteritis (GCA)**, **retinal detachment (RD)**, **acute angle closure glaucoma (AACG)**, **orbital cellulitis**, **orbital compartment syndrome**, and concerns after orbital trauma.

## OPHTHALMIC EXAMINATION

A basic ophthalmic examination includes measurement of visual acuity, pupillary assessment, review of extraocular movements, and confrontational visual fields. A color vision test can narrow a differential diagnosis involving the optic nerve. If tonometry is available, intraocular pressure (IOP) should be measured. A fundus examination can be performed with a direct or an indirect ophthalmoscope, and examination should be performed with a slit lamp if available. A dilated examination should be avoided if there is suspicion of **AACG** or injury to the iris. In addition, a patient should not be pharmacologically dilated if serial neurologic examinations and pupillary assessments are required because this will interfere with monitoring.

The hospitalized patient may present unique obstacles to ophthalmic examination. For a bed-bound inpatient, there is limited mobility for the slit lamp and the fundus will be limited to 20-diopter (D) examinations, which have increased range of peripheral fundus visualization, but lack the detail of a 90-D examination.

When assessing visual function, a focused ocular review of systems should include visual acuity, diplopia, photophobia, photopsia (flashing lights), ocular pain, or headaches. The timeline of symptom onset and duration should be quantified; review ocular history including trauma, surgery, history of ocular disease, and contact lens wear; evaluate family history of ophthalmic conditions, especially those with a strong inheritance pattern such as macular degeneration and glaucoma.

# OCULAR EMERGENCIES

The following highlights the treatment of ocular emergencies that may arise in the hospitalized patient (Table 16.1). Early recognition and treatment is critical for preserving visual function. Sudden vision loss is always an alarming symptom, and the diagnosis should further be triaged with description of pain or no pain and history of trauma.

# SUDDEN VISION LOSS WITHOUT PAIN

## Central Retinal Artery Occlusion

CRAO is an **ophthalmic emergency** analogous to a stroke of the eye.[1,2] The central retinal artery is a branch of the ophthalmic artery, the first branch of the internal carotid artery, and it supplies the inner layer of the retina. Loss of central retinal artery blood supply causes retinal ischemia and subsequent vision loss. The incidence of CRAO is estimated to be 0.85/100 000 population per year and occurs most often in elderly populations, especially patients with cardiovascular risk factors including coronary artery disease, hypertension, hyperlipidemia, and previous stroke.[3,4] There are three subclassifications of nonarteritic **CRAO**:

1. Nonarteritic transient: secondary to thromboembolic causes

2. Nonarteritic permanent: secondary to arterial inflammation

3. Nonarteritic permanent with cilioretinal sparing: approximately 30% to 50% of patients have a cilioretinal artery, a branch of the short posterior ciliary artery that supplies the fovea responsible for fine central vision.[1,5] The cilioretinal artery is sometimes spared in **CRAO**, and patients with this anatomic variant sometimes have better visual outcomes.

**TABLE 16.1** • Summary of Ophthalmic Emergencies

| Ophthalmic Emergency | Common Clinical Features | Summary of Treatment |
|---|---|---|
| Transient monocular blindness, "amaurosis fugax" | • Transient (seconds-minutes), painless vision loss<br>• Monocular | • Screening and treatment of stroke risk factors<br>• Carotid endarterectomy (surgical indications under debate) |
| Permanent central retinal artery occlusion | • Sudden, nonremitting, painless vision loss<br>• Monocular | • Screening and treatment of stroke risk factors<br>• Carotid endarterectomy<br>• Ongoing areas of research: treatments to increase retinal perfusion |
| Giant-cell arteritis | • Sudden, nonremitting, painless vision loss<br>• Monocular<br>• Systemic features: jaw claudication, temporal or occipital headache, scalp tenderness, weight loss<br>• High association with polymyalgia rheumatic<br>• Elevated ESR > 50 | • High-dose glucocorticoids: pulse vs nonpulse, long taper required<br>• Glucocorticoid-sparing agents: tocilizumab (FDA approved), MTX, other agents for ongoing research |
| Retinal detachment | • Sudden, painless<br>• Most often spontaneous, may be from trauma<br>• New-onset floaters, photopsia, visual field loss<br>• Increased risk with myopia | • Surgical management |
| Acute angle closure glaucoma | • Painful<br>• Fixed, mid-dilated pupil<br>• Conjunctival injection<br>• Blurry vision with halos around lights<br>• High intraocular pressure<br>• Systemic: gastrointestinal distress, headache | • Intraocular pressure–lowering agents |
| Orbital cellulitis | • Painful, sudden vision loss<br>• Proptosis<br>• Chemosis (conjunctival edema), lid edema<br>• Limited extraocular movements<br>• History of sinusitis | Broad-spectrum intravenous antibiotics<br>CT scan for periosteal abscess, abscess drainage |
| Orbital compartment syndrome | • Proptosis<br>• High intraocular pressure<br>• Limited extraocular movements<br>• Most commonly caused by retrobulbar hemorrhage | • Surgical management: decompression with lateral canthotomy or cantholysis |
| Ruptured globe | • History of penetrating trauma to eye<br>• Shallow anterior chamber<br>• Irregularly shaped pupil<br>• Vitreous hemorrhage | • Surgical management |
| Orbital wall fractures and entrapment | • Tenderness of orbital rim<br>• Bony step-offs<br>• Ptosis<br>• Enophthalmos or exophthalmos | • Surgical management |

Abbreviations: CT, computed tomography; ESR, erythrocyte sedimentation rate; FDA, U.S. Food and Drug Administration; MTX, methotrexate.

The following sections describe nonarteritic transient **CRAO** (**transient monocular blindness [TMB]**), nonarteritic permanent **CRAO**, and **GCA**, the most common type of arteritic **CRAO**.

## Nonarteritic Transient Central Retinal Artery Occlusion: Transient Monocular Blindness

**TMB** is less specifically called "amaurosis fugax." **TMB** is considered a transient ischemic attack (TIA) of the eye. It is an important warning sign that must be addressed immediately because it frequently precedes permanent vision loss from **CRAO** (see Section "Nonarteritic Permanent Central Retinal Artery Occlusion") or a larger stroke.[6] When studied, the risk of progression to permanent visual loss after **TMB** was 1% to 2% per year; and the risk of stroke or death after **TMB** was 3% to 5% per year.[6,7]

Vision loss in **TMB** is painless, lasts seconds to minutes, and then reverses. Patients often describe dark or hazy vision, often altitudinal, in one eye.[6,8] Most commonly, the vision loss is caused by a retinal embolus from the ipsilateral internal carotid artery. Patients with a high degree of internal carotid artery stenosis are at greatest risk of these atherothromboemboli.[4,9] Other causes include thrombosis in the posterior ciliary artery or central retinal vein, embolism from atrial fibrillation, internal carotid artery dissection, vascular malformations, and fibromuscular dysplasia.[6,8]

**TMB** requires urgent evaluation for underlying cardiovascular causes. In elderly populations, causes of retinal emboli may include carotid artery occlusion, other atherosclerotic large-vessel disease, or from cardiac abnormalities. The workup for **TMB** should include a complete ophthalmoscopic examination, imaging of the carotids, echocardiogram, and laboratory testing. Funduscopy will evaluate for primary ocular etiologies of **TMB**. Retinal emboli may be directly viewed on funduscopy, although these are transient and often may not be apparent.[9] Fundoscopy may also reveal cotton wool spots, retinal hemorrhages, retinal whitening, or dilated retinal veins.[8] A carotid ultrasound is vital in the workup of **TMB** to evaluate for arterial stenosis and dissection, and it should be performed regardless of whether there was evidence of embolism on funduscopic examination. Several studies have demonstrated significant stenosis in patients with **CRAO** or stroke. In the Northern Manhattan Stroke Study (NOMASS), 7% of patients with first-time strokes had carotid stenosis greater than 60%; and in a large retrospective chart review of 43 patients with **CRAO**, 14% of patients had stenosis greater than 50%.[10,11] If carotid Doppler has equivocal results and there is a high suspicion for carotid stenosis in a symptomatic patient with **TMB**, then further imaging studies such as magnetic resonance angiography or computed tomography (CT) angiography may be warranted.[12] For elderly patients, a full review of systems and a laboratory workup with complete blood count, erythrocyte sedimentation rate (ESR), and C-reactive protein (CRP) measurements can help evaluate for **GCA**. If a cause cannot be identified from these measures, then echocardiography, particularly using the transesophageal approach, may be helpful to evaluate other embolic sources.[6,9]

The treatment of **TMB** is multifaceted. It involves balancing maximal medical therapy to reduce cardiovascular risk factors and possible need for surgical intervention. The need for surgical revascularization with carotid endarterectomy (CEA) or carotid artery stenting after **TMB** is debated.[12] Of note, the risk of progression to stroke after **TMB** is about half the risk of stroke after a hemispheric TIA, and the strokes after **TMB** tend to be less disabling.[7] As a result, there is a concern about whether conservative medical management is more appropriate. The North American Symptomatic Carotid Endarterectomy Trial (NASCET) and the European Carotid Surgery Trial (ECST) were two large and influential trials to investigate indications for CEA.[13,14] NASCET recommends CEA for **TMB** patients with >70% carotid stenosis and at least one risk factor for stroke, including age 75 years or older, male sex, history of hemispheric TIA or stroke, history of intermittent claudication, absence of collateral circulation, and internal carotid artery stenosis 80% to 99%.[7] ECST also supported CEA for patients with high-grade symptomatic carotid stenosis.[15]

Medical management for patients after **TMB** primarily focuses on reducing cardiovascular risk factors with antiplatelet therapy,[16-20] antihypertensives,[21-23] cholesterol-lowering medications,[24] and treatment of any comorbid condition such as atrial fibrillation. In addition, lifestyle modification is stressed, including smoking cessation, limiting alcohol intake, and increasing daily exercise.

## Nonarteritic Permanent Central Retinal Artery Occlusion

Nonarteritic permanent **CRAO** comprises most of **CRAO** cases. Vision loss is sudden, painless, and monocular. The **CRAO** is most often caused by an embolus to the central retinal artery.[2] Visual acuity should be measured on presentation and is often very poor in the involved eye. In a survey of 260 patients with **CRAO**, 80% of patients had a visual acuity of 20/400 or worse.[25]

Platelet fibrin thrombi, cholesterol, and calcium emboli have been observed on ophthalmoscopy. Cholesterol emboli, called Hollenhorst plaques, appear as small, yellow plaques, whereas calcium emboli appear white.[5] However, emboli are not directly observed in every case of **CRAO**. For example, in a retrospective study of 89 patients, emboli were only seen in 15 of 89 patients.[26] Therefore, it is most important to treat on the basis of the entire clinical picture.

In an observational study of patients with **CRAO**, 90% of patients had a cherry-red spot at presentation.[27] Other acute funduscopic findings included retinal opacity in the posterior pole, retinal arterial attenuation, optic disc edema, and optic disc pallor.[5,27] Chronic changes observed include optic atrophy, retinal arterial attenuation, cilioretinal collaterals, and macular retinal pigment epithelial changes.[27]

An evaluation for atherosclerotic risk factors should be undertaken after the acute stage of **CRAO**, including a history of cardiovascular disease, diabetes, hypertension, hyperlipidemia, previously **TMB** or TIA, and smoking.[1,5] As in the workup of **TMB**, carotid Doppler test should be obtained. In addition, fluorescein angiography is used to evaluate the retinal vessels. In **CRAO**, it will show vascular filling defects or delayed filling of the affected vessels.[5]

Timeline of treatment is critical to treatment efficacy. In a 2004 study, **CRAO** was induced in 38 elderly rhesus monkeys with hypertension and atherosclerosis, and the rate of ischemia was measured.[28] In the first 97 minutes after **CRAO**, researchers found no detectable retinal damage. After 240 minutes, the effects of ischemia were irreversible. The study demonstrates the importance of early intervention in **CRAO**. However, the timeline may not apply exactly to humans. In the study of rhesus monkeys, the researchers had a controlled environment and were able to induce a complete **CRAO**. In patients, emboli do not always cause a 100% occlusion, and the timeline to irreversible vision loss may therefore be slightly extended.[29]

The best treatment regimen for **CRAO** is debated, and visual outcomes are overall poor.[2] Most patients have a final acuity of counting fingers or worse even after treatment.[25,26,30] There has been extensive research regarding treatment of **CRAO**; however, the data have several limitations. **CRAO** is not very common, and studies have small sample sizes.[31] Many studies use two or more treatments, and it is difficult to make comparisons between different multistep treatment regimens.[3] A 2009 Cochrane review regarding **CRAO** treatment found only two studies designed as randomized controlled trials design, and these studies' conclusions were limited by a small sample size and not having visual acuity as an end point measurement.[2]

There is question in the literature about the utility of intervention because some studies show spontaneous improvements in visual acuity that parallel recovery in patients who underwent treatment. In a retrospective study of all **CRAO** treatment strategies, 18% of patients had spontaneous visual acuity improvement of two or more Snellen lines, which was not significantly different from the visual acuity improvement in treated patients.[26] In a meta-analysis with 396 patients who received no treatment after **CRAO**, 17% had spontaneous visual recovery.[32] Conversely, there are studies that show significant recovery in treatment patients over controls. For example, one case report cites a patient who improved from no light perception to 20/200 visual acuity after treatment, and provides an argument that all patients should be treated, regardless of baseline visual acuity, because there is a chance for improvement.[3]

The primary treatments and clinical trials that have been evaluated are detailed here and summarized in Table 16.2. Therapies aim to increase retinal perfusion through vasodilation, means to lower the IOP, and thrombolysis.

Pentoxifylline, carbogen, and hyperbaric oxygen have all been used to promote retinal vasodilation. It is believed that vasodilation will increase retinal blood flow, enhance tissue perfusion, and overall improve oxygenation after **CRAO**. Pentoxifylline and other methylxanthine derivatives have vasodilator properties and inhibit platelet aggregation.[33] Research is mixed. A 2009 Cochrane review about the methylxanthine

| **TABLE 16.2 • Therapeutics for Central Retinal Artery Occlusion** | |
|---|---|
| Standard Treatment | • No treatment (may see spontaneous recovery) <br> • Carotid endarterectomy |
| **Ongoing Areas of Research: Overall Goal to Increase Retinal Perfusion** | |
| Promote retinal vasodilation | • Pentoxifylline and other methylxanthine derivatives <br> • Carbogen <br> • Hyperbaric oxygen |
| Intraocular pressure reduction | • Sublingual isosorbide dinitrite <br> • Ocular massage <br> • Intravenous acetazolamide <br> • Intravenous mannitol or glycerol <br> • Topical glaucoma eye drops <br> • Anterior chamber paracentesis |
| Thrombolytic therapy | • Tissue plasminogen activator: intra-arterial to ophthalmic artery vs intravenous |

derivatives pentoxifylline, propentofylline, and pentifylline did not find support regarding their ability to improve clinical outcome after acute ischemic stroke.[33] In a randomized controlled trial specifically addressing patients with **CRAO**, central retinal artery blood flow was monitored after treatment with 1800 mg of pentoxifylline daily. The pentoxifylline-treated group had increased peak systolic and end diastolic flow velocity, although conclusions about these results are limited because of the small sample size (10 patients) and no correlation made to final visual acuity after treatment.[34]

Carbogen is an inhaled mixture of 4% to 7% carbon dioxide and 93% to 96% oxygen. Carbogen administration varies in different studies. In one protocol, it was administered for 10 minutes every hour during the day and 10 minutes every 4 hours at night for a total duration of 48 to 72 hours.[1] Carbon dioxide is administered to prevent and potentially reverse oxygen-induced vasoconstriction. It has been shown to dilate retinal arterioles and therefore increase oxygen delivery to retinal tissue.[26] Documented arteriolar response varies in the literature. For example, one study measuring the change in arterial caliber in healthy participants given first 100% oxygen and then a carbogen mixture (95% oxygen and 5% carbon dioxide) did not demonstrate responsive vasodilation.[35] Another similar study had consistent results; however, researchers did measure increased arterial flow velocity, which could correlate with improved retinal perfusion.[36]

Hyperbaric oxygen is administered after **CRAO** to increase the partial pressure of oxygen delivered to the ischemic retinal tissue. On average, protocols administer 2 to 2.5 atmospheres hyperbaric oxygen for approximately 90 minutes.[1] There have been several promising studies regarding this treatment. In a 2011 case study, 8 of 11 patients treated with hyperbaric oxygen after **CRAO** had visual acuity improvement of two lines or more.[37] In a retrospective study of patients with **CRAO**, those who received five sessions of hyperbaric oxygen treatment along with hemodilution had significantly better visual outcomes than did the patients who underwent only hemodilution.[29]

IOP reduction is another goal of CRAO treatment. Ocular perfusion pressure is equal to the mean arterial pressure minus the IOP. Therefore, by decreasing the IOP, ocular perfusion pressure should increase.[1] Means to increase ocular perfusion pressure include sublingual isosorbide dinitrite, ocular massage, intravenous (IV) acetazolamide, IV mannitol or glycerol, and topical glaucoma medications. Anterior chamber paracentesis can also be used to reduce IOP. Acetazolamide reduces the production of aqueous humor to reduce IOP. A typical dose is 500 IV one-time stat injection or 250 mg four times a day for 24 hours.[1] One study examined the effect of acetazolamide on retinal blood flow in 10 healthy participants and found a significant reduction in IOP as well as a significant increase in retinal blood flow 30 minutes and 60 minutes after acetazolamide administration.[38] IV acetazolamide is used preferentially over topical glaucoma medications for emergency situations because it has a faster onset of action than that of topical drops.[1]

Ocular massage is a readily accessible means to decrease IOP that can be performed quickly in an emergency.[39] In addition to decreasing IOP, ocular massage may assist in physically dislodging the embolus so it can pass through the ophthalmic circulation.[2] Intermittent pressure is applied through the closed eye for 15 to 30 minutes.[1,30] The combination of ocular massage and 500 mg of IV acetazolamide can rapidly bring IOP to as low as 5 mm Hg, and it is a frequently used treatment for acute CRAO that can be administered in any clinical setting.[30]

Anterior chamber paracentesis is another means to rapidly reduce pressure in acute CRAO; however, this method is more limiting because it requires an ophthalmologist. With this technique, 0.1 to 0.2 mL of aqueous humor is removed from the anterior chamber.[1,2] In addition to IOP decrease, it is hypothesized that the distortion of the globe promotes further dilation of the retinal arteries.[1] Evidence in the literature of the efficacy of anterior chamber paracentesis in CRAO is mixed. In one retrospective study covering 89 cases of CRAO, statistical analysis did not find significant visual acuity changes after anterior chamber paracentesis when compared with control eyes.[26] However, a similar study performed 10 years ago found a significant visual acuity improvement of two or more Snellen lines after anterior chamber paracentesis compared with controls.[40]

The most current research for CRAO has focused on the efficacy of thrombolytic therapy with tissue plasminogen activator (tPA).[1,31] Thrombolytic agents for CRAO are delivered intravenously or intra-arterially by catheterizing the ophthalmic artery.[1] The literature has preference for intra-arterial administration, because it is more direct and limits systemic bleeding risk.[30] Treatment should be reserved for patients who present a few hours after the CRAO onset and are low-risk candidates for thrombolytic therapy, which has serious risks of bleeding.

Although several studies have suggested that thrombolysis may improve the visual outcome of CRAO, the treatment remains controversial. A 2007 review of 35 studies about thrombolysis identified visual acuity improvement after thrombolytic treatment in most studies.[31] The review included both intra-arterial and IV administration of thrombolytic agents. A meta-analysis of 16 studies in 2000 that specifically investigated intra-arterial thrombolysis determined that thrombolytic therapy might provide a "marginal benefit" over other treatment practices. However, the review noted a lack of randomized controlled trials limiting the ability to make clinical recommendations.[30] Two subsequent recently published randomized trials do not show as promising an effect. The EAGLE (European Assessment Group for Lysis in the Eye) study in 2010 enrolled 82 patients with CRAO for 20 hours or less and compared an intra-arterial tPA-treated group to a "conservative" treatment group that received multimodal treatment with isovolemic hemodilution, ocular massage, timolol 0.5% drop, and IV acetazolamide 400 mg.[41] The study did not find a significant difference in visual acuity improvement between the two groups and the tPA group had a higher risk of complications from treatment, so the study was discontinued early. A randomized controlled trial in 2011 compared an IV tPA–treated group with a control group treated with IV saline.[42] Two of eight participants in the tPA group had three-line visual acuity improvement 1 week after tPA. Although this was not a significant difference from the control group, the researchers noted that these two patients were the only ones treated within 6 hours of the CRAO onset. The result emphasizes the importance of rapid time to treatment. This observation was consistent with the findings from a 2015 meta-analysis, which identified a benefit from tPA treatment if it was administered earlier than 4.5 hours after CRAO.[32]

Long-term treatment of CRAO should address underlying risk factors that predispose patients to additional future cardiovascular events such as stroke or myocardial infarction.[1,2,30] These include dietary modifications, increasing exercise, smoking cessation, antiplatelet therapy, statins, and antihypertensive medication (see Section on Nonarteritic Transient Central Retinal Artery Occlusion: Transient Monocular Blindness).

## Giant-Cell Arteritis

It is critical to rule out GCA in the geriatric patient who presents with sudden onset monocular vision loss. GCA is a medium- and large-vessel vasculitis that mainly affects the thoracic aorta and its branches, most often extending to the cranial arteries.[43] It primarily affects white individuals 50 years or older with a 3:1 female-to-male predominance. Incidence increases with age and peaks between the ages of 70 and 80 years.[43,44]

Early intervention with high-dose glucocorticoids (GCs) is crucial to prevent future ischemic events.[45] Ischemic visual complications have been reported in 30% to 50% of patients, with vision loss in 15% to 25%, and these changes are often irreversible.[45-47] If treatment is not initiated early, there is a high risk of vision loss quickly extending to the second eye.[48] In about 80% of **GCA** cases with vision loss, visual complications are secondary to anterior ischemic optic neuropathy: arteritis of the posterior ciliary arteries disrupts blood flow to the optic nerve head.[46,47,49] Less commonly, vision loss in **GCA** is caused by direct inflammation of the central retinal artery (arteritic **CRAO**) or cilioretinal artery, ischemic retrobulbar neuritis, or stroke in the vertebrobasilar territory.[43,46,47,49]

The clinical presentation of **GCA** is varied and can make diagnosis a challenge. Most often, patients report visual symptoms related to ischemic complications of **GCA**. Vision loss is typically sudden, painless, unchanging, and monocular at onset, although there is a risk of bilateral involvement if treatment is not initiated in a timely manner.[43,49] Patients may report the "feeling of a shade covering one eye."[48] In one study in which half of all patients with **GCA** had ocular manifestations, the early ocular symptoms included vision loss of varying severity in 98%, **TMB** in 30%, ocular pain in 8%, and diplopia in 6%.[47]

Ocular symptoms are accompanied by one or more systemic and inflammatory symptoms of **GCA**. A new-onset, continuous temporal or occipital headache that interferes with sleep is most common and reported in two-thirds of patients with **GCA**.[48] Temporal artery changes are also notable. In one review of patients with **GCA**, temporal artery tenderness was observed in 48% of patients, absent artery pulsations in 15%, and arterial thickening in 15%.[45] Patients may also have scalp tenderness, jaw claudication from ischemia to the muscles of mastication, generalized malaise, anorexia, weight loss, low-grade fever, musculoskeletal pains, and otalgia.[43,45,46,48]

In addition to these symptoms, there is a high association of polymyalgia rheumatica (PMR) with **GCA**. In one report, one-fifth of patients with PMR have symptoms of **GCA** and half of all patients with **GCA** have clinical features of PMR.[43] PMR is a rheumatologic condition characterized by proximal musculoskeletal stiffness, pains, and weakness most frequently involving the neck, shoulders, and hips.[46] The American College of Rheumatology (ACR) classification for **GCA** is as follows[50]:

1. Age at disease onset greater than or equal to 50 years

2. New-onset headache or new type of localized pain in the head

3. Temporal artery tenderness to palpation or decreased pulsation, unrelated to arteriosclerosis of cervical arteries

4. Elevated ESR $> 50$ mm

5. Arterial biopsy demonstrating necrotizing arteritis, characterized by predominance of mononuclear cell infiltrates or a granulomatous process with multinucleated giant cells

Meeting three or more of these criteria is associated with a 93.5% sensitivity and 91.2% specificity for diagnosis of **GCA**.

To assess the ACR criteria and gain information about overall prognosis, diagnostic workup for **GCA** includes detailed history taking for classic symptoms, ophthalmic examination, laboratory testing for inflammatory markers, and a temporal artery biopsy. Laboratory studies should include platelets, ESR and CRP measurements, other rheumatologic testing, and evaluations of renal, liver, and thyroid function.[5,46] Elevated ESR, CRP, and thrombocytosis are associated with **GCA**.[51] On physical examination, the temporal artery should be palpated, examining for hardening, tenderness, or decreased pulsation. A full cranial nerve examination should be conducted, because cranial nerve palsies are often manifested. The face and scalp should be examined for any tenderness or necrosis. A musculoskeletal examination will evaluate for proximal muscle weakness and muscular tenderness.[5,46,48] A full ophthalmic examination is also warranted. Funduscopic examination will reveal "chalky white" optic nerve edema, secondary to anterior ischemic optic neuropathy.[48] Optic atrophy occurs with time and will be observed in follow-up examinations. In most cases, fluorescein angiography will show occlusion of the posterior ciliary arteries and delayed choroidal filling.[47]

A temporal artery biopsy is the gold standard diagnostic test for **GCA**.

Classic histologic findings include transmural inflammation of the arterial wall with multinucleated giant cells, lymphocytes, and macrophages, thickening and disruption of the internal elastic lamina, and muscle necrosis.[5,43,46,48] The vasculitis has a segmental distribution along the artery, termed skip lesions, and, therefore, a significant length of temporal artery is required for diagnosis.[5] Imaging modalities, including ultrasonography, high-resolution magnetic resonance imaging, CT, and CT angiography have been studied as adjunctive tools for identifying the inflammatory changes in the temporal arteries and other involved vessels with promising findings.[46] These modalities are useful noninvasive measures to assist with early diagnosis. In a large meta-analysis including a total of 2036 patients with **GCA**, color duplex ultrasound repeatedly demonstrated a hypoechoic halo around the lumen of the temporal artery, indicating arterial wall edema and inflammation.[52] This finding had a high specificity (82%) for **GCA**, although a lower sensitivity (69%). Ultrasound also identified areas of arterial stenosis of occlusion that assisted with diagnosis. High-resolution magnetic resonance imaging also has high specificity for **GCA** diagnosis. Areas of bright enhancement demonstrate inflammation of multiple cranial arteries in patients with clinically diagnosed **GCA**.[53]

Treatment for **GCA** should be initiated immediately on the basis of high clinical suspicion. Although biopsy is the gold standard for diagnosis, treatment with high-dose GCs should be given before obtaining a biopsy because of the time-sensitive nature of the disease with high risk of worsening, irreversible vision loss, or fatal ischemic sequelae such as stroke or myocardial infarction if treatment is delayed.[54] High-dose GC therapy is required initially to control severe inflammation, followed by a slow taper of steroid dose over a period of 1 to 2 years as clinically tolerated.[55]

The initial GC dose is generally reported to be 40 to 60 mg/d of prednisone or an equivalent; however, higher doses—often 1 g/d—are used if vision loss is present.[48,55] GC is continued for 2 to 4 weeks and slowly decreased after correction of ESR and CRP levels, and control of reversible symptoms is identified.[48] It is recommended to decrease the dose every 1 to 2 weeks by no more than 10% of the total daily dose. Tapering should be modified depending on the patient's clinical status and measures of ESR/CRP.

Current research about **GCA** management is focused on reducing the time course of GC therapy, because long-term treatment with GCs poses several significant risk factors for elderly patients. Treatment with GCs for 1 to 2 years increases the risk of osteoporosis and subsequent fractures, diabetes mellitus, infection, cataract progression, hypertension, myopathy, and gastrointestinal bleeding in a patient population that is already vulnerable to these factors because of advancing age.[54] In one study, the median time from initiation of GC therapy to the first GC-related adverse event was 1.1 years, which falls within the average window of treatment duration.[56] The percentage of patients treated for **GCA** with subsequent GC-related adverse effects is as high as 80%.[57] In patients with preexisting cardiovascular risk factors such as diabetes mellitus, hypertension, or osteoporosis, long-term GC treatment poses an even greater risk, and alternate modalities of inflammatory suppression may be safer and more efficacious for this high-risk group.[58] Furthermore, evaluation of other treatment modalities can have benefit for patients who are unable to fully taper the GC dose. Approximately 50% of patients have a clinical flare during taper, particularly during the first 12 to 16 months when prednisone dose reaches 5 to 10 mg/d, and some patients have multiple relapses requiring higher and longer courses of GCs.[48,56,57]

IV pulse steroids and a few days of IV GCs before initiation of high-dose oral prednisone is one method being investigated to reduce the duration of GC therapy and improve clinical outcomes.[55] In a randomized controlled trial with 27 patients, all patients were initiated on prednisone 40 mg/d. The experimental group was also given 15 mg/kg daily dose of IV methylprednisolone for 3 days at the initiation of GC treatment, whereas a control group received saline injections.[59] Researchers found that the experimental group tolerated a faster GC taper with less relapses, with a tapered dose of 5 mg/d of prednisone by 36 weeks, and effects sustained at 52- and 78-week follow-ups. Comparatively, a larger randomized controlled trial that studied pulse GC at a lower dose of 240 mg IV for 3 days did not find a significant difference in long-term oral GC requirements or GC-related side effects.[60]

GC-sparing treatment with other immunosuppressive agents has also been studied to reduce long-term GC needs while maintaining control of disease activity (Table 16.3).[54] Agents researched include methotrexate (MTX), anti-tumor necrosis factor (TNF)-alpha agents, mycophenolate mofetil, cyclophosphamide, tocilizumab, leflunomide, and antiplatelet agents. Key studies regarding these medications are described subsequently.

MTX, a dihydrofolate reductase inhibitor, is the most studied GC-sparing regimen for patients with **GCA**. There have been several randomized controlled trials conducted for MTX use, and many studies found that administering MTX in the early

| **TABLE 16.3** • Summary of Therapeutics for giant-cell arteritis | |
|---|---|
| Standard treatment | • High-dose steroids with prolonged taper ± intravenous pulse steroids |
| Ongoing research: glucocorticoid-sparing agents | • Tocilizumab (FDA approved)<br>• Methotrexate<br>• Infliximab, adalimumab, rituximab, etanercept<br>• Mycophenolate mofetil<br>• Leflunomide<br>• Cyclophosphamide |

Abbreviations: FDA, U.S. Food and Drug Administration.

stages of GCA treatment can shorten GC treatment duration.[54] A 2007 meta-analysis of three double-blind, randomized controlled trials enrolling a total of 161 patients with GCA investigated the use of weekly MTX in combination with GC treatment.[58] The analysis identified a 35% reduced risk of first relapse, 51% reduced risk of second relapse, and overall reduction in cumulative GCs needed for treatment. MTX doses in the three studies ranged from 7.5 to 15 mg/wk, with increased doses of MTX given as clinically indicated to the maximum dose of 15 mg/wk.[57,61,62] Although the meta-analysis indicates a potential benefit of combined MTX and GC therapy, the reduced cumulative GC administered has not been correlated with a reduction in GC-related complications.[54] Further research is also needed regarding the specific use of MTX in GC-resistant patients with high relapse rates and those patients with preexisting conditions placing them at high risk for long-term GC treatment.[48,55]

Anti-TNF-α agents, infliximab, adalimumab, rituximab, and etanercept, have all been researched regarding their role in treating GC-refractory disease. Their use has been advocated because GCA is an inflammatory state involving overexpression of cytokines, and TNFα has specifically been found in 60% of cells within inflamed arteries.[54,63] When anti-TNF-α agents have been studied for their application at the initiation of GC treatment, studies overall did not find improved clinical outcomes.[63-66] For example, a 2002 double-blind randomized controlled trial investigating the use of infliximab alongside GC therapy did not result in improved clinical outcomes regarding relapse or GC taper. The study was discontinued early because the infliximab group encountered a higher rate of infections (71%) compared with placebo group (56%).[63] However, there has been promise for the use of anti-TNF-α agents started midway through GCA treatment in the subgroup of patients with GC resistance or complications.[67,68] In a 2008 double-blind randomized controlled trial, etanercept was studied in patients with GCA who had GC-related adverse effects or were unable to taper the GC dose after 10 months of treatment.[67] The etanercept-treated group had a significantly lower cumulative GC dose at the end of 1 year compared with the control group. There was a strong trend toward decreased relapses in the etanercept-treated group, with 50% achieving disease control compared with 22% in the control group.

Tocilizumab, an IL-6 receptor antibody, is the only U. S. Food and Drug Administration (FDA)-approved GC-sparing regimen to date. Its use was proposed for use in GCA after elevated levels of IL-6 were found in both GCA and PMR.[54] Research results have been overall positive, although currently limited by small sample sizes. In a case study of three patients with multiple relapses of GCA on GC therapy, all patients had beneficial clinical responses when GC therapy was combined with tocilizumab 8 mg/kg every 4 weeks for 6 months.[69] A retrospective study of seven patients with GC-resistant GCA found that all patients were able to taper GCs without relapse after the initiation of tocilizumab treatment.[70]

Mycophenolate mofetil inhibits inosine monophosphate dehydrogenase required in purine synthesis, and there is early evidence from case reports to suggest that it has a benefit for patients with GCA having contraindications to prolonged GC use. In a small 2013 case series, mycophenolate mofetil enabled three high-risk patients to taper GC treatment at a faster rate.[71] Larger scale research is needed to expand on these findings. Leflunomide inhibits dihydroorotate dehydrogenase to decrease pyrimidine synthesis. The active metabolite of leflunomide inhibits dendritic cell maturation, thereby decreasing cytokine production and the inflammatory response that is involved in the pathology of GCA. Studies of leflunomide combined with GC treatment for GCA found that patients were able to reduce GC dose and showed clinical improvement.[72,73] Adverse effects of leflunomide are largely tolerable compared with other GC-sparing agents and include rash, diarrhea, and malaise.

Cyclophosphamide is a strong immunosuppressive alkylating agent that works by cross-linking DNA. Research supports its efficacy when used in patients with GCA who have unremitting disease that is not responsive to GC treatment alone.[74-76] However, the use of cyclophosphamide is limited by a high risk of side effects.[55] In most studies investigating the use of cyclophosphamide for GCA, trials were stopped early as a result of complications such as acute hepatitis, neutropenia, pancytopenia, and aplastic crisis.[74,75] As a result, cyclophosphamide is not advised as a first-line GC-sparing agent. If it is used, it should be administered with mesna, which binds toxic metabolites excreted into the urinary system and prevents serious complications including hemorrhagic cystitis and risk of transitional cell bladder carcinoma. Weekly laboratory monitoring for renal, hepatic, and hematologic functions should be maintained for the first month of treatment.[75]

## Retinal Detachment

RD is a cause of painless, sudden visual disturbance that requires early surgical intervention. In RD, the neurosensory retina separates from the underlying retinal pigment epithelium, which separates the retinal photoreceptor cells from their blood supply and results in ischemic injury and vision loss. RD subtypes include the following:

1. Rhegmatogenous: most common subtype, involves a break in the retinal leads subretinal fluid accumulation between the retina and retinal pigment epithelium.

2. Tractional: epiretinal tissue, such as fibrovascular membranes, pulls the retina away from the retinal pigment epithelium.

3. Exudative: damaged blood–retinal barrier from retinal or choroidal pathology allows for fluid accumulation in the space between the retina and the retinal pigment epithelium.

**RD** may be spontaneous or secondary to trauma, with spontaneous being more common. In one survey of rhegmatogenous **RD**, the incidence of nontraumatic **RD** was 11 per 100 000 population and traumatic **RD** was 1.4 per 100 000 population.[77] Patients who are myopic are at increased risk for rhegmatogenous **RD** because their globes are elongated and at risk for lattice degeneration: retinal thinning and atrophy.[78] Areas of the retina with lattice degeneration are more likely to tear and are associated with rhegmatogenous **RD** in up to 66% of cases.[78] The prevalence of **RD** also increases with age. The elderly are particularly susceptible to rhegmatogenous **RD** because vitreous thinning and lattice degeneration of the retina are also associated with aging.[79] Other risk factors for **RD** include family history and previous **RD**, with 15% of patients with **RD** in one eye reported to develop it in the other.[80] In studies of patients with blunt orbital trauma, **RD** may be an immediate consequence of trauma (12%) or occur up to 1 year after injury (80%).[81]

The symptoms of **RD** include new-onset floaters, photopsia, and visual field loss often described as a curtain or shadow moving across the visual field. Vision loss is often painless and acute. On the basis of the location and extent of detachment, pupillary examination may demonstrate an afferent pupillary defect. Diagnosis is strongly based on this clinical presentation and followed by a 360° funduscopic examination. Funduscopy can reveal retinal breaks or vitreous hemorrhage overlying the detachment. Ultrasound is another useful diagnostic tool that can be used quickly for diagnosis at bedside.[78,82,83]

There is no medical management for **RD**. Prompt **ophthalmology** referral is therefore important for any patient presenting with the clinical signs of **RD**. Surgical management includes techniques such as pars plana vitrectomy, scleral buckling, or pneumatic retinopexy. The type and timeline of surgical management is determined on the basis of factors including the type of **RD**, location, size, and surgical preference/experience.[81,84,85]

# SUDDEN VISION LOSS WITH PAIN

## Acute Angle Closure Glaucoma

**AACG** is another **ophthalmic emergency**. It occurs after an acute, complete closure of the anterior chamber angle (the angle between the iris and the cornea) at the location where the aqueous humor drains from the eye.[86] Subsequent aqueous humor accumulation leads to a rapid rise in IOP.[87] Prompt recognition and treatment with IOP-lowering agents within hours of onset is essential for preserving visual function.[88,89] Without prompt treatment, high IOP is transferred to the optic nerve, restricts blood supply, and causes optic nerve atrophy with irreversible vision loss.[87] It is important to recognize that the much more common type of glaucoma is primary open-angle glaucoma, which is painless.

Patients with susceptible anatomy for **AACG** include those with hyperopia and shallow anterior chambers. It is more often identified in women, the elderly, and patients of Asian heritage.[90] The elderly are more susceptible to **AACG** because of cataracts and age-related posterior segment changes.[88,90] In patients with susceptible anatomy, pupillary dilation from medications or dim lighting can cause "pupillary block," in which the dilated iris blocks aqueous flow.[91] Alternatively, some medications may affect a shallow anterior chamber angle by causing movement of the ciliary body, anterior movement of the lens, and other anatomic changes.

Medications that have been implicated in **AACG** include topical mydriatics, adrenergic agonists, selective serotonin reuptake inhibitors, topiramate, anticholinergics, and drugs with anticholinergic side effects including antihistamines and tricyclic antidepressants.[87,91-93] Prescription or over-the-counter medication is linked to about one-third of **AACG** cases.[93] Pilocarpine, although used for glaucoma treatment as a miotic agent to increase aqueous humor outflow, has also been implicated in some cases of **AACG** because it can cause anterior lens movement.[88,93]

Ocular symptoms of **AACG** include pain, conjunctival injection, blurry vision, and halos seen around lights.[86,87] Extraocular symptoms are commonly associated, including frontal headache and gastrointestinal distress including nausea, vomiting, and abdominal pain.[87] Diagnosis of **AACG** is made on the basis of clinical presentation, understanding circumstances surrounding symptom onset, recent medication use, and IOP measurements. The normal range for IOP is between 10 and 21 mm Hg. In **AACG**, IOP is typically higher than 40 mm Hg.[88,91] If there is no available method for IOP measurement, palpation of the globe can be used to emergently gain an understanding of the IOP. The affected globe will be firm compared with the unaffected eye. Diagnosis also involves assessment of the anterior chamber angle. An ophthalmologist can view the anterior chamber angle with gonioscopy. In an emergency, any provider can perform the "oblique flashlight test" to assess anterior chamber depth.[87,91,94] A penlight is shined across the anterior chamber at an angle parallel to the iris, in the direction pointing toward the nose. The anterior chamber angle is wide if the entire iris is illuminated, and it is shallow if a shadow is seen on the nasal side of the iris.

Fast treatment of **AACG** with IOP-lowering agents has been associated with good visual acuity outcomes.[87,90,95] Topical IOP-lowering agents include β-blockers, α-2 agonists, prostaglandin analogs, and carbonic anhydrase inhibitors. Because topical agents are systemically absorbed, β-blockers should be avoided in patients with reactive airway disease or cardiac conduction abnormality. Acetazolamide, a carbonic anhydrase inhibitor, can be given in oral or in IV form. Acetazolamide is contraindicated in patients with sulfa allergies or with sickle-cell disease; mannitol is an alternative agent that can be used. In addition to pressure-lowering agents, topical corticosteroids may be administered to reduce corneal inflammation. Topical pilocarpine can be used to induce pupillary constriction.

There are various published protocols regarding timing and order of administration of IOP-lowering agents.[88] In general, oral and topical agents should be given in combination when diagnosis is made. The IOP should be repeated every hour, and medical therapy should be continued until IOP is within normal range. In one study, IOP was sufficiently reduced with a mean time of 3 hours after treatment initiation.[88] At the same time as IOP is corrected, analgesics and antiemetics should be administered to manage the symptomatology of AACG.

Definitive, long-term treatment for **AACG** is performed with surgical iridectomy or laser peripheral iridotomy (LPI), which reduces the pressure differential across the iris to maintain a normal IOP.[96] LPI is the preferred, because it has reduced risk and can be performed quickly.[88] LPI is indicated after IOP is controlled and corneal edema has begun to subside; however, it may be needed in the acute phase of **AACG** if medical management is not successful.[39,97] The contralateral eye should also be treated with LPI as a preventive measure to reduce risk of **AACG**.[86] The patient should continue long-term follow-up with an ophthalmologist for regular IOP checks.

## Orbital Cellulitis

**Orbital cellulitis** describes infection of the orbital structures posterior to the orbital septum and presents the risk of irreversible vision loss and sometimes even death if untreated. The majority of cases are linked to bacterial extension from sinusitis.[98,99] Bacteria can enter the valveless venous system or spread across bony walls, particularly relevant for ethmoid sinusitis in which infection can spread across the thin lamina papyracea causing a subperiosteal abscess.[99] Other sources of infection include spread from other periorbital structures (ie, face, eyelids, and lacrimal sac), dental infections, foreign bodies after trauma, surgery, bacteremia with septic embolization, endophthalmitis, or dacryoadenitis.

The clinical presentation of **orbital cellulitis** includes acute, painful vision loss, proptosis, chemosis (conjunctival edema), lid edema, and restriction of extraocular movements because of both pain and inflammation.[99] Patients have symptoms compatible with acute infection, including fever and leukocytosis. **Orbital cellulitis** should be distinguished from the more benign preseptal cellulitis, which does not present with proptosis, ocular movement restriction, or vision changes.

Imaging with CT of the orbits and sinuses is critical to diagnosis, allowing localization of a sinus infection and assessment of the degree of orbital inflammation.[98] If there is no sinusitis, then evaluation into an alternative underlying cause should take place, because it will direct medical management.

The treatment of **orbital cellulitis** involves early, broad-spectrum IV antibiotic coverage. The most common organisms isolated in adults include *Hemophilus influenzae*, *Moraxella catarrhalis*, anaerobes, and *Staphylococcus* and *Streptococcus* species.[100-102] Compared with **orbital cellulitis** in children, adults are more likely to be infected with multiple organisms, and coverage for both aerobic and anaerobic pathogens is critical. Antibiotic choices should be based on local sensitivities and modified depending on tissue cultures and clinical improvement after treatment.

In addition to antibiotic therapy, if a subperiosteal abscess is identified on CT, the abscess may need to be drained.[98,103] If there is poor clinical improvement despite 24 to 36 hours of antibiotics or sight-threatening clinical findings on presentation, sinus drainage may be needed to minimize and prevent long-term complications.

## Orbital Compartment Syndrome

**Orbital compartment syndrome** involves an acute increase in orbital pressure within the contents of a restricting orbital space: the rigid bony walls surrounding the globe and retrobulbar contents as well as the orbital septum and eyelids forming an anterior boundary. Because of the restricting orbital anatomy, the globe cannot compensate for an increase in volume and IOP rises in the confined orbital space. With rising pressure, there is decreased vascular perfusion to the globe, retinal vessels, and optic nerve.[80,104-106] Permanent visual loss can occur after 60 to 100 minutes of increased IOP and ischemia.[107]

The clinical presentation of **orbital compartment syndrome** includes proptosis, decreased extraocular movements, acute and painful vision loss, an afferent pupillary defect, increased IOP, and a tense globe on palpation.[104,106] Diagnosis is largely clinical, because urgent intervention is needed and cannot wait for imaging studies.[107]

In the diagnosis of **orbital compartment syndrome**, consideration should be made for evaluating the cause of the increased orbital volume. Causes of compartment syndrome include **orbital cellulitis**, intraorbital abscess, orbital emphysema (air in orbital soft tissues), orbital tumors, progressive orbital edema associated with trauma or surgery, and retrobulbar hemorrhage.[107]

Retrobulbar hemorrhage (also known as retrobulbar hematoma) is the most common cause of compartment syndrome. It involves hemorrhage into the potential space surrounding the globe.[104] Retrobulbar hemorrhage may occur after blunt or penetrating trauma to the globe, orbital or endoscopic sinus surgery, retrobulbar injection, or it can occur spontaneously in patients with coagulopathy or venous anomalies.[80,105,106,108] Elderly patients on blood thinners are at an increased risk for **orbital compartment syndrome**. For patients with spontaneous retrobulbar hemorrhage, bleeding disorder workup with coagulation studies is recommended to identify the underlying cause.[107]

The treatment of **orbital compartment syndrome**, regardless of cause, involves immediate decompression with lateral canthotomy and cantholysis.[80] Lateral canthotomy has high success rates for reducing IOP; and with early intervention, there is a good prognosis for visual recovery.[106] For example, in a case report of acute retrobulbar hemorrhage after a punch to the eye, diagnosis was made within 3 hours and urgent treatment, including lateral canthotomy, was performed soon after diagnosis with recovery of visual acuity 9 days after presentation.[109] In the interim before the procedure, medical management with IOP-lowering topical or oral agents can be given (see Section "Acute Angle Closure Glaucoma").[80,106]

# OCULAR TRAUMA

The **geriatric** population is at risk for trauma after mechanical falls or syncope at home. It is important for the general medicine practitioner to quickly identify the signs of traumatic ocular injury and facilitate early **ophthalmology** referral and intervention. The management of ocular trauma is primarily surgical and is briefly highlighted in this section.

# RUPTURED GLOBE

It is imperative to rule out a **ruptured globe** for any patient who has sustained blunt or penetrating trauma to the orbit. A **ruptured globe** involves a full-thickness scleral or corneal laceration and poses a high risk of complications including expulsion of orbital contents and endophthalmitis.[80] A ruptured globe most frequently occurs anteriorly where the sclera is the thinnest, but it can also occur posteriorly and have a less obvious clinical presentation. Patients with a previous history of ophthalmic surgery have a higher risk of **ruptured globe** after trauma, and this is pertinent to the evaluation of a **geriatric** patient who is likely to have undergone a cataract extraction or other ocular surgery.

After trauma, patients with a **ruptured globe** may experience decreased vision. On physical examination, they may have subconjunctival hemorrhage, a shallow anterior chamber, limited extraocular movements, an irregularly shaped pupil that will peak toward the site of rupture, exposed brownish red uveal tissue, and vitreous hemorrhage.[80,105] IOP measurements will be low. Of note, direct tonometry and palpation of the globe should be avoided when there is suspicion for **ruptured globe** because of risk of expulsion of intraocular contents. CT should be performed to evaluate for foreign bodies and other surrounding injuries; however, this imaging is secondary to the need for urgent surgical exploration if there is a high suspicion of a **ruptured globe**.[105]

A protective eye shield should be placed, and **ophthalmology** should be consulted immediately. The patient should be instructed to avoid Valsalva maneuvers or any high-pressure maneuver such as sneezing with the mouth closed. Prophylactic systemic antibiotics, often cefazolin or vancomycin combined with a fourth-generation fluoroquinolone, should be given to decrease the risk of endophthalmitis.[80]

# ORBITAL WALL FRACTURES AND ENTRAPMENT

Blunt trauma to the orbit yields the risk of orbital wall, which may compromise surrounding orbital contents such as the extraocular muscles. Physical examination of a patient after blunt orbital trauma should focus on signs of orbital floor fracture, including tenderness surrounding the orbital rim, bony step-offs, subcutaneous emphysema, ptosis, exophthalmos, enophthalmos, hypesthesia in the distribution of V2, diplopia, and vision changes.[105,110-112] Diplopia may be due to extraocular muscle or soft-tissue entrapment, and extraocular movements should be observed. Nearby associated orbital injuries, including injury to the lacrimal system and globe, should also be ruled out. In addition to these clinical signs, coronal CT scans are critical for diagnosis of orbital floor fractures and help guide the need for early or late surgical intervention.[110,112]

Early surgical intervention for orbital fractures is indicated if there are clinical signs of entrapment—restricted and painful extraocular motility, nausea, vomiting, and bradycardia.[112-114] Patients with a positive oculocardiac reflex, which is stimulation of increased vagal tone as a result of orbital soft-tissue entrapment, need urgent management to prevent dangerous outcomes including bradycardia, syncope, and heart block.[110] Of note, the **geriatric** population rarely experiences tissue entrapment because they have more brittle bones that have a tendency to cause tissue prolapse instead of entrapment. Patients with **orbital wall fractures** should be careful to avoid Valsalva maneuvers and should be instructed to sneeze with their mouth open and avoid nose blowing.[111] There is debate whether prophylactic systemic antibiotics should be given.

Patients with orbital floor fracture who do not meet criteria for urgent surgical intervention typically have surgery postponed after a 1- to 2-week period of observation. This period permits resolution of periorbital edema and hemorrhage for better physical examination to evaluate whether there are indications for surgery which include large fractures, enophthalmos, hypoglobus, or diplopia in primary gaze.[112,114]

# FUTURE AREAS OF UNCERTAINTY

For all the **ophthalmic emergencies** described, continuing research is needed to improve potential vision-saving treatments. For **TMB** and **CRAO**, ongoing research focuses on the indications for medical versus surgical management with carotid artery stenosis. **CRAO**, in particular, has poor visual outcomes, and clinical research has been limited by small case studies. There will be ongoing investigation regarding the best methods for regaining retinal perfusion after **CRAO** and avoiding cell damage. GCA is another emergency with potential for poor visual outcomes, and future studies will continue to investigate the best glucocorticoid regimens and alternatives to glucocorticoid therapy.

# CONCLUSIONS

A wide array of **ophthalmic emergencies** may present in the hospitalized **geriatric** patient. High suspicion should be held for these conditions when patients complain of sudden vision changes or severe eye pain. Urgent intervention and **ophthalmology** consultation is essential for preventing irreversible visual damage.

# SUMMARY

The review highlights common **ophthalmic emergencies** seen in the hospitalized **geriatric** patient. It describes key features of the ophthalmic examination, early identification, and treatment of **ophthalmic emergencies**, including transient monocular loss of vision with risk of future ischemic complications, **central retinal artery occlusion, giant-cell arteritis, retinal detachment, acute angle closure glaucoma, orbital cellulitis**, and orbital trauma. Research is ongoing regarding the best techniques to maximize visual outcome for these conditions. The benefits of surgical versus medical management for TMB and **central retinal artery occlusion** are debated. Currently, patients with **central retinal artery occlusion** have low potential for visual recovery; and to change this potential, there is significant ongoing research into novel medical approaches, including the use of thrombolytics, pentoxifylline to promote vasodilation, and hyperbaric oxygen to enhance oxygenation of damaged retinal tissue. GCA is another emergency with potential for poor visual outcome; and mainstream management at this time dictates prolonged steroid regimens, which have their own significant side effects. Current therapeutic research is investigating optimal glucocorticoid regimens as well as newer therapeutic advances for alternatives to glucocorticoid therapy, such as tocilizumab and methotrexate. For all the **ophthalmic emergencies** described, high suspicion should be held for these conditions when patients complain of sudden vision changes or severe eye pain. Urgent intervention and **ophthalmology** consultation are essential for preventing irreversible visual damage.

## References

1. Cugati S, Varma DD, Chen CS, et al. Treatment options for central retinal artery occlusion. *Curr Treat Options Neurol.* 2013;15:63-77.
2. Fraser SG, Adams W. Interventions for acute nonarteritic central retinal artery occlusion. *Cochrane Database Syst Rev.* 2009:CD001989.
3. Rumelt S, Dorenboim Y, Rehany U. Aggressive systematic treatment for central retinal artery occlusion. *Am J Ophthalmol.* 1999;128:733-738.
4. Kvickström P, Lindblom B, Bergström G, et al. Amaurosis fugax: risk factors and prevalence of significant carotid stenosis. *Clin Ophthalmol.* 2016;10:2165-2170.
5. Varma DD, Cugati S, Lee AW, et al. A review of central retinal artery occlusion: clinical presentation and management. *Eye (Lond).* 2013;27:688-697.
6. Kappelle LJ, Donders RCJM, Algra A. Transient monocular blindness. *Clin Exp Hypertens.* 2006;28:259-263.
7. Benavente O, Eliasziw M, Streifler JY, et al. Prognosis after transient monocular blindness associated with carotid-artery stenosis. *N Engl J Med.* 2001;345:1084-1090.

8. Biousse V, Trobe JD. Transient monocular visual loss. *Am J Ophthalmol*. 2005;140:717-721.

9. Kramer M, Goldenberg-Cohen N, Shapira Y, et al. Role of transesophageal echocardiography in the evaluation of patients with retinal artery occlusion. *Ophthalmology*. 2001;108:1461-1464.

10. White H, Boden-Albala B, Wang C, et al. Ischemic stroke subtype incidence among whites, blacks, and Hispanics: the Northern Manhattan Study. *Circulation*. 2005;111:1327-1331.

11. Leavitt JA, Larson TA, Hodge DO, et al. The incidence of central retinal artery occlusion in Olmsted County, Minnesota. *Am J Ophthalmol*. 2011;152:820.e2-823.e2.

12. Litsky J, Stilp E, Njoh R, et al. Management of symptomatic carotid disease in 2014. *Curr Cardiol Rep*. 2014;16:462.

13. North American Symptomatic Carotid Endarterectomy Trial Collaborators. Beneficial effect of carotid endarterectomy in symptomatic patients with high-grade carotid stenosis. *N Engl J Med*. 1991;325:445-453.

14. European Carotid Surgery Trialists' Collaborative Group. Randomised trial of endarterectomy for recently symptomatic carotid stenosis: final results of the MRC European Carotid Surgery Trial (ECST). *Lancet*. 1998;351:1379-1387.

15. Rothwell PM, Warlow CP; European Carotid Surgery Trialists' Collaborative Group. Prediction of benefit from carotid endarterectomy in individual patients: a risk-modelling study. *Lancet*. 1999;353:2105-2110.

16. Antithrombotic Trialists' Collaboration. Collaborative meta-analysis of randomised trials of antiplatelet therapy for prevention of death, myocardial infarction, and stroke in high risk patients. *BMJ*. 2002;324:71-86.

17. Diener HC, Bogousslavsky J, Brass LM, et al. Aspirin and clopidogrel compared with clopidogrel alone after recent ischaemic stroke or transient ischaemic attack in high-risk patients (MATCH): randomised, doubleblind, placebo-controlled trial. *Lancet*. 2004;364:331-337.

18. Diener HC, Cunha L, Forbes C, Sivenius J, Smets P, Lowenthal A. European stroke prevention study. 2. Dipyridamole and acetylsalicylic acid in the secondary prevention of stroke. *J Neurol Sci*. 1996;143:1-13.

19. Sacco RL, Diener HC, Yusuf S, et al. Aspirin and extended-release dipyridamole versus clopidogrel for recurrent stroke. *N Engl J Med*. 2008;359:1238-1251.

20. Wang Y, Pan Y, Zhao X, et al. Clopidogrel with aspirin in acute minor stroke or transient ischemic attack. *N Engl J Med*. 2013;369:11-19.

21. Lawes CMM, Bennett DA, Feigin VL, et al. Blood pressure and stroke: an overview of published reviews. *Stroke*. 2004;35:776-785.

22. Neal B, MacMahon S, Chapman N, et al; Blood Pressure Lowering Treatment Trialists' Collaboration. Effects of ACE inhibitors, calcium antagonists, and other blood-pressure-lowering drugs: results of prospectively designed overviews of randomised trials. *Lancet*. 2000;356:1955-1964.

23. Semplicini A, Calò L. Administering antihypertensive drugs after acute ischemic stroke: timing is everything. *CMAJ*. 2005;172:625-626.

24. Karam JG, Loney-Hutchinson L, and McFarlane SI; Stroke Prevention by Aggressive Reduction in Cholesterol Levels (SPARCL) Investigators. High-dose atorvastatin after stroke or transient ischemic attack: the stroke prevention by aggressive reduction in cholesterol levels (SPARCL) investigators. *J Cardiometab Syndr*. 2008;3:68-69.

25. Hayreh SS, Zimmerman MB. Central retinal artery occlusion: visual outcome. *Am J Ophthalmol*. 2005;140:376-391.

26. Atebara NH, Brown GC, Cater J. Efficacy of anterior chamber paracentesis and carbogen in treating acute nonarteritic central retinal artery occlusion. *Ophthalmology*. 1995;102:2029-2035.

27. Hayreh SS, Zimmerman MB. Fundus changes in central retinal artery occlusion. *Retina Phila Pa*. 2007;27:276-289.

28. Hayreh SS, Zimmerman MB, Kimura A, et al. Central retinal artery occlusion. Retinal survival time. *Exp Eye Res*. 2004;78:723-736.

29. Menzel-severing J, Siekmann U, Weinberger A, et al. Early hyperbaric oxygen treatment for nonarteritic central retinal artery obstruction. *Am J Ophthalmol*. 2012;153:454.e2-459.e2.

30. Beatty S, Au Eong KG. Acute occlusion of the retinal arteries: current concepts and recent advances in diagnosis and management. *J Accid Emerg Med*. 2000;17:324-329.

31. Biousse V, Calvetti O, Bruce BB, et al. Thrombolysis for central retinal artery occlusion. *J Neuroophthalmol.* 2007;27:215-230.

32. Schrag M, Youn T, Schindler J, et al. Intravenous fibrinolytic therapy in central retinal artery occlusion: a patient-level meta-analysis. *JAMA Neurol.* 2015;72:1148-1154.

33. Bath PMW, Bath-Hextall FJ. Pentoxifylline, propentofylline and pentifylline for acute ischaemic stroke. *Cochrane Database Syst Rev.* 2004:CD000162.

34. Incandela L, Cesarone MR, Belcaro G, et al. Treatment of vascular retinal disease with pentoxifylline: a controlled, randomized trial. *Angiology.* 2002;53(suppl 1):S31-S34.

35. Deutsch TA, Read JS, Ernest JT, et al. Effects of oxygen and carbon dioxide on the retinal vasculature in humans. *Arch Ophthalmol.* 1983;101:1278-1280.

36. Arend O, Harris A, Martin BJ, et al. Retinal blood velocities during carbogen breathing using scanning laser ophthalmoscopy. *Acta Ophthalmol (Copenh).* 1994;72:332-336.

37. Cope A, Eggert JV, O'Brien E. Retinal artery occlusion: visual outcome after treatment with hyperbaric oxygen. *Diving Hyperb Med.* 2011;41:135-138.

38. Rassam SM, Patel V, Kohner EM. The effect of acetazolamide on the retinal circulation. *Eye (Lond).* 1993;7:697-702.

39. Lam AKC, Chen D. Effect of ocular massage on intraocular pressure and corneal biomechanics. *Eye (Lond).* 2007;21:1245-1246.

40. Magargal LE, Goldberg RE. Anterior chamber paracentesis in the management of acute nonarteritic central retinal artery occlusion. *Surg Forum.* 1977;28:518-521.

41. Schumacher M, Schmidt D, Jurklies B, et al. Central retinal artery occlusion: local intra-arterial fibrinolysis versus conservative treatment, a multicenter randomized trial. *Ophthalmology.* 2010;117:1367.e1-1375.e1.

42. Chen CS, Lee AW, Campbell B, et al. Efficacy of intravenous tissue-type plasminogen activator in central retinal artery occlusion: report from a randomized, controlled trial. *Stroke.* 2011;42:2229-2234.

43. Salvarani C, Pipitone N, Versari A, et al. Clinical features of polymyalgia rheumatica and giant cell arteritis. *Nat Rev Rheumatol.* 2012;8:509-521.

44. Gonzalez-gay MA, Vazquez-Rodriguez TR, Lopez-Diaz MJ, et al. Epidemiology of giant cell arteritis and polymyalgia rheumatica. *Arthritis Rheum.* 2009;61:1454-1461.

45. Ezeonyeji AN, Borg FA, Dasgupta B. Delays in recognition and management of giant cell arteritis: results from a retrospective audit. *Clin Rheumatol.* 2011;30:259-262.

46. Paraskevas KI, Boumpas DT, Vrentzos GE, et al. Oral and ocular/orbital manifestations of temporal arteritis: a disease with deceptive clinical symptoms and devastating consequences. *Clin Rheumatol.* 2007;26:1044-1048.

47. Hayreh SS, Podhajsky PA, Zimmerman B. Ocular manifestations of giant cell arteritis. *Am J Ophthalmol.* 1998;125:509-520.

48. Salvarani C, Cantini F, Hunder GG. Polymyalgia rheumatic and giant-cell arteritis. *Lancet.* 2008;372:234-245.

49. González-gay MA, García-porrúa C, Llorca J, et al. Visual manifestations of giant cell arteritis. Trends and clinical spectrum in 161 patients. *Medicine (Baltimore).* 2000;79:283-292.

50. Hunder GG, Bloch DA, Michel BA, et al. The American College of Rheumatology 1990 criteria for the classification of giant cell arteritis. *Arthritis Rheum.* 1990;33:1122-1128.

51. Foroozan R, Danesh-Meyer H, Savino PJ, et al. Thrombocytosis in patients with biopsy-proven giant cell arteritis. *Ophthalmology.* 2002;109:1267-1271.

52. Karassa FB, Matsagas MI, Schmidt WA, Ioannidis JP. Meta-analysis: test performance of ultrasonography for giant-cell arteritis. *Ann Intern Med.* 2005;142:359-369.

53. Bley TA, Weiben O, Uhl M, et al. Assessment of the cranial involvement pattern of giant cell arteritis with 3T magnetic resonance imaging. *Arthritis Rheum.* 2005;52:2470-2477.

54. Frohman L, Wong ABC, Matheos K, et al. New developments in giant cell arteritis. *Surv Ophthalmol.* 2016;61:400-421.

55. Watelet B, Samson M, de Boysson H, et al. Treatment of giant-cell arteritis, a literature review. *Mod Rheumatol.* 2017;27:747-754.

56. Proven A, Gabriel SE, Orces C, et al. Glucocorticoid therapy in giant cell arteritis: duration and adverse outcomes. *Arthritis Rheum.* 2003;49:703-708.

57. Jover JA, Hernández-García C, Morado IC, et al. Combined treatment of giant-cell arteritis with methotrexate and prednisone. a randomized, double-blind, placebo-controlled trial. *Ann Intern Med.* 2001;134:106-114.

58. Mahr AD, Jover JA, Spiera RF, et al. Adjunctive methotrexate for treatment of giant cell arteritis: an individual patient data meta-analysis. *Arthritis Rheum.* 2007;56:2789-2797.

59. Mazlumzadeh M, Hunder GG, Easley KA, et al. Treatment of giant cell arteritis using induction therapy with high-dose glucocorticoids: a double-blind, placebo-controlled, randomized prospective clinical trial. *Arthritis Rheum.* 2006;54:3310-3318.

60. Chevalet P, Barrier JH, Pottier P, et al. A randomized, multicenter, controlled trial using intravenous pulses of methylprednisolone in the initial treatment of simple forms of giant cell arteritis: a one year follow-up study of 164 patients. *J Rheumatol.* 2000;27:1484-1491.

61. Hoffman GS, Cid MC, Hellmann DB, et al. A multicenter, randomized, double-blind, placebo-controlled trial of adjuvant methotrexate treatment for giant cell arteritis. *Arthritis Rheum.* 2002;46:1309-1318.

62. Leon L, Rodriguez-Rodriguez L, Morado I, et al. Treatment with methotrexate and risk of relapses in patients with giant cell arteritis in clinical practice. *Clin Exp Rheumatol.* 2018;36(2)(suppl 111):121-128.

63. Hoffman GS, Cid MC, Rendt-zagar KE, et al. Infliximab for maintenance of glucocorticosteroid-induced remission of giant cell arteritis: a randomized trial. *Ann Intern Med.* 2007;146:621-630.

64. Visvanathan S, Rahman MU, Hoffman GS, et al. Tissue and serum markers of inflammation during the follow-up of patients with giant-cell arteritis–a prospective longitudinal study. *Rheumatol (Oxf).* 2011;50:2061-2070.

65. Seror R, Baron G, Hachulla E, et al. Adalimumab for steroid sparing in patients with giant-cell arteritis: results of a multicentre randomised controlled trial. *Ann Rheum Dis.* 2014;73:2074-2081.

66. Samson M, Espigol-Frigole G, Terrades-Garcia N, et al. Biological treatments in giant cell arteritis and Takayasu arteritis. *Eur J Intern Med.* 2018;50:12-19.

67. Martínez-taboada VM, Rodríguez-valverde V, Carreño L, et al. A double-blind placebo controlled trial of etanercept in patients with giant cell arteritis and corticosteroid side effects. *Ann Rheum Dis.* 2008;67:625-630.

68. Cantini F, Niccoli L, Salvarani C, et al. Treatment of longstanding active giant cell arteritis with infliximab: report of four cases. *Arthritis Rheum.* 2001;44:2933-2935.

69. Beyer C, Axmann R, Sahinbegovic E, et al. Anti-interleukin 6 receptor therapy as rescue treatment for giant cell arteritis. *Ann Rheum Dis.* 2011;70:1874-1875.

70. Unizony S, Arias-urdaneta L, Miloslavsky E, et al. Tocilizumab for the treatment of large-vessel vasculitis (giant cell arteritis, Takayasu arteritis) and polymyalgia rheumatica. *Arthritis Care Res (Hoboken).* 2012;64:1720-1729.

71. Sciascia S, Piras D, Baldovino S, et al. Mycophenolate mofetil as steroid-sparing treatment for elderly patients with giant cell arteritis: report of three cases. *Aging Clin Exp Res.* 2012;24:273-277.

72. Adizie T, Christidis D, Dharmapaliah C, et al. Efficacy and tolerability of leflunomide in difficult-to-treat polymyalgia rheumatica and giant cell arteritis: a case series. *Int J Clin Pract.* 2012;66:906-909.

73. Diamantopoulos AP, Hetland H, Myklebust G. Leflunomide as a corticosteroid-sparing agent in giant cell arteritis and polymyalgia rheumatica: a case series. *Biomed Res Int.* 2013;2013:120638.

74. De boysson H, Boutemy J, Creveuil C, et al. Is there a place for cyclophosphamide in the treatment of giant-cell arteritis? A case series and systematic review. *Semin Arthritis Rheum.* 2013;43:105-112.

75. Quartuccio L, Maset M, De Maglio G, et al. Role of oral cyclophosphamide in the treatment of giant cell arteritis. *Rheumatol (Oxford).* 2012;51:1677-1686.

76. Loock J, Henes J, Kötter I, et al. Treatment of refractory giant cell arteritis with cyclophosphamide: a retrospective analysis of 35 patients from three centres. *Clin Exp Rheumatol.* 2012;30:S70-S76.

77. Haimann MH, Burton TC, Brown CK. Epidemiology of retinal detachment. *Arch Ophthalmol.* 1982;100:289-292.

78. Mitry D, Charteris DG, Fleck BW, Campbell H, Singh J. The epidemiology of rhegmatogenous retinal detachment: geographical variation and clinical associations. *Br J Ophthalmol.* 2010;94:678-684.

79. Johnston PB. Traumatic retinal detachment. *Br J Ophthalmol.* 1991;75:18-21.

80. Romaniuk VM. Ocular trauma and other catastrophes. *Emerg Med Clin North Am.* 2013;31:399-411.

81. Ersanli D, Sonmez M, Unal M, et al. Management of retinal detachment due to closed globe injury by pars plana vitrectomy with and without scleral buckling. *Retina Phila Pa*. 2006;26:32-36.

82. Yoonessi R, Hussain A, Jang TB. Bedside ocular ultrasound for the detection of retinal detachment in the emergency department. *Acad Emerg Med*. 2010;17:913-917.

83. Blaivas M, Theodoro D, Sierzenski PR. A study of bedside ocular ultrasonography in the emergency department. *Acad Emerg Med*. 2002;9:791-799.

84. Heimann H, Bartz-schmidt KU, Bornfeld N, et al. Scleral buckling versus primary vitrectomy in rhegmatogenous retinal detachment: a prospective randomized multicenter clinical study. *Ophthalmology*. 2007;114:2142--2154.

85. Rouberol F, Denis P, Romanet JP, et al. Comparative study of 50 early-or late-onset retinal detachments after open or closed globe injury. *Retina Phila Pa*. 2011;31:1143-1149.

86. Emanuel ME, Parrish RK, Gedde SJ. Evidence-based management of primary angle closure glaucoma. *Curr Opin Ophthalmol*. 2014;25:89-92.

87. Dargin JM, Lowenstein RA. The painful eye. *Emerg Med Clin North Am*. 2008;26:199-216.

88. Choong YF, Irfan S, Menage MJ. Acute angle closure glaucoma: an evaluation of a protocol for acute treatment. *Eye (Lond)*. 1999;13:613-616.

89. Khaw PT, Shah P, Elkington AR. Glaucoma–1: diagnosis. *BMJ*. 2004;328:97–99.

90. Wright C, Tawfik MA, Waisbourd M, et al. Primary angle-closure glaucoma: an update. *Acta Ophthalmol (Copenh)*. 2016;94:217-225.

91. Razeghinejad MR, Myers JS, Katz LJ. Iatrogenic glaucoma secondary to medications. *Am J Med*. 2011;124:20-25.

92. Gordon-Bennett P, Ung T, Stephenson C, et al. Misdiagnosis of angle closure glaucoma. *BMJ*. 2006;333:1157-1158.

93. Lachkar Y, Bouassida W. Drug-induced acute angle closure glaucoma. *Curr Opin Ophthalmol*. 2007;18:129-133.

94. Shikino K, Hirose Y, Ikusaka M. Oblique flashlight test: lighting up acute angle-closure glaucoma. *J Gen Intern Med*. 2016;31:1538.

95. David R, Tessler Z, Yassur Y. Long-term outcome of primary acute angle-closure glaucoma. *Br J Ophthalmol*. 1985;69:261-262.

96. He M, Friedman DS, Ge J, et al. Laser peripheral iridotomy in primary angle-closure suspects: biometric and gonioscopic outcomes: the Liwan eye study. *Ophthalmology*. 2007;114:494-500.

97. Fleck BW, Wright E, Fairley EA. A randomised prospective comparison of operative peripheral iridectomy and Nd:YAG laser iridotomy treatment of acute angle closure glaucoma: 3 year visual acuity and intraocular pressure control outcome. *Br J Ophthalmol*. 1997;81:884-888.

98. Davis JP, Stearns MP. Orbital complications of sinusitis: avoid delays in diagnosis. *Postgrad Med J*. 1994;70:108-110.

99. Tomaç S, Turgut S. Orbital cellulitis and irreversible visual loss owing to acute sinusitis. *Ann Ophthalmol (Skokie)*. 2006;38:131-133.

100. Chang CH, Lai YH, Wang HZ, et al. Antibiotic treatment of orbital cellulitis: an analysis of pathogenic bacteria and bacterial susceptibility. *J Ocul Pharmacol Ther*. 2000;16:75-79.

101. Connell B, Kamal Z, McNab AA. Fulminant orbital cellulitis with complete loss of vision. *Clin Exp Ophthalmol*. 2001;29:260-261.

102. Baker AS. Role of anaerobic bacteria in sinusitis and its complications. *Ann Otol Rhinol Laryngol Suppl*. 1991;154:17-22.

103. Harris GJ. Age as a factor in the bacteriology and response to treatment of subperiosteal abscess of the orbit. *Trans Am Ophthalmol Soc*. 1993;91:441-516.

104. Carrim ZI, Anderson IWR, Kyle PM. Traumatic orbital compartment syndrome: importance of prompt recognition and management. *Eur J Emerg Med*. 2007;14:174-176.

105. Bord SP, Linden J. Trauma to the globe and orbit. *Emerg Med Clin North Am*. 2008;26:97-123.

106. Shek KC, Chung KL, Kam CW, et al. Acute retrobulbar haemorrhage: an ophthalmic emergency. *Emerg Med Australas*. 2006;18:299-301.

107. Lima V, Burt B, Leibovitch I, et al. Orbital compartment syndrome: the ophthalmic surgical emergency. *Surv Ophthalmol*. 2009;54:441-449.

108. Sullivan TJ, Wright JE. Non-traumatic orbital haemorrhage. *Clin Exp Ophthalmol.* 2000;28:26-31.

109. Vassallo S, Hartstein M, Howard D, et al. Traumatic retrobulbar hemorrhage: emergent decompression by lateral canthotomy and cantholysis. *J Emerg Med.* 2002;22:251-256.

110. Burnstine MA. Clinical recommendations for repair of isolated orbital floor fractures: an evidence-based analysis. *Ophthalmology.* 2002;109:1207-1210.

111. Joseph JM, Glavas IP. Orbital fractures: a review. *Clin Ophthalmol Auckl.* 2011;5:95-100.

112. Cole P, Boyd V, Banerji S, et al. Comprehensive management of orbital fractures. *Plast Reconstr Surg.* 2007;120:57S-63S.

113. Rinna C, Ungari C, Saltarel A, et al. Orbital floor restoration. *J Craniofac Surg.* 2005;16:968-972.

114. Burnstine MA. Clinical recommendations for repair of orbital facial fractures. *Curr Opin Ophthalmol.* 2003;14:236-240.

# Therapeutic Advances in Advanced Care Planning

# The Family Meeting as a Therapeutic Intervention

Maria Torroella Carney, MD and Tara Liberman, DO

# CHAPTER 17

## BACKGROUND

In the book entitled *How to Care for Aging Parents*, Virginia Morris describes the importance of **family meetings** as a means of holding crucial conversations.[1] As one ages and new stages are faced, it is important to address how and where one wants to live and what is most important during this stage. Literature has shown that many diverse patient populations have benefited from having the ability to communicate their wishes.[2,3] Indeed, there is increasing evidence that **family meetings** improve clinical outcomes.[4] **Acute care** hospitals provide care for older adults who have complex medical needs and fluctuating caregiving demands. It is often with an acute illness in a hospital setting that one's ability to live independently can be threatened. It is in this **acute care** setting that the family meeting is most needed and is recommended to be used to involve family members in future planning.[3] The family meeting is, therefore, a form of therapeutic intervention to be used during a patient's hospital stay.

**Communication** with an interdisciplinary and comprehensive approach is vital to providing assessment and treatment guidance to the hospitalized older adult. A family meeting is an interventional tool that can and should be used for hospitalized older adults with complex and serious illness. This chapter introduces the family meeting as a medical intervention. It describes its purpose, challenges, and also provides education on how to execute a family meeting. This intervention can be used to involve a family early in a patient's care.

### Purpose

The family meeting typically involves the patient (if able to participate), caregiver, healthcare surrogate, family/loved ones, and healthcare professionals.[5] The purpose is to establish a level of understanding of the patient's current medical conditions, treatment options, and prognosis. Also, it is important to address caregiving needs, goals of care, expectations for patient and family, and facilitation of discharge planning.[6]

Although the family meeting is also a method for clinical team members to understand all the issues involving a patient, family, and loved ones, it serves to clarify the past, ease the present, and protect the future.[7] **Family meetings** are often a means to identify barriers to care and discharge planning. They provide a method to build consensus and/or come to a compromise between patient, family, and the healthcare team.[8]

**Family meetings** are not only for situations when a serious decision needs to be made but also when there is a change in a patient's status; when a patient or family believes a meeting would be beneficial; when there is conflict between family members or family members and the healthcare team; and when the patient, family, or healthcare team believes that the goals of care should change.[9]

Once a family meeting has been conducted, it is important that the events and decisions made be documented and communicated with other healthcare team members.[10,11] The family meeting is an intervention; it impacts the hospitalization course, treatment, and discharge plans, as well as patient and family satisfaction.

# AREAS OF UNCERTAINTY

Meetings are often needed to establish care plans. However, there are challenges to holding **family meetings**. Some families are unable or unwilling to participate, and there may be limited availability of space and time to conduct an adequate family meeting. These can contribute to delays in decision making. Furthermore, a growing number of individuals are aging away from their children or may not have support at all, adding to the complexity in the development of an appropriate treatment plan.

# THERAPEUTIC ADVANCES

## The Family Meeting

**Family meetings** can be effective and are especially vital for patients who are critically ill or facing serious illness.[9,12,13] Traditionally, physicians interact with families in a clinician-to-patient manner with outcomes focused on diagnosis and disease management. **Family meetings** are similar to this traditional format in some respect.[10,14] However, **family meetings** differ from clinician-to-patient meetings in that family group dynamics can be complex and affect how the meetings progress and their outcomes. **Family meetings** take time to prepare, coordinate, and execute. They require specific skills to be conducted well and, hence, are not done as frequently as may be needed. Evidence suggests that **communication** with families, in general, is often less than desirable.[10,13,15-20] These meetings can be difficult depending on family histories, group dynamics, complexity of decisions, and medical resources available.[9] Therefore, utilization of **family meetings** on a more routine basis has the potential to improve **communication** for the most vulnerable and seriously ill older adults.

## Why, Who, and Where

Like any other therapeutic intervention, a successful family meeting should follow a structured format to help minimize barriers and maximize therapeutic goals. First and foremost, one must know and understand why the meeting is being held, who will be joining, and where and when it will take place. The primary reason for a family meeting is to facilitate **communication** between the healthcare team, decision makers, and caregivers.

The next step is to clarify who should participate. Ask patients who they would like to be present with them. If the patient is unable to participate or lacking capacity, invite the next of kin, the healthcare proxy, caregivers, or surrogate decision makers to be present along with the interdisciplinary healthcare team. Determine where and when the meeting will take place and inform all participants. The medical team can invite other specialists and determine a mutually convenient time for all. It may also be beneficial for the patient and family to have a nurse, case manager, social worker, and/or hospital chaplain included in the meeting.[21]

Once the "who" has been clarified, a location that can accommodate all must be identified.[5] A private, quiet room is the ideal place because emotions are more easily expressed and difficult questions can be asked and addressed appropriately. A private room often depends on its availability and the ability of a patient with decision-making capacity to leave the bedside. In the event a patient is unable to leave the bedside, accommodations to hold the meeting must be made. Nonetheless, once the location has been agreed on and invitations extended, preparation for the meeting can begin.

## Preparation

A family meeting requires a leader. Although no literature examines who is best suited for this role, the family meeting leader will require group facilitation skills, counseling skills, knowledge of medical and prognostic information, and a willingness to provide decision-making guidance.[22]

Preparing for a family meeting is almost as important as holding the meeting. It requires time, attention, and facilitation skills. In preparation for a family meeting, one needs to review the patient's history, health data, medical opinions, and treatment options. It is most ideal to discuss the case with all the team members for a comprehensive understanding of the patient's situation. Once the information is gathered, one should synthesize the information and be prepared to offer an independent determination of treatment, impact on function and quality of life, and estimation of the patient's longevity. A premeeting with the healthcare team may be necessary to align the agenda and goals of the family meeting (Table 17.1).

One suggestion for executing a successful family meeting includes minimizing distractions. Have phones on silent mode and adjust calendars so there are no interruptions. It is a good practice to anticipate questions the family may have and to

| **TABLE 17.1 • Family Meeting Preparation** |
| --- |
| Review history, data, opinions, and treatment options |
| Discuss with all team members<br>Synthesize all this information and make an independent determination of the treatment and test impact on function, quality of life, and longevity of patient. |
| Prepare to lead the meeting or designate a meeting leader<br>Need group facilitation skills, counseling skills, knowledge of medical and prognostic information, and willingness to provide decision-making guidance |
| Invitations |
| Setting |
| Premeeting meeting |

Derived from DeLisser HM. How to run a family meeting. Decision Support in Medicine. 2017. Available at: http://www.cancertherapyadvisor.com/critical-care-medicine/how-to-run-a-family-meeting/article/584833/. Accessed September 14, 2018.

have water and tissues available. Meeting with a family is an opportunity to establish trust, maximize **communication**, and manage expectations. Adequate preparation will help meet these goals.

## The Meeting

On starting a family meeting, introductions set the tone. As the leader of the meeting, it is important to be sure that all attendees are present and feel comfortable. Respectful introductions help establish trust and build relationships; thank everyone for attending and explain the goal of the meeting. For example, "We are meeting to discuss Ms MK's situation and determine best next steps in her care." Before proceeding to share information, establish a connection by asking the patient and/or family to tell you "a bit about the patient." It is important to also assess what the patient and/or family understands by asking "What do you understand is happening and why are you hospitalized?" Let the participants explain where they are in their knowledge and provide support for when the patient and family are correct, such as, "You are correct in what you understand." Or clarify when family descriptions are inaccurate by saying, "In addition to what you said, there are some other things you should know."[23] It is from this point that you begin to explain the clinical situation and clarify the medical status. The information shared often includes diagnosis, prognosis, therapy, and discharge plans and needs (Table 17.2). Many family members want to know more details about prognosis; this is an opportunity to answer questions and support emotions. It is important to be as truthful as possible; this may include a nonspecific answer such as "I don't know." You may be able to provide more specific information such as "based on all the information we have available." Sometimes when bad news is being provided, a warning shot is advised, such as "I'm afraid I have some bad news." Ranges of prognosis may need to be provided (eg, days to weeks or months to years; Table 17.3). Caregiving needs are one aspect of the discussions

| TABLE 17.2 • The Family Meeting Infrastructure |
| --- |
| Why are you meeting? |
| Where? |
| Who? |
| Introduction and relationship building |
| Determine what the patient/family already know |
| Review medical status and respond to emotions |
| Recognize when there is no consensus |
| Summarize and wrap-up |

Derived from Hudson P, Quinn K, O'Hanlon B, et al. Family meetings in palliative care: multidisciplinary clinical practice guidelines. *BMC Palliat Care*. 2008;7:12; DeLisser HM. How to run a family meeting. Decision Support in Medicine. 2017. Available at: http://www.cancertherapyadvisor.com/critical-care-medicine/how-to-run-a-family-meeting/article/584833/. Accessed September 14, 2018.

| TABLE 17.3 • Examples of Statements of Prognoses |
| --- |
| The patient will likely die in the next 24-48 hours despite receiving maximum intensive care. |
| The patient will likely not survive to be discharged from the intensive care unit. |
| The patient will likely not survive to be discharged from the hospital. |
| The patient may be able to be discharged from the hospital, but she/he is not likely to survive for more than a few days or weeks, and caregiving needs will be increased. |
| The patient may be able to be discharged from the hospital, but she/he is not likely to survive for more than a few weeks or months, and caregiving needs will be significant. |

From DeLisser HM. How to run a family meeting. Decision Support in Medicine. 2017. Available at: http://www.cancertherapyadvisor.com/critical-care-medicine/how-to-run-a-family-meeting/article/584833/. Accessed September 14, 2018.

that must be addressed;[6] therefore, nurses should be engaged and empowered to be involved in **family meetings**.[7] A social worker or case manager can be a vital resource to highlight this aspect of medical care.[8,21] Often, patients need increased supervision and assistance with their activities of daily living not previously required before their hospitalization; the family and support system need to fully understand this change.

After listening to the family and understanding the medical information, this may be the point at which to recommend treatment options consistent with the goals of care.[5,23] Questions that should be asked include, "Will the patient continue with life-prolonging care (eg, utilization of all available resources), limited care (care short of intensive care unit stay), or comfort focused care?," as described by Angelo Volandes in The Conversation.[24] Alternatively, another format to use when discussing serious information or breaking bad news is the SPIKES protocol[15] (Table 17.4).

| TABLE 17.4 • SPIKES | |
| --- | --- |
| 1 | Setting |
| 2 | Patient perspective |
| 3 | Invitation |
| 4 | Knowledge share |
| 5 | Emotions-respond to emotions |
| 6 | Support |

Adapted from Buckman R. Breaking bad news: a six-step protocol. In: *How to Break Bad News: A Guide for Health Care Professionals*. Baltimore, MD: The John Hopkins University; 1992:65-97.

At the end of the meeting, summarize the consensus and compromises met, and how the treatment plan and future should proceed.[23] Write down the decisions on a paper and provide it to the patient and family. This step is important because the patient and family are often overwhelmed, so being able to read the decisions later will be beneficial. Furthermore, documentation in the patient's chart of the discussion and its outcomes is needed.[10,11]

## When There Is No Consensus?

Occasionally, families and healthcare professionals may not come to an agreement, which can prolong hospitalization and be burdensome for all involved. Trying to understand the family issues may help uncover barriers to the decision-making process. Without expressing frustration or anger, respectfully end the meeting if a consensus has not been developed after 1 hour and make plans for another meeting and/or mediation.[5] Social work, chaplaincy, ethics committee, hospital attorney, administration, and palliative care team involvement can also assist in reaching a consensus.[8]

## Challenges

Some unique and challenging situations need special attention. **Family meetings** are often needed to establish care plans; however, some families are unable or unwilling to participate, and this can contribute to delays in decision making. Currently, there is a growing population of individuals aging alone, who have caregiving and decision-making needs.[25] These individuals are highly vulnerable and represent a challenge that will be faced by healthcare providers when trying to establish **family meetings** for decision making. It is for this reason that the earlier a family meeting can occur in a patients' trajectory of illness, the better. Take any opportunity to involve family members when possible because relationships can change, and it allows families to establish goals of care over time.

As the aging population grows, more individuals are aging away from their children; this inevitably leads to the need for additional healthcare professionals equipped to manage chronic, complex, and serious illness. Social workers and case managers help patients and families navigate healthcare and community support services, and chaplains provide benefit to patients and families who are struggling with emotional and spiritual suffering and decisions.[8,21] Although these support roles are highly beneficial, they may be a limited resource depending on the institution.

The availability of a private and comfortable location to conduct a family meeting is also a challenge. In addition, the ability to schedule the time, location, and availability of all participants requires administrative support, or if done by the clinical team, may impact their clinical care time. This is a very real challenge in the ability to hold more **family meetings**, so although they are highly beneficial, the ability to coordinate them takes effort. It is best to identify an efficient process of scheduling **family meetings** in your individual setting.

Another struggle often faced is limiting a family meeting to 1 hour, and it is important to state this to all participants before the meeting starts. Have an agenda prepared, and as the meeting progresses, give updates on time. Unfortunately, more than one meeting might be necessary to make decisions about important changes to a patient's care plan. Of note, there is no literature to support when a family meeting is most optimally held, such as at the beginning of a hospitalization, in the middle, or before discharge. Research in the area of family meeting utilization would help further the evidence behind using **family meetings** as an intervention.

# CONCLUSIONS

The family meeting is an increasingly important component of a patient's care plan. The population is aging and living longer with complex medical conditions. Critical decisions around the health care of this age group must involve the support of an interdisciplinary team and is essential to providing appropriate care. **Family meetings** have shown to improve outcomes and patient satisfaction, and, therefore, should be viewed as a medical intervention.[26,27]

Having a structured approach to guide **family meetings** is imperative. This chapter provides guidelines for the healthcare team. Limitations of the family meeting are noted, and more research on **family meetings** with the complex older adult population in the hospital setting, not just in the intensive care unit, is needed. It is vital that the medical team and the patient, as well as the patient's family, have the opportunity to share their perspectives to make decisions for further treatment and discharge planning. The family meeting becomes an increasingly important component of care as health care becomes more complex, with an emphasis on the need for advanced care planning, complex discharge planning, and caregiving.

# SUMMARY

**Acute care** hospitals provide care for older adults who have complex medical needs and fluctuating caregiving demands. Often, one's ability to live independently can be threatened when faced with an acute illness in a hospital setting. It is in this **acute care** setting that the family meeting is most needed and recommended for treatment planning.

Meetings are often needed to establish care plans. However, there are challenges to holding **family meetings**. Some families are unable or unwilling to participate, and there may be limited availability of space and time to conduct an adequate family meeting. These can contribute to delays in decision making.

A family meeting is, therefore, a form of therapeutic intervention to be used during a patient's hospital stay. This chapter highlights the importance of **family meetings** as a means of medical intervention; describing the purpose, challenges, and education on carrying out the intervention. The primary reason for a family meeting is to facilitate **communication** between the healthcare team, decision makers, and caregivers. Participants should prepare ahead and a successful family meeting should follow a structured format to help minimize barriers and maximize therapeutic goals, including why the meeting is being called, who will participate, and when/where it will be held. A structured format allows for information to be shared from care provider to patient/family, including diagnosis, prognosis, therapy, and discharge plans and needs. At the end of the meeting, a summary should be provided.

The population is aging and therefore these meetings need to become more common. The family meeting is an increasingly important component of a patient's care plan for those living longer and with complex medical conditions. **Family meetings** have shown improved outcomes and patient satisfaction, and therefore, should be viewed as a medical intervention.

## References

1. Morris V. *How to Care for Aging Parents*. 3rd ed. New York, NY: Workman Publishing Company; 2014.
2. Holroyd-Leduc J, Resin J, Ashley L, et al. Giving voice to older adults living with frailty and their family caregivers: engagement of older adults living with frailty in research, health care decision making, and in health policy. *Res Involv Engagem*. 2016;2:23.
3. Bradway C, Hirschman KB. Working with families of hospitalized older adults with dementia: caregivers are useful resources and should be part of the care team. *Am J Nurs*. 2008;108:52-60; quiz 61.
4. Lilly CM, De Meo DL, Sonna LA, et al. An intensive communication intervention for the critically ill. *Am J Med*. 2000;109:469.
5. Curtis JR, Patrick DL, Shannon SE, et al. The family conference as a focus to improve communication about end-of-life care in the intensive care unit: opportunities for improvement. *Crit Care Med*. 2001;29(2 suppl):N26-N33.
6. McMillan SC. Interventions to facilitate family caregiving at the end of life. *J Palliat Med*. 2005;8(suppl 1):3132-3139.
7. Meeker MA, Waldrop DP, Seo JY. Examining family meeting at end of life: The Model of Practice in a Hospice Inpatient Unit. *Palliat Support Care*. 2015;13:1283-1291.

8. Gay EB, Pronovost PJ, Bassett RD, et al. The intensive care unit family meeting: making it happen. *J Crit Care.* 2009;24:629.e1.

9. Joshi R. Family meetings: an essential component of comprehensive palliative care. *Can Fam Physician.* 2013; 59:637-639.

10. Ambuel B. Conducting a family conference. In: Weissman DE, Ambuel B, Hallenbeck J, eds. *Improving End-of-life Care: A Resource Guide for Physician Education.* 3rd ed. Milwaukee, WI: The Medical College of Wisconsin; 2001.

11. Nelson JE, Walker AS, Luhrs CA, et al. Family meeting made simpler. A tool kit for the ICU. *J Crit Care.* 2009;4:626.e7-626.e14.

12. Hudson PL, Girgis A, Mitchell GK, et al. Benefits and resource implications of family meetings for hospitalized palliative care patients. *BMC Palliat Care.* 2015;14;1-9.

13. Hudson P, Quinn K, O'Hanlon B, et al. Family meetings in palliative care: multidisciplinary clinical practice guidelines. *BMC Palliat Care.* 2008;7:12.

14. Lipkin M, Putnam S, Lazare A. *The Medical Interview.* New York: Springer-Verlag; 1995.

15. Buckman R. Breaking bad news: a six-step protocol. In: *How to Break Bad News: A Guide for Health Care Professionals.* Baltimore, MD: The John Hopkins University Press; 1992:65-97.

16. Levy MM. End-of-life care in the intensive care unit: can we do better? *Crit Care Med.* 2001;29:N56.

17. Hanson LC, Danis M, Garrett J. What is wrong with end-of-life care? Opinions of bereaved family members. *J Am Geriatr Soc.* 1997;45:1339.

18. Abbott KH, Sago JG, Breen CM, et al. Families looking back: one year after discussion of withdrawal or withholding of life-sustaining support. *Crit Care Med.* 2001;29:197.

19. Baker R, Wu AW, Teno JM, et al. Family satisfaction with end-of-life care in seriously ill hospitalized adults. *J Am Geriatr Soc.* 2000;48:S61.

20. Ahrens T, Yancey V, Kollef M. Improving family communications at the end of life: implications for length of stay in the intensive care unit and resource use. *Am J Crit Care.* 2003;12:317.

21. Shaw DJ, Davidson J, Smilde RE, et al. Multidisciplinary team training to enhance family communication in the ICU. *Crit Care Med.* 2014;42:265.

22. Hwang DY, Yagoda D, Perrey HM, et al. Consistency of communication among intensive care unit staff as perceived by family members of patients surviving to discharge. *J Crit Care.* 2014;29:134.

23. DeLisser HM. How to run a family meeting. Decision Support in Medicine. 2017. Available at: http://www.cancertherapyadvisor.com/critical-care-medicine/how-to-run-a-family-meeting/article/584833/. Accessed September 14, 2018.

24. Volandes AE. *The Conversation: A Revolutionary Plan for End-of-life Care.* New York, NY: Bloomsbury; 2015.

25. Carney MT, Jujiwara J, Emmert BE, et al. Elder orphans hiding in plain sight: a growing vulnerable population. *Curr Gerontol Geriatr Res.* 2016;2016:11.

26. Lilly CM, Sonma LA, Haley KJ, et al. Intensive communication: four-year follow-up from a clinical practice study. *Crit Care Med.* 2003;31(5 suppl):394.

27. Dowdy MD, Robertson C, Bader JA. A study of proactive ethics consultation for critically and terminally ill patients with extended length of stay. *Crit Care Med.* 1998;26:252.

# Index

Note: Page numbers followed by *f*, *t* indicate material in figures and tables respectively.